Common Pitfalls in Cerebrovascular Disease

Case-Based Learning

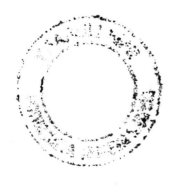

Common Pitfalls in Cerebrovascular Disease

Case-Based Learning

Edited by

José Biller MD FACP FAAN FANA FAHA
Professor and Chairman, Department of Neurology, Loyola University Chicago Stritch School of Medicine, Maywood, IL, USA

José M. Ferro MD PhD
Professor of Neurology and Head, Department of Neurosciences (Neurology), University of Lisbon; Hospital de Santa Maria, Lisbon, Portugal

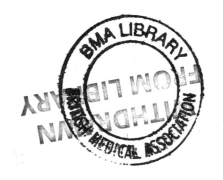

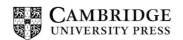

CAMBRIDGE
UNIVERSITY PRESS

CAMBRIDGE
UNIVERSITY PRESS

University Printing House, Cambridge CB2 8BS, United Kingdom

Cambridge University Press is part of the University of Cambridge.

It furthers the University's mission by disseminating knowledge in the pursuit of education, learning and research at the highest international levels of excellence.

www.cambridge.org
Information on this title: www.cambridge.org/9780521173650

© Cambridge University Press 2015

First published 2015

Printed in the United Kingdom by Bell and Bain Ltd

A catalog record for this publication is available from the British Library

Library of Congress Cataloging in Publication data
Common pitfalls in cerebrovascular disease : case-based learning / edited by José Biller, José M. Ferro.
   p. ; cm.
Includes bibliographical references and index.
ISBN 978-0-521-17365-0 (paperback)
I. Biller, José, editor. II. Ferro, José M., editor.
[DNLM: 1. Cerebrovascular Disorders–diagnosis–Case Reports. 2. Cerebrovascular Disorders–therapy–Case Reports. WL 355]
RC388.5
616.8′1–dc23
2015003681

ISBN 978-0-521-17365-0 Paperback

It is a great joy to dedicate this book to my wife Rhonda for her unfailing patience and encouragement; my children Sofia, Gabriel, and Rebecca; my step-children Adam and Emily; and the priceless gift of my grandchildren Selim, Ira, and Oz.

José Biller

I wish to dedicate this book to my clinical teachers in Neurology – Francisco Pinto, Miller Guerra and João AF Lobo Antunes.

José M. Ferro

Contents

Contributors

Paul D. Ackerman MD
Chief Resident, Department of Neurosurgery, Loyola University Chicago Stritch School of Medicine, Maywood, IL, USA

José Biller MD FACP FAAN FANA FAHA
Professor and Chairman, Department of Neurology, Loyola University Chicago Stritch School of Medicine, Maywood, IL, USA

James R. Brorson MD
Associate Professor, Department of Neurology, University of Chicago, Chicago, IL, USA

Katharina Maria Busl MD MS
Assistant Professor, Department of Neurological Sciences, and Attending Neurointensivist, Section of Neurocritical Care, Rush University Medical Center, Chicago, IL, USA

Patrícia Canhão MD PhD
Associate Professor, Department of Neurosciences (Neurology), Hospital de Santa Maria, University of Lisbon, Lisbon, Portugal

Leanne K. Casaubon MD MSc FRCPC DABPN
Director, TIA and Minor Stroke (TAMS) Unit, Toronto Western Hospital; Assistant Professor, Department of Neurology, University of Toronto, Toronto, Canada

Hugues Chabriat MD PhD
Professor of Neurology, Department of Neurology, CERVCO and DHU NeuroVasc, Hôpital Lariboisière, APHP; INSERM U 1161, Université Denis Diderot, Paris, France

Gabrielle deVeber MD
Staff Neurologist, Department of Neurology, The Hospital for Sick Children; Professor, Department of Paediatrics, University of Toronto, Toronto, Canada

José M. Ferro MD PhD
Professor of Neurology and Head, Department of Neurosciences (Neurology), University of Lisbon; Hospital de Santa Maria, Lisbon, Portugal

Murray Flaster MD PhD
Associate Professor, Department of Neurology, Loyola University Chicago Stritch School of Medicine, Maywood, IL, USA

Ana Catarina Fonseca MD PhD MPH
Department of Neurosciences (Neurology), Hospital de Santa Maria, University of Lisbon, Lisbon, Portugal

Ruth Geraldes MD MSc
Neuroanatomy Invited Teacher, Anatomy Department, Lisbon Medical School, Lisbon University; Neurology Consultant, Department of Neurosciences (Neurology), Hospital de Santa Maria, Lisbon, Portugal

Raquel Gil-Gouveia MD MMed
Headache Center, Neurology Department, Hospital da Luz; Department of Neurosciences (Neurology), Hospital de Santa Maria, Lisbon, Portugal

Dominique Hervé MD
Department of Neurology, CERVCO and DHU NeuroVasc, Hôpital Lariboisière, APHP; INSERM U 1161, Université Denis Diderot, Paris, France

Alejandro Hornik MD
Neurointensivist, Medical Director Teleneurology, Southern Illinois Healthcare, USA

Manoelle Kossorotoff MD
Department of Child Neurology, Hôpital Necker Enfants-Malades; INSERM U 1140, French Center for Pediatric Stroke, Paris, France

Christopher M. Loftus MD
Professor of Neurosurgery and Neurology and Chair, Department of Neurosurgery, Loyola University Chicago Stritch School of Medicine, Maywood, IL, USA

Demetrius K. Lopes MD
Associate Professor of Neurosurgery and Radiology, Director, Rush Center for Neuroendovascular Surgery, Rush University Medical Center, Chicago, IL, USA

Erwin Z. Mangubat MD MPH
Neuroendovascular Fellow, Rush University Medical Center, Chicago, IL, USA

Sarkis Morales-Vidal MD
Assistant Professor, Department of Neurology, Loyola University Chicago Stritch School of Medicine, Maywood, IL, USA

David D. Pasquale MD
Assistant Professor of Radiology and Neurological Surgery, Loyola University Chicago Stritch School of Medicine, Maywood, IL, USA

Shyam Prabhakaran MD MS FAHA FANA
Associate Professor of Neurology, Northwestern University Feinberg School of Medicine, Chicago, IL, USA

Christopher P. Robinson DO MS
Co-Chief Resident, Department of Neurology, Loyola University Chicago Stritch School of Medicine, Maywood, IL, USA

Jordan Rosenblum MD
Professor of Radiology and Neurology and Chief, Section of Neuroradiology, Loyola University Chicago Stritch School of Medicine, Maywood, IL, USA

Sean Ruland DO
Associate Professor of Neurology, Loyola University Chicago Stritch School of Medicine, Maywood, IL, USA

Arash Salardini MBBS
Instructor, Department of Neurology, Yale School of Medicine, New Haven, CT, USA

Michael J. Schneck MD
Professor of Neurology and Neurosurgery, Loyola University Chicago Stritch School of Medicine, Maywood, IL, USA

Adriane J. Sinclair MD
Division of Neurology, The Hospital for Sick Children, Toronto, Canada

Aneesh B. Singhal MD FAAN FAHA
Associate Professor of Neurology, Harvard Medical School, Vice-Chair of Neurology, Quality and Safety, Massachusetts General Hospital, Boston, MA, USA

David A. Stidd MD MS
Neuroendovascular Fellow, Rush University Medical Center, Chicago, IL, USA

Ana Verdelho MD PhD
Dementia Unit, Hospital do Mar; Invited Professor of Neurology, Department of Neurosciences, Hospital de Santa Maria, University of Lisbon, Lisbon, Portugal

Preface

We are humbled and honored to follow in the footsteps of our esteemed colleagues Valerie Purvin and Aki Kawasaki's *Common Neuro-Ophthalmic Pitfalls – Case-Based Teaching* (Cambridge University Press, 2009) and Alberto J. Espay and Anthony E. Lang's *Common Movement Disorders Pitfalls – Case Based Learning* (Cambridge University Press, 2012). Today more than ever, despite the caprice of technology innovation in the digital age, experience with specific clinical problems and the clinical-case study, remains among the best and most suitable methods of learning and continuing professional development.

The discipline of Cerebrovascular Disease has grown into an exciting and therapeutically oriented discipline. Over the past two decades, there has been an explosion of new and innovative medical, surgical, and endovascular therapies for a variety of ischemic and hemorrhagic cerebrovascular disorders. In this volume on Cerebrovascular Diseases, one of the most specialized interdisciplinary and applied area of the modern clinical neurosciences, a deliberate attempt has been made to streamline the presentation of clinically relevant topical material by bridging theory and practice, with an aim to strike a balance between readability and completeness including a fairly comprehensive list of relevant references given at the end of each chapter.

This volume goes beyond the scope and configuration of classic neurology or cerebrovascular texts, and is intended for the instruction of neurology and neurosurgery residents, stroke fellows, practicing general neurologists, neurohospitalists, hospitalists, and emergency medicine specialists. We also aim to serve the experienced and busy adult and child stroke specialist and general neurologists. We are hopeful that the readership will find this volume informative, reliable, and intellectually stimulating, and we welcome criticisms for any potential distortions.

In daily clinical experience, patients do not present with known diagnoses, thus, in cerebrovascular disease, as in neurology in general, diagnosis is built upon details found by thorough and probing clinical examination artfully distinguishing between *looking* and *seeing*. As such, this special volume on *Pitfalls in Cerebrovascular Disease – Case Based Learning* includes 18 chapters encompassing an array of ischemic and hemorrhagic cerebrovascular disorders. The book begins with thorough discussions on transient ischemic attacks in adults and children. This is followed by an insightful discussion on different aspects of cerebrovascular imaging challenges and potential pitfalls. The next chapters address comprehensive discussions on antithrombotic and thrombolytic therapy in the context of atrial fibrillation, other cardiovascular disorders, recurrent atherothrombotic cerebrovascular disease, and hyperacute ischemic stroke management. Detailed accounts in the management of selective disorders with modern endovascular interventions, carotid artery revascularization procedures, and the conundrum of closure in patients with stroke and patent foramen ovale is covered in the next chapters. Subsequent chapters deal with pitfalls and tips in the diagnosis and management of cerebral vasculitis, cerebrovascular causes of *thunderclap headaches*, reversible cerebral vasoconstriction syndromes, moyamoya disease and other non-atherosclerotic cerebral vasculopathies, as well as vascular cognitive impairment. Later chapters deal with critical accounts on pitfalls in diagnosis and management of subarachnoid hemorrhage and intracerebral hemorrhage, to conclude with an artful and cogent discussion of pitfalls, tips, and potential fallacies in managing patients with cerebrovascular disease or rather their often over utilized ancillary tests.

We wish to thank all the contributing authors for their kindness and collegiality in giving of their time, effort and expertise to the preparation of this volume. We are deeply indebted to Nicholas Dunton, LailaGrieg-Gran, Jenny Slater and other members of the editorial staff at Cambridge University Press for their gracious support. Our thanks are due to Linda Turner for her forbearance and her efficient secretarial and administrative expertise. Last but not least, we wish to express our appreciation to the patients in our care.

Transient ischemic attacks and stroke mimics and chameleons

Ana Catarina Fonseca

In most cases the diagnosis of transient ischemic attacks (TIAs) and strokes is straightforward. However, there are non-vascular disorders that can present with neurologic deficits that simulate cerebrovascular disease (mimics), and TIAs and strokes that can present in unusual ways that resemble something else (chameleons) (Tables 1.1 and 1.2). In this chapter, eight clinical scenarios highlight some of the most common stroke or TIA mimics and chameleons. Careful history gathering thorough clinical examination, and appropriate imaging tests are needed to identify these mimics and chameleons.

Case 1. Patient with focal neurologic deficits

Case description

A 72-year-old man was found by his wife lying on the ground. She noticed he was rather sleepy, did not answer questions, and was unable to move his right side. She had last seen him well 20 minutes earlier. Past medical history was remarkable for arterial hypertension, dyslipidemia, and a left middle cerebral artery (MCA) stroke 2 years earlier. He had recovered with only minor sequelae in performing fine movements with his right hand.

When he arrived at the emergency department, half an hour later, he was awake, had a global aphasia, right central facial paresis, right-sided hemiparesis (Medical Research Council grade 3), and bilateral Babinski signs. The National Institutes of Health Stroke Scale (NIHSS) score was 12. According to his wife, he was improving clinically. He had no lateral tongue biting, urinary or fecal incontinence, or trauma. He was afebrile. Blood pressure was 160/70 mmHg. Blood glucose, full blood count, electrolytes, C-reactive protein (CRP), INR, and a PTT were unremarkable. Brain computed tomography scan (CT scan) showed an old left insular infarct (Figure 1.1). Otherwise, the CT was unremarkable without signs of an acute infarct.

As he was leaving the CT-scan room, he had brief involuntary movements of the right hemibody, with twitching of the right side of the face, and right gaze deviation. The involuntary movements lasted for approximately 20 seconds. Brain magnetic resonance imaging (MRI) with diffusion-weighted imaging (DWI) and apparent diffusion coefficient (ADC) sequences showed no evidence of acute ischemic lesions.

Diagnostic reasoning

In the emergency department, physicians have to decide promptly what is the most probable diagnosis and what the next action will be. When our patient arrived at the emergency department, his neurologic examination and presentation were compatible with an acute ischemic stroke of the left MCA territory. He had sudden onset of focal neurologic deficits and had multiple vascular risk factors. As the patient was last seen without symptoms within 50 minutes before arriving at the emergency department, the patient was well within the 4.5 hour time window from symptom onset or from last seen well to administer intravenous thrombolysis with recombinant tissue plasminogen activator (tPA). The CT was also unremarkable for acute ischemic stroke and excluded other disorders that could mimic an acute ischemic stroke such as primary central nervous system (CNS) tumors, metastasis, brain abscess, or hemorrhages.

However, the adventitious movements experienced by the patient as he was leaving the CT-scan

Common Pitfalls in Cerebrovascular Disease: Case-Based Learning, ed. José Biller and José M. Ferro. Published by Cambridge University Press. © Cambridge University Press 2015.

Table 1.1 Examples of TIA and stroke mimics

- Intracranial mass lesions (tumors)
- Intracranial infection (abscess, encephalitis)
- Subdural hematoma
- Seizures and Todd's paralysis
- Acute peripheral vestibulopathy (benign paroxysmal positional vertigo [BPPV] or acute labyrinthitis)
- Transient global amnesia
- Peripheral neuropathies including Bell's palsy
- Migraine with aura including sporadic or familial hemiplegic migraine
- Metabolic disturbances that may cause new neurologic deficits or re-expression of previous deficits (hypoglycemia, non-ketotic hyperglycemia, hyponatremia, hypoxia, hepatic encephalopathy, Wernicke–Korsakoff syndrome, alcohol and drug intoxication, systemic infection)
- Mitochondrial encephalomyopathy, lactic acidosis, and stroke-like episodes (MELAS)
- Psychiatric disorders (conversion disorder, anxiety or panic attacks, malingering)
- Acute demyelination (multiple sclerosis)
- Alternating hemiplegia
- Syncope
- Retinal/ocular pathology

Table 1.2 Examples of TIA and stroke chameleons

- Bilateral thalamic infarcts
- Cortical stroke or TIA
- Limb shaking TIA
- Capsular warning syndrome
- Bilateral occipital strokes or TIAs
- Lateral medullary strokes or TIAs

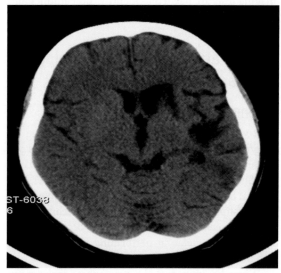

Figure 1.1 Brain CT scan showing an old infarct in the left middle cerebral artery territory.

room raised concerns for a possible seizure secondary to an acute ischemic stroke, or a seizure with a Todd's paralysis since the very onset. Partial or secondary generalized seizures may occur in the acute phase of ischemic stroke. Initially described in the nineteenth century by Robert Bentley Todd, Todd's paralysis refers to a post-seizure event, defined as a transient weakness and depression of motor ability lasting hours to days. It usually affects one or more limbs and follows a focal seizure, or more rarely a generalized tonic-clonic seizure [1]. Sometimes, there may be other neurologic signs such as aphasia, neglect, or psychosis depending on the epileptic focus and surrounding focal areas involved. Therefore, features of post-seizure Todd's paralysis may be similar to an acute ischemic stroke. Several clinical series present unwitnessed or unrecognized seizures with the post-ictal state misdiagnosed as stroke being the most common stroke mimic.

Some small series suggest that patients with structural lesions, such as those with previous brain infarcts and the elderly, may be more likely to have transient focal weakness following a seizure. Although there is no consensus regarding the pathophysiology of Todd's paralysis, hypotheses regarding its pathogenesis include: neuronal desensitization, neurotransmitter depletion, active suppression and exhaustive neuronal firing, and localized cerebral hypoperfusion resulting from motor cortex exhaustion.

A detailed description of the onset of symptoms is critical to distinguish between Todd's paralysis and an acute ischemic stroke. However, patients are often unable to report onset of symptoms either because they are aphasic or unaware of their deficits. In these cases, accompanying family members may provide valuable information. However, in our patient, symptom onset was not witnessed, and doubts regarding the precise diagnosis remained. This diagnostic uncertainty has a clear repercussion in management, as interventional stroke therapies have potential serious side effects such as intracranial bleeding. Also, although patients with seizures at stroke onset were excluded from thrombolytic trials due to the possibility of confusion with Todd's paralysis, case series suggest that thrombolysis could be useful if there is evidence of a new ischemic stroke. Therefore, it is currently recommended by the European Stroke Organisation that intravenous tPA may be used in patients with seizures at stroke onset, if the neurologic deficit is related to acute cerebral ischemia (Class IV, Good Clinical Practice – GCP) [2]. Guidelines from the American Heart Association/American Stroke Association (AHA/ASA) [3] state that "intravenous tPA is reasonable in patients with a seizure at the time of onset of stroke, if evidence suggests that residual impairments are secondary to stroke and not a postictal phenomenon" (Class IIa, Level of Evidence C).

The elderly have a high incidence of epilepsy that may be related to cerebrovascular disease [4]. In our patient, there were subtle symptoms in favor of a seizure with Todd's paralysis such as his sleepiness, his neurologic improvement, and the past history of a cortical infarct.

However, our patient was found lying on the floor with an acute focal neurologic deficit. He had multiple vascular risk factors including hypertension, dyslipidemia, and a previous stroke, all of which could have been in favor of a new stroke. However, our patient did not have a prior history of seizures.

In these situations, MRI with DWI/ADC sequences can be useful to exclude the presence of acute cerebral lesions not yet detectable with a CT scan. DWI/MRI is the most useful exam to differentiate between an acute ischemic stroke and stroke mimics. Of note, there are reports of hyperintensities on brain DWI/MRI in Todd's postepileptic paralysis described as gyriform cortical hyperintensities that do not necessarily reflect ongoing seizure activity. These image changes are not associated with a particular vascular distribution, and rather reflect the epileptic foci and surrounding tissue.

Brain CT angiography may be an indirect useful modality in differentiating Todd's paralysis from early seizure and ischemia by detection of intracranial occlusions, which would favor a diagnosis of an ischemic lesion [5]. Electroencephalography (EEG) does not help in differentiating these entities, as focal slowing and epileptiform activity can occur in both acute ischemia and in the post-seizure period.

Tip

An adequate clinical history that properly characterizes time of symptom onset is critical to distinguish TIA or stroke from other pathologies that can also present with focal neurologic deficits.

Case 2. Headache and hemiparesis

Case description

A 21-year-old woman noticed that upon standing up from a chair, her left side became weak and numb. One hour later, she had a throbbing left-sided headache and felt nauseous. She had a history of recurring unilateral throbbing headaches of moderate intensity accompanied by nausea, photophobia, and sonophobia. Headaches were severe enough to interfere with her daily activities. One year earlier, she had a similar episode of headache, preceded by a feeling of heaviness of the right arm which subsided in a few hours. Her sister and mother had a similar history of headaches and occasional weakness. On admission, her blood pressure was 105/60 mmHg. When she arrived at the emergency department she had a left central facial paresis, a left hemiparesis (Medical Research Council grade 4), and left hemisensory loss. Blood glucose was 110 mg/dL. Brain MRI was unremarkable. The headache resolved within 3 hours, but her left hemiparesis persisted for 5 more hours.

Diagnostic reasoning

The young age of our patient and the lack of traditional vascular risk factors raised the possibility of an alternative diagnosis to a TIA. TIAs are rare in young patients without vascular risk factors. The presence of recurrent transient neurologic deficits followed by an evanescent headache led to the diagnosis of migraine with aura. Migraines usually start in the first or second decades of life. Our patient had a past history of pulsatile, moderate intensity, unilateral headaches with nausea and photophobia that suggest a diagnosis of migraines [6]. Migraine is a common disorder that can be accompanied by aura in about a third of patients. Migraines with aura can present with neurologic symptoms resembling a TIA or stroke. An aura is defined as transient focal neurologic symptoms that usually precede, or sometimes accompany, the headache. The symptoms usually last minutes and are fully reversible, and are usually followed by a headache and other associated migrainous symptoms [7]. However, the headache may sometimes be absent masking the correct diagnosis. The typical migraine aura is most commonly visual, but it may also be characterized by sensory, speech, or language difficulties. Visual symptoms may be characterized by positive features such as zigzag lines or flickering spots with or without negative features such as scotomata. Basilar migraine may present with double vision, unsteadiness, fainting, or losing consciousness. Retinal or ophthalmic migraine typically affects only one eye. Whenever the aura includes weakness as a symptom, it is classified as hemiplegic migraine, as in our patient. Distinguishing motor from sensory auras can be challenging at times. The motor aura should be a clearly characterized motor deficit such as weakness with difficulty moving one hand, arm, or leg. Some patients with a sensory aura may report dropping objects. A population-based epidemiological survey found a prevalence of 0.005% for hemiplegic migraine [8]. Patients with hemiplegic migraine may, in addition to motor aura, have any of the aura symptoms of migraines with aura or basilar migraine [7]. Most patients also have attacks of migraines with typical aura – without weakness. The most common accompanying aura symptom besides weakness in these patients is sensory. The typical sensory aura is characterized by tingling involving one of the digits that gradually progresses to involve other digits, up to the arm, and then affects the face, tongue, and later the body and leg. The different aura symptoms progress slowly over 20–30 minutes and occur successively, mainly in the following order: visual, sensory, motor, aphasic, and basilar disturbances.

Migraine aura is considered to be caused by cortical spreading depression, which is characterized by a brief neuronal excitation that initiates a depolarization wave that moves across the cortex followed by a prolonged inhibition of neuronal activity [9]. Hemiplegic migraine can occur as a sporadic or a familial disorder.

Patients with sporadic hemiplegic migraine lack a family history of at least one affected first-degree or second-degree relative. The sporadic and hemiplegic migraine forms have a similar prevalence of 0.002–0.003%. Familial hemiplegic migraine (FHM) is dominantly inherited. The presence of similar symptoms in both her sister and mother suggest this type of inheritance in our patient. FHM1 is caused by mutations in the *CACNA1A* gene located in chromosome 19, FHM2 by mutations in the *ATP1A2* gene located in chromosome 1, and FHM3 by mutations in the *SCN1A* gene located in chromosome 2. All the involved genes take part in ion transport. Both sporadic and familial forms of hemiplegic migraine have similar clinical presentations. The mean frequency of episodes is approximately three per year; the frequency and severity tend to decrease with advancing age.

Imaging and cerebrospinal fluid (CSF) studies done during or after an episode of migraine are unremarkable, except in FHM1 where cerebellar atrophy may be present.

Headache is a common feature of acute ischemic stroke. Twenty-seven percent of patients experience a headache at stroke onset. Sometimes, headache in patients with stroke may point to a cervical artery dissection as the cause. There is also a specific type of stroke related to migraine – migrainous infarction. In migrainous infarction the symptoms associated with the typical aura are not fully reversible. The International Classification of Headache Disorders, 3rd Edition (ICHD-3) beta version defines migrainous infarction as one or more otherwise typical auras persisting beyond one hour with neuroimaging confirmation of an ischemic infarction in the affected territory [6]. Meningitis and intracranial venous thrombosis may also present with headaches and focal neurologic deficits, but usually other diagnostic clues are present.

Tip

Diagnosis of hemiplegic migraine relies on a careful description of the aura and on the exclusion of other symptomatic causes. The diagnosis is often made only after recurrent, stereotypic attacks.

Case 3. Sudden memory impairment

Case description

A 65-year-old woman was admitted to hospital due to a sudden onset of memory impairment. Early in the morning, she telephoned her husband telling him she had vertigo and was not feeling well. Five minutes later, when her husband found her, she made him repeat questions: Where am I? What happened? What am I doing here? What day is this? Although he answered appropriately, she did not seem to remember his answers, as she repeated the same questions over and over again. She also did not remember what she had done the day before. This episode lasted 5 hours, with a gradual improvement in her ability to recall information. During the episode, she never lost contact with her husband. He did not notice any involuntary movements or automatisms. When she was seen at the emergency department, she was able to recall new information. However, she could not remember what had happened early in the day. She had a past history of hypertension and was under treatment with lisinopril. There was no history of recent head trauma. She did not take any drugs or new medications. On admission, she was afebrile. Blood pressure was 113/70 mmHg. Neurologic examination was unremarkable, including her ability to recall new information, tested by the three-word test/word list and evocation of recent events. Blood glucose was 120 mg/dL. Brain MRI with DWI and ADC sequences were unremarkable. EEG showed focal slowing or epileptiform activity. Follow-up brain MRI with diffusion sequence performed 3 days later showed a rounded image restriction in the CA1 segment of the right hippocampus (Figure 1.2). She did not have further symptoms.

Diagnostic considerations

This sudden impairment of memory is consistent with transient global amnesia (TGA). The incidence of TGA ranges between 3 and 8 per 100 000 people per year [10]. TGA is characterized by sudden onset of anterograde and retrograde amnesia lasting for up to 24 hours, but usually lasting substantially less. There should be no loss of personal identity, personality, language, or visuospatial functions during the amnestic episode. Also, no other neurologic deficits, recent head trauma, or signs of a seizure should be present. After the episode, anterograde memory returns to normal, but the patient may never remember what happened during the period of amnesia. TGA most commonly occurs in patients in their sixth or seventh decade of life. Headaches, dizziness, or nausea may be present during an episode of TGA. Strenuous physical activities or strong emotional events may antedate onset

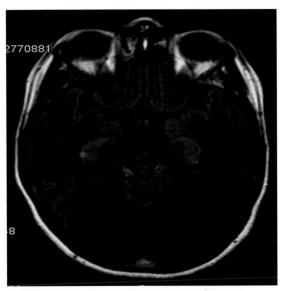

Figure 1.2 Brain MRI showing a rounded image in the CA1 segment of the right hippocampus.

of symptoms [11]. Neuroimaging studies following an acute TGA event show transient perturbation of specific hippocampal circuits involved in memory processing. Focal diffusion lesions can be selectively detected in the CA1 field of the hippocampal cornu ammonis on brain MRI with DWI/ADC when done approximately 72 hours after symptom onset.

Although migraine, focal ischemia, venous flow abnormalities, and epileptic phenomena have been implicated in the pathophysiology of TGA, the factors triggering these unique events remain unknown. Recent data suggest that the vulnerability of the CA1 neurons to metabolic stress plays an important role in the pathophysiological cascade, leading to an impairment of hippocampal function during TGA [12].

There are cases of transient amnesia due to focal seizure activity also known as transient epileptic amnesia. Transient epileptic amnesia has clinical presentation similar to TGA episodes and tends to occur in the morning hours, but it can be distinguished by the shorter duration and repeated amnestic periods.

TIAs or strokes with memory impairment are rare. Every region of the limbic system involved in memory processing may be damaged by strokes, but very rarely in isolation. The combination of amnesia with other acute associated neurologic deficits often leads to the suspicion of a cerebrovascular event in these patients [13].

Tip

TGA leads to an isolated temporary memory impairment that can last up to 24 hours.

Case 4. Focal neurologic deficits due to metabolic disturbances

Case description

A 60-year-old woman was admitted to hospital half an hour after her husband noticed increased somnolence, confusion, and decreased strength in her left arm and leg. She had taken her medications during the morning and had gone jogging. Two hours later, her husband found her to be somnolent, with confused speech and difficulty moving her left arm and leg. She had a past history of diabetes mellitus type 2 and ischemic heart disease; she was on metformin, glibenclamide, aspirin, and bisoprolol. Upon admission, neurologic examination showed impaired alertness, confusion, and left hemiparesis (Medical Research Council grade 3). Blood glucose level was 50 mg/dL. She immediately received intravenous 10% glucose. Brain CT scan was unremarkable. Approximately 20 minutes following correction of her blood glucose levels, she started to improve, and made a complete recovery 5 hours after symptom onset. It was later determined that the patient had taken a higher dose of glibenclamide.

Diagnostic considerations

Hypoglycemia and less often hyperglycemia (blood glucose concentration >400 mg/dL) can cause focal neurologic deficits that can mimic a TIA or stroke [14]. Hypoglycemia is a very important differential diagnosis of TIA and stroke. Generally defined as a blood glucose level <70 mg/dL (3.9 mmol/L), it is more common among patients with diabetes mellitus. However, any patient can have hypoglycemia. Causes of hypoglycemia include medications (insulin or sulfonylureas), exercise, fasting, alcohol, insulin secreting tumors, and endocrine disorders such as Addison's disease. In our patient, a personal history of diabetes mellitus and antidiabetic medications namely with sulfonylureas (glibenclamide) should lead to the suspicion of a broad differential diagnosis including hypoglycemia. Glucose is an obligate metabolic fuel for the brain under physiologic conditions, and it is essential for brain metabolism as the brain cannot synthesize glucose or store more than a few minutes' supply as glycogen. Therefore, the brain needs a continuous arterial supply of glucose. As the plasma glucose concentration falls, blood-to-brain glucose transport becomes insufficient to support brain energy metabolism and function. If hypoglycemia is severe and prolonged and remains untreated, it can lead to a life-threatening situation. Acute effects of hypoglycemia are primarily neurologic. Symptoms of hypoglycemia are initially related to catecholamine release, and later, if untreated, due to neuroglycopenia. Autonomic symptoms include tachycardia, diaphoresis, tremor, anxiety, and hunger. These symptoms are important warnings; however, they may be lacking, for example, among diabetic patients with autonomic insufficiency or in patients on beta-blockers like our patient. Beta-blockers may mask the sympathetic nervous system manifestations of hypoglycemia, and therefore, patients may manifest only symptoms of neuroglycopenia. Neuroglycopenic symptoms are usually present when levels of blood glucose are <50 mg/dL (<2.8 mmol/L). However, these thresholds are dynamic, and in patients with poorly controlled diabetes mellitus, these thresholds are shifted to higher blood glucose concentrations. Neuroglycopenic symptoms include impairment of consciousness that can progress to coma if untreated, confusion, abnormal behaviors, seizures, headaches, and focal neurologic symptoms [15]. Therefore, measurement of blood glucose levels should be part of the initial evaluation of all patients presenting with focal neurologic deficits. Focal neurologic deficits in hypoglycemia may include aphasia, homonymous hemianopsia, hemisensory deficits, hemiparesis, unilateral hyperreflexia, and Babinski sign(s). Both the American Heart Association (AHA) and the European Stroke Organisation (ESO) recommend determination of blood glucose concentration in their guidelines for the evaluation of stroke patients [1,2]. When hypoglycemia is detected, treatment should be started as soon as possible. Both intravenous dextrose and infusion of 10–20% glucose can be used to correct hypoglycemia. Thiamine, 100 mg intravenously or intramuscularly, is given to patients with alcohol dependence to prevent Wernicke's encephalopathy before administering glucose. If intravenous therapy is not possible, subcutaneous or intramuscular glucagon may be used. For non-hypoglycemic patients, excessive dextrose-containing fluids have the potential to exacerbate cerebral injury. Therefore, normal saline is more appropriate if rehydration is required. Of note, there can be a delay of hours to days between correction of blood glucose concentration and improvement of neuroglycopenic symptoms. If abnormalities persist longer than 30 minutes following glucose administration and hypoglycemia has not recurred, other causes should be investigated with brain imaging and appropriate laboratory evaluation.

Imaging abnormalities in patients with hypoglycemia are uncommon but very variable, weakly associated with the neurologic deficits, and about a fifth may mimic an acute ischemic stroke. Diffuse and extensive injury observed on DWI with MRI predicts a poor neurologic outcome in patients with hypoglycemic injuries [16].

Other metabolic disturbances that may account for focal neurologic deficits include hyponatremia, hypernatremia [17], and hepatic encephalopathy [18].

Tip

Always check blood glucose concentration in patients presenting with impaired consciousness or focal neurologic symptoms.

Case 5. Recurrent stroke?

Case description

A 78-year-old woman was admitted to hospital due to worsening left-sided hemiparesis. Past medical history was remarkable for diabetes mellitus, dyslipidemia, atrial fibrillation, hypertension, and a right MCA infarct 2 years earlier. She was on metformin, simvastatin, enalapril, and warfarin. As a result of her stroke, she had a left hemiparesis (Medical Research Council grade 4) that allowed her to do most of her daily activities. On the day before admission, her son noticed she was more sleepy and confused, and on the day of admission, he noticed she had increased difficulty moving her left side, shortness of breath, and cough. On admission, she was afebrile. Respiratory rate was 20 cycles per minute. Blood pressure was 137/72 mmHg. Oxygen saturation was 92% on room air. Her breath sounds were decreased over the left lung base. She was somnolent and had a left hemiparesis with a left Babinski sign. There was a neutrophilic leukocytosis. CRP was 7 mg/dL. Blood glucose concentration was 233 mg/dL. Electrolytes and renal function tests were unremarkable. INR was 2.3. Chest X-ray showed consolidation of the left lung base. Brain MRI showed an old right MCA infarct with no new acute lesions on DWI or ADC sequences. She received antibiotics for community-acquired pneumonia,

and her neurologic deficits returned to baseline after 3 days.

Diagnostic considerations

In our patient it was important to consider if the patient had a new stroke. The presence of vascular risk factors, such as hypertension, dyslipidemia, and atrial fibrillation, a previous stroke, and worsening of previous neurologic deficits suggested the possibility of a new stroke. Moreover, the patient was on warfarin, raising concerns for a possible intracranial hemorrhage, one of the most feared complications of anticoagulants. Furthermore, elderly patients with motor deficits may also suffer frequent falls, and when under anticoagulant therapy, they are at increased risk of having subdural hematomas caused by rupture of intracranial bridging veins. Chronic subdural hematomas may present weeks to months after mild head trauma although a history of head trauma may not be remarkable. The neurologic examination showed she had worsening of her previous neurologic deficits, apparently without new neurologic signs. She also had symptoms of a respiratory infection such as cough and shortness of breath. Many times, elderly patients lack fever or other clear signs of infections, and an underlying infection may present as an acute confusional state or worsening of previous neurologic deficits. While a systemic infection can account for re-expression of previous focal neurologic deficits, sepsis by itself may be a risk factor for stroke, as it can induce a hypercoagulable state or be associated with infective embolism. In our patient's brain, MRI with DWI/ADC sequences showed no new lesions, and her physical examination, blood analysis, and chest X-ray confirmed she had pneumonia. Few scientific studies have directly analyzed the underlying reasons why metabolic insults may cause re-expression of neurologic deficits in patients with previous stroke. The most common culprits include urinary tract infections, pneumonia, hypoxia, hyponatremia, medication overdose, hypoglycemia, and non-ketotic hyperglycemia. All patients evaluated for a possible acute stroke require a set of laboratory tests, including a complete blood count, basic metabolic profile, coagulation studies, urinalysis, toxicology screen when appropriate, and chest X-rays. The laboratory tests assist in identifying stroke mimics, determine whether patients may be eligible for intravenous thrombolysis, and also assist in screening for conditions that may influence stroke outcomes.

Two main hypotheses have been preferred regarding the re-expression of neurologic symptoms in patients with previous strokes:

1. Pathways formed during stroke recovery may be more susceptible to intercurrent metabolic derangements.
2. The penumbral region may be more susceptible to intercurrent metabolic changes than healthy tissue.

Tip

Metabolic insults may cause re-expression of neurologic deficits in a patient with previous stroke. Patients usually regain their baseline status following correction of the precipitating insult.

Case 6. Difficulty in using hand

Case description

A 28-year-old woman was admitted to hospital due to decreased right-hand strength. She had been well on the previous day. However, upon awakening she noticed difficulty performing some activities with her right hand. Past medical history was unremarkable. Blood pressure on admission was 120/90 mmHg. Neurologic examination disclosed paresis of the right hand with impaired extension of the fingers and dorsiflexion of the right hand, and decreased sensation on the dorsum of the first and second digits of the right hand. The rest of the neurologic examination including muscle stretch reflexes was unremarkable. Brain MRI with DWI/ADC sequences did not disclose acute ischemic lesions.

Diagnostic considerations

Focal neurologic deficits may have other causes than stroke. Our patient had a right radial neuropathy. The signs and symptoms included wrist drop, finger extension weakness, thumb abduction weakness, and sensory loss over the dorsal web between the thumb and index finger. Patients with radial nerve compression at the spinal groove of the humerus may wake up with a wrist drop after a sound sleep. The triceps reflex is often intact. Sometimes, there may be a history of alcohol intoxication. Patients undergoing surgical procedures may also present with mononeuropathies due to compression during limb positioning. In these instances, the ulnar and peroneal nerves are more commonly affected.

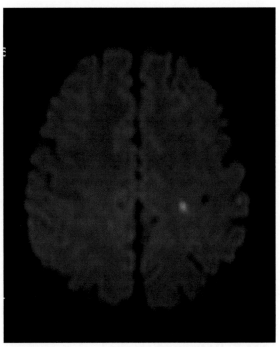

Figure 1.3 Brain diffusion-weighted MRI showing restriction in the left precentral gyrus.

Isolated monoparesis is the main clinical presentation in 5% of all strokes [19]. Cortical strokes may be distinguished from a radial neuropathy due to weakness or sensory changes outside of the territory of the radial nerve and alteration in muscle tone and muscle stretch reflexes. Sometimes, the differential diagnosis may be challenging, and in these instances, brain MRI can be quite useful (Figure 1.3). Strokes simulating a radial neuropathy often involve the "hand-knob" area of the cerebral cortex [20]. This omega-shaped region within the precentral gyrus referred to as the cortical "hand-knob" is the site of hand motor function.

Electromyography (EMG) with nerve conduction studies may be unremarkable in the first 2 to 3 weeks after symptom onset, and therefore may not be helpful for differential diagnosis in the acute phase. In most cases, radial neuropathy improves spontaneously after 6 to 8 weeks.

Tip

It is important to perform a thorough neurologic examination in patients presenting with focal neurologic deficits and establish if the pattern of neurologic deficit suggests a particular lesion site.

Case 7. Shaking movements of the left hemibody

Case description

A 57-year-old man was admitted to hospital due to involuntary "shaking" movements of his left hemibody. He had had several previous episodes, which were only noticed when standing or walking. These "non-marching" involuntary and non-rhythmic shaking movements lasted an average of 2 minutes, and simultaneously involved the upper and lower limbs. There was no alteration in the level of consciousness. He had a personal history of hypertension, dyslipidemia, and smoking, and was under treatment with losartan. On admission, blood pressure was 120/90 mmHg. Neurologic examination was unremarkable, except for a right carotid bruit. Brain MRI showed old watershed infarcts between the right anterior cerebral artery (ACA) and right MCA and between the right MCA and the right posterior cerebral artery (PCA) (Figure 1.4).

Carotid Doppler ultrasound showed a subtotal stenosis of the right internal carotid artery (ICA) (Figure 1.5), later confirmed by magnetic resonance angiography.

Transcranial Doppler (TCD) showed a post-occlusive flow on the right MCA. Interictal EEG showed no epileptiform activity.

The patient was started on aspirin and simvastatin. A right carotid endarterectomy was performed and the patient did not have further symptoms.

Diagnostic considerations

Transient ischemic attacks usually present with neurologic deficits such as loss of muscular strength, reduced sensation, speech and/or language disturbances, or loss of vision. However, they can also present with unusual symptoms such as involuntary movements. Limb shaking TIA, first described by C. Miller Fisher in 1962, has been associated with severe ICA stenosis. Limb shaking TIAs manifest as rhythmic or arrhythmic involuntary hyperkinesias affecting the hand, arm, leg, hand–arm, or hand–arm–leg unilaterally. The movements can be mistaken for focal motor seizures; however, there is no Jacksonian march or involvement of the face. The involuntary movements usually have a low frequency (about 3 Hz), and are frequently described as shaking, jerking, twitching, or trembling [21]. There may also be other associated symptoms

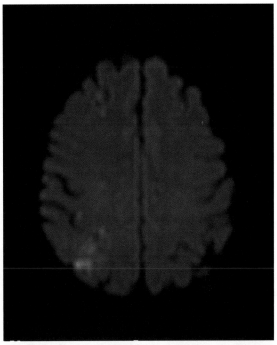

Figure 1.4 Brain MRI in DWI sequence showing watershed infarcts between the right anterior cerebral artery and right middle cerebral artery and between the right middle cerebral artery and the right posterior cerebral artery.

including ataxia, myoclonus, or dystonic limb posturing. Transient aphasia and/or dysarthria, ipsilateral hemiparesis, and numbness of the shaking extremity may also be present. Symptoms are often precipitated by postural changes such as standing or hyperextending the neck, and relieved by sitting or lying down.

The mechanism underlying limb shaking TIA is considered to be hypoperfusion. The critical ICA stenosis leads to decreased blood supply to watershed territories. The involuntary movements are provoked by maneuvers that further compromise cerebral hypoperfusion [22]. Additional studies suggest reduced vasomotor reactivity of corresponding cerebral territories. Some case reports have had normal carotid angiographies; in these instances, ACA stenosis, small vessel disease, and thalamic and midbrain infarction have been reported in association with limb shaking TIAs. Limb shaking TIAs have also been associated with moyamoya disease, and in these instances they can be elicited by hyperventilation.

EEG in patients with limb shaking TIAs does not show epileptiform activity. Some patients have contralateral slowing in the EEG.

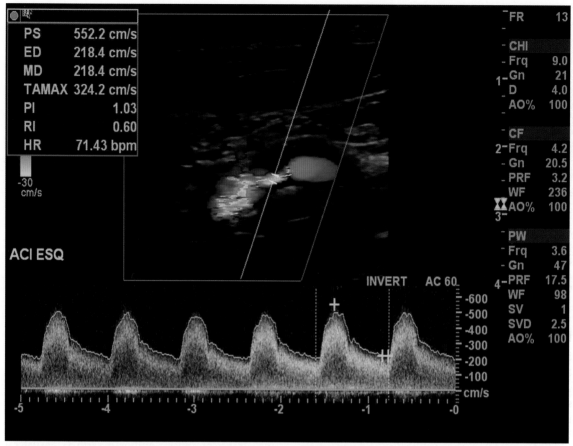

Figure 1.5 Carotid Doppler ultrasound showing stenosis of the right internal carotid artery.

It is important to recognize limb shaking TIAs as they are generally associated with a high-grade carotid artery stenosis that may benefit from reperfusion procedures.

Hemiballismus, chorea, or unilateral dyskinesis may result from acute vascular lesions in the subthalamic nucleus or connections.

Tip

TIAs and strokes may present with less frequent symptoms such as involuntary movements.

Case 8. Altered mental state

Case description

A 55-year-old man was admitted to the hospital due to increased somnolence. His wife noticed he did not wake up in the morning, and he had been sleeping for 10 hours. She attempted to wake him up but he did not react. Past medical history was remarkable for hypertension, diabetes mellitus, and cigarette smoking. He was on metformin and ramipril. There was no history of drug abuse, alcohol intake, or recent head trauma. Blood pressure was 155/90 mmHg. Heart rate was 74 beats per minute. On admission he was somnolent, reacting only to vigorous verbal stimuli. He had bilateral miotic pupils and upward gaze palsy. Blood glucose was 90 mg/dL. Brain MRI with DWI disclosed paramedian bilateral thalamic infarcts (Figure 1.6). Cerebral angiography showed a stenosis of the medial and upper third of the basilar artery with occlusion of the left PCA. EEG showed a pattern of sleep with abnormal architecture with increased stage 1 and reduced stage 2 sleep; neither slow wave sleep nor sleep spindles were registered.

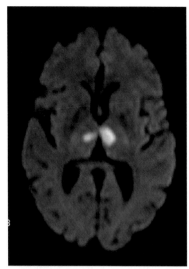

Figure 1.6 Brain MRI with DWI showing paramedian bilateral thalamic infarcts.

Diagnostic considerations

Stroke may present with impaired consciousness. In these cases, it may be initially difficult to differentiate strokes from other pathologies such as postictal states, non-convulsive status epilepticus, encephalitis, or metabolic disturbances. A stroke leading to impaired consciousness involves either the brainstem, the diencephalon, or multiple regions in both cerebral hemispheres. Coma is frequently found in basilar artery occlusion. One of the stroke subtypes that can also present with disturbed consciousness is bilateral paramedian thalamic infarcts caused by occlusion of the artery of Percheron. The Percheron artery is a rare variant of the paramedian branches of the PCA which supplies the paramedian areas of the thalami and upper midbrain [23]. In a registry of 2750 patients with bilateral thalamic stroke, it was reported in 0.6% of the patients [24]. Bilateral paramedian thalamic infarcts typically present with decreased level of consciousness, sleep disturbances, vertical gaze palsy, and memory impairment [25,26]. On presentation to the emergency room, the patient may be comatose or hypersomnolent without other localizing neurologic signs. The cognitive impairment becomes apparent when the decreased level of consciousness improves. This is one of the locations known as "strategic infarcts," which represent single stroke locations that can lead to dementia. Patients with bilateral

paramedian thalamic infarcts frequently have sleep disturbances as the paramedian thalamus has a dual role in the maintenance of wakefulness and promotion of non-REM sleep. The thalamus is also essential in the production of spindles and slow wave activity. The usual changes associated with bilateral paramedian thalamic infarcts include increased stage 1, decreased stage 2, variable decreases in stages 3 and 4, and unchanged REM sleep [27].

Tip

Patients with bilateral paramedian thalamic infarcts may present comatose or hypersomnolent, without other localizing neurologic features.

References

1. Widdess-Walsh P, Devinsky O. Historical perspectives and definitions of the postictal state. *Epilepsy Behav* 2010;19:96–9.

2. European Stroke Organisation (ESO) Executive Committee; ESO Writing Committee. Guidelines for management of ischaemic stroke and transient ischaemic attack 2008. *Cerebrovasc Dis* 2008;25(5):457–507.

3. Jauch EC, Saver JL, Adams HP Jr., Bruno A, Connors JJ, et al. American Heart Association Stroke Council; Council on Cardiovascular Nursing; Council on Peripheral Vascular Disease; Council on Clinical Cardiology. Guidelines for the early management of patients with acute ischemic stroke: a guideline for healthcare professionals from the American Heart Association/American Stroke Association. *Stroke* 2013;44:870–947.

4. Theodore WH. The postictal state: effects of age and underlying brain dysfunction. *Epilepsy Behav* 2010;2:118–20.

5. Mathews MS, Smith WS, Wintermark M, Dillon WP, Binder DK. Local cortical hypoperfusion imaged with CT perfusion during postictal Todd's paresis. *Neuroradiology* 2008;50:397.

6. Headache Classification Committee of the International Headache Society (IHS). The International Classification of Headache Disorders, 3rd edition (beta version). *Cephalalgia* 2013;33:629–808.

7. Russell MB, Ducros A. Sporadic and familial hemiplegic migraine: pathophysiological mechanisms, clinical characteristics, diagnosis, and management. *Lancet Neurol* 2011;10:457–70.

8. Thomsen LL, Eriksen MK, Roemer SF, Andersen I, Olesen J, Russel MB. A population-based study of familial hemiplegic migraine suggests revised diagnostic criteria. *Brain* 2002;125:1379–91.

9. Tfelt-Hansen PC. History of migraine with aura and cortical spreading depression from 1941 and onwards. *Cephalalgia* 2010;30:780–92.

10. Quinette P, Guillery-Girard B, Dayan J, de la Sayette V, Marquis S, Viader F, Desgranges B, Eustache F. What does transient global amnesia really mean? Review of the literature and thorough study of 142 cases. *Brain* 2006;129:1640–58.

11. Bartsch T, Deuschl G. Transient global amnesia: functional anatomy and clinical implications. *Lancet Neurol* 2010;9:1205–14.

12. Bartsch T, Butler C. Transient amnestic syndromes. *Nat Rev Neurol* 2013;9:86–97.

13. Lim C, Alexander MP. Stroke and episodic memory disorders. *Neuropsychologia* 2009;47:3045–58.

14. Yong AW, Morris Z, Shuler K, Smith C, Wardlaw J. Acute symptomatic hypoglycaemia mimicking ischaemic stroke on imaging: a systemic review. *BMC Neurol* 2012;12:139.

15. Suh SW, Hamby AM, Swanson RA. Hypoglycemia, brain energetics, and hypoglycemic neuronal death. *Glia* 2007;55:1280–6.

16. Wallis WE, Donaldson I, Scott RS, Wilson J. Hypoglycemia masquerading as cerebrovascular disease (hypoglycemic hemiplegia). *Ann Neurol* 1985;18:510–12.

17. Amort M, Fluri F, Schafer J, Weisskopf F, Katan M, Burrow A, Bucher HC, Bonati LH, Lyrer PA, Engelter ST. Transient ischemic attack versus transient ischemic attack mimics: frequency, clinical characteristics and outcome. *Cerebrovasc Dis* 2011;32:57–64.

18. Cadranel JF, Lebiez E, Di Martino V, Bernard B, El Koury S, Tourbah A, Pidoux B, Valla D, Opolon P. Focal neurological signs in hepatic encephalopathy in cirrhotic patients: an underestimated entity? *Am J Gastroenterol* 2001;96:515–18.

19. Maeder-Ingvar M, van Melle G, Bogousslavsky J. Pure monoparesis: a particular stroke subgroup? *Arch Neurol* 2005;62:1221–4.

20. Gass A, Szabo K, Behrens S, Rossmanith C, Hennerici M. A diffusion-weighted MRI study of acute ischemic distal arm paresis. *Neurology* 2001;57:1589–94.

21. Ali S, Khan MA, Khealani B. Limb-shaking transient ischemic attacks: case report and review of literature. *BMC Neurol* 2006;26(6):5.

22. Tatemichi TK, Young WL, Prohovnik I, Gitelman DR, Correll JW, Mohr JP. Perfusion insufficiency in limb-shaking transient ischemic attacks. *Stroke* 1990;21:341–7.

23. Amin OS, Schwani SS, Zangana HM, Hussein EM, Ameen NA. Bilateral infarction of paramedian thalami: a report of two cases of artery of Percheron occlusion and review of the literature. *BMJ Case Rep* 2011doi:10.1136/bcr.09.2010.3304.

24. Kumral E, Evypan D, Balkir K, Kutluhan S. Bilateral thalamic infarction. Clinical, etiological and MRI correlates. *Act Neurol Scand* 2001;103:35–42.

25. Bogousslavsky J, Van Melle G, Regli F. The Lausanne Stroke Registry: analysis of 1000 consecutive patients with first stroke. *Stroke* 1988;19:1083–92.

26. Bogousslavsky J, Regli F, Uske A. Thalamic infarcts: clinical syndromes, etiology and prognosis. *Neurology* 1988;38:387.

27. Bassetti C, Mathis J, Gugger M, Lovblad KO, Hess CW. Hypersomnia following paramedian thalamic stroke: a report of 12 patients. *Ann Neurol* 1996;39:471–80.

Chapter

2

Recognizing transient ischemic attacks in children and young adults

Adriane J. Sinclair, Leanne K. Casaubon, and Gabrielle deVeber

Introduction

Transient ischemic attacks (TIAs) occur in all age groups including infants, children [1], young adults, and the elderly. The age definition of "young adult" varies in the stroke literature. For the purpose of this chapter, we will generally be referring to children and young adults between 1 and 50 years of age. The definition of a transient ischemic attack has evolved from the original "time-based" definition to a "tissue-based" definition [2]. In the time-based definition, a transient ischemic attack was defined as any focal ischemic cerebral event with symptom duration of <24 hours. A transient ischemic attack is now defined as a transient episode of neurologic dysfunction caused by focal brain, spinal cord, or retinal ischemia without corresponding acute infarction on imaging studies. This tissue-based definition recognizes the risk of permanent brain injury, even with symptom duration of less than 1 hour.

A transient ischemic attack is considered a medical emergency and early recognition and diagnosis are crucial due to the risk of subsequent arterial ischemic stroke. In the adult population, the risk of stroke following a TIA is 10–15% at 3 months, with half of strokes occurring in the first week following a TIA [2]. Early treatment can significantly reduce this risk [3,4]. Transient ischemic attack diagnosis is primarily based on a comprehensive history and clinical assessment. Unfortunately, diagnostic delays of 24 hours or more commonly occur in childhood arterial ischemic stroke (AIS) [5] and this is also likely true for TIA. A number of factors may lead to delayed recognition of TIA and AIS in children and young adults. There is a lack of awareness of the occurrence of TIA in the young. There is also a high frequency of TIA and AIS mimics and symptoms may not be correctly attributed to cerebral

ischemia [6,7]. Additionally, neuroimaging may be delayed and/or the type of neuroimaging performed may be inadequate to confirm a diagnosis of AIS. In a young child general anesthesia is usually required to perform magnetic resonance imaging (MRI) of the brain and this may contribute to delays. Worldwide, resource availability is probably the greatest challenge.

Case 1

Case description

A 10-year-old Caucasian boy presented to the emergency department with an episode the previous day of left hand numbness. He had also reported numbness at the corner of his mouth on the left side and his parents had noticed that his speech was slurred. The symptoms came on suddenly and concurrently, and lasted approximately 10 minutes. Neurological examination in the emergency department after his symptoms resolved was normal. A brain computed tomography (CT) scan was performed; it was normal and hence he was discharged home. Over the next 6 months he had five further episodes. In three of the episodes he again reported numbness of the left hand with or without associated numbness of the left arm and face. However, in two episodes he had isolated right hand numbness. The symptom duration was 10–30 minutes. There was no associated alteration in awareness or headache. Between episodes he had occasional mild frontal headaches. There had been no decline in school performance or changes in behavior.

Due to a suspicion that these events were seizures, an electroencephalogram (EEG) was requested; however, this was normal. Four months after his initial event, brain magnetic resonance imaging (MRI) and

---

Common Pitfalls in Cerebrovascular Disease: Case-Based Learning, ed. José Biller and José M. Ferro. Published by Cambridge University Press. © Cambridge University Press 2015.

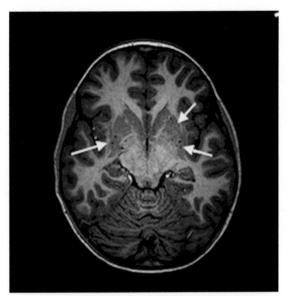

Figure 2.1 Flow voids in the basal ganglia are demonstrated bilaterally on axial T1 MRI (see arrows). This is representative of hypertrophy of the basal ganglia perforator arteries.

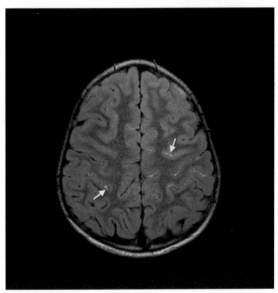

Figure 2.2 Unenhanced MRI axial FLAIR sequence demonstrates leptomeningeal high signal or "ivy" sign (most prominent on left hemisphere) (see arrows). Although the pathogenesis of the ivy sign is uncertain, it is thought to represent slow flow in engorged pial vessels.

MR angiography (MRA) were performed. The MRI did not demonstrate evidence of recent or old cerebral infarction or hemorrhage. However, hypertrophy of the basal ganglia perforator arteries and leptomeningeal high signal on fluid-attenuated inversion recovery

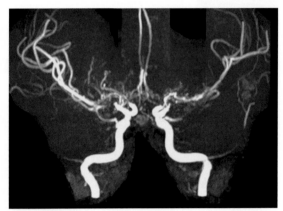

Figure 2.3 Magnetic resonance angiography of the anterior circulation demonstrates bilateral stenosis of the terminal internal carotid arteries with flow gaps in the proximal middle and anterior cerebral arteries as well as hypertrophied perforator arteries.

sequence known as "ivy" sign were present (Figures 2.1 and 2.2) [8]. The MRA revealed bilateral narrowing of the terminal portions of the internal carotid arteries and the proximal segments of the middle cerebral (M1) and anterior cerebral (A1) arteries, respectively (Figure 2.3). Conventional cerebral angiography confirmed the findings seen on MRA and demonstrated greater than 75% stenosis of the M1 segments bilaterally. Further investigations including transthoracic echocardiography, renal ultrasound scan with Doppler, and prothrombotic testing did not reveal any abnormalities. Neuropsychological testing demonstrated a normal cognitive profile.

A diagnosis of moyamoya disease was made and the patient was commenced on low dose (3 mg/kg/day) aspirin. No further transient ischemic attacks occurred within the subsequent 2–3 months. However, due to the ongoing risk of cerebral ischemia and the potential for cognitive decline in moyamoya [9], a neurosurgical assessment was requested. The neurosurgeon counseled the family regarding surgery and shortly thereafter, bilateral indirect revascularization surgery was performed. One brief TIA occurred 2 weeks following surgery; however, to date he has had no further TIAs and follow-up MRI again did not show evidence of deep white matter or vascular territorial infarction. He remains on aspirin.

Discussion

Potential difficulties in the recognition of TIAs in children are highlighted by this case. This child's

Table 2.1 Differential diagnosis of transient ischemic attack in children and young adults

Hemiplegic migraine: familial or spontaneous

Migraine with other focal neurological auras

Focal seizures +/− postictal (Todd's) paresis

Functional disorder

Brain tumor with hemorrhage

Demyelination

Acute cerebellar ataxia of childhood

Peripheral vestibulopathies

Metabolic or toxic conditions: MELAS, hypoglycemia, hypocalcemia

Peripheral nerve or nerve root disorders with unilateral focal deficits

Posterior reversible encephalopathy syndrome (PRES)

Syncope

Channelopathies: alternating hemiplegia of childhood and episodic ataxia

MELAS: mitochondrial encephalomyopathy with lactic acidosis and stroke-like events.

initial event was incorrectly thought to be a focal seizure. Other common differential diagnoses of TIA are listed in Table 2.1. Analysis of the clinical characteristics of focal seizures and TIAs assists in differentiation between these two entities. Both seizures and TIAs have a sudden onset, although an aura may precede a focal seizure. The duration of a focal seizure (usually <1 minute) is typically shorter than a TIA, although both can be of very short duration. In this case the events lasted 10–30 minutes and this is more consistent with TIAs. Sensory symptoms during seizures are usually "positive" type symptoms such as tingling or pins and needles rather than the "negative" symptoms of numbness or sensory loss as seen in this child. Focal seizures are stereotyped and alternating sides are uncommon in focal epilepsy, secondary to a structural lesion. The alternating of sides in this case was in keeping with the finding of a bilateral arteriopathy. The frequency of events is also an important consideration. If episodes occur very often with full neurologic recovery, then this would favor a diagnosis of focal epilepsy.

This case also highlights the need for early MRI brain and cerebral vascular imaging. Due to the delayed recognition that this child was having TIAs, and possibly due to the false reassurance provided by the CT brain, MRI brain and vascular imaging were not performed until 4 months after symptom onset. Brain CT may miss 50–80% of childhood strokes that are later confirmed on MRI. [10,11] Also, as seen in this case, CT will not detect certain characteristic imaging features of moyamoya that can be seen on MRI. Vascular imaging was critical as the finding of an arteriopathy supported a clinical diagnosis of recurrent TIAs and guided further investigations and management. As arteriopathies such as moyamoya are very important causes of cerebral ischemia in childhood, vascular imaging must be strongly considered in all children with suspected TIA or AIS. Other risk factors for stroke in children and young adults are outlined in Table 2.2.

The term moyamoya describes a progressive arteriopathy involving the terminal portions of the internal carotid arteries and their branches with hypertrophy of the deep perforating arteries [12]. Moyamoya *disease* is the term used when moyamoya occurs in isolation without associated medical conditions including sickle cell disease or syndromes such as neurofibromatosis type 1 or Down syndrome. In moyamoya, cerebral ischemia is thought to occur secondary to both chronic hypoperfusion and thromboembolism. Characteristic of moyamoya, cerebral ischemia may be precipitated by hyperventilation induced by crying, blowing, physical exertion, or ingestion of a hot meal, therefore a history of precipitating factors should be sought. Spontaneous TIAs can also occur, as seen in this child.

Pediatric guidelines suggest using aspirin as initial therapy for children with moyamoya, although the level of evidence is low [13,14]. Anticoagulation is generally avoided because of concerns about bleeding, a common form of stroke in adults with moyamoya. Children with moyamoya should be promptly referred to a neurosurgeon with expertise in moyamoya. Revascularization surgery may be indicated, particularly if there are recurrent clinical symptoms presumed secondary to cerebral ischemia or if abnormalities have been demonstrated on cerebral blood flow studies such as single photon emission tomography (SPECT) with acetazolamide, or cerebrovascular reactivity study with hypercarbia challenge [15]. Revascularization surgery results in improvement in clinical symptoms in approximately 90% of children [16]. Direct (in older children) or indirect revascularization procedures may be performed. The timing of surgery and the surgical approach depend on a number of factors and although proposed guidelines exist [17], decisions are best made

15

Table 2.2 Risk factors and etiologies of TIA and AIS in children and young adults

	Children	Young adults
Arteriopathies	Inflammatory arteritis (e.g., transient cerebral arteriopathy; post-varicella angiopathy; bacterial meningitis; HIV; other infections) Moyamoya Cervicocephalic arterial dissection Radiation-induced vasculopathy Reversible cerebral vasoconstriction syndrome	Inflammatory arteritis (e.g., Takayasu's, hepatitis B and C, HIV) Moyamoya Cervicocephalic arterial dissection Reversible cerebral vasoconstriction syndrome Radiation-induced vasculopathy Atherosclerosis Small vessel disease
Cardiac	Congenital heart disease Acquired heart disease Cardiac surgery or catheterization Mechanical circulatory support devices Patent foramen ovale	Acquired heart diseases (cardiomyopathy, ischemic heart disease) Congenital heart disease Cardiac surgery or catheterization Mechanical circulatory support devices Patent foramen ovale
Hematological	Prothrombotic disorders Sickle cell disease	
Vascular risk factors promoting atherosclerosis	Hypertension (rare)	Hypertension Diabetes mellitus Dyslipidemia Obesity Smoking
Other	Migraine with aura Illicit drugs Alcohol abuse Obstructive sleep apnea Oral contraceptive pill Pregnancy Inborn errors of metabolism (rare)	

on a case-by-case basis in a center with expertise in moyamoya.

Case 2

Case description

A 5-year-old girl presented to the emergency department after having acute onset of left-sided weakness at school. Her past medical history was significant for an uncomplicated chicken pox infection 2 months prior. While sitting in the classroom, her teacher noticed that she was unable to move her left arm, was drooling from the left corner of her mouth, and was unable to walk. An ambulance was called and she was taken to the emergency department. On examination there it was described that she could "barely" move the left arm and leg and there was a clear left facial droop in the upper motor neuron distribution.

It was also suspected that she had diminished sensation down the left side in the same distribution as her motor weakness. She made a full recovery within 3 hours and was discharged from hospital. The following day she returned to the emergency department after having a near identical episode, again with complete recovery. A brain MRI was performed and this demonstrated diffusion restriction in the right middle cerebral artery (MCA) territory (involving the cortex and basal ganglia) consistent with acute infarction (Figure 2.4). The MRA demonstrated occlusion of the proximal right MCA and probable narrowing of the proximal portion of the right anterior cerebral artery (ACA). She was commenced on intravenous unfractionated heparin and as a part of standard neuroprotective care, close attention was given to maintenance of normal blood pressure, temperature, glucose, and hydration status. There was vigilant clinical monitoring for seizures.

The following day, while in hospital, she had an episode that consisted first of drooling from the left corner of the mouth and involuntary flexion of the left arm. This lasted 1 minute and was followed by moderate left arm and leg weakness. The weakness resolved within 15 minutes. It was uncertain whether or not altered awareness was present at the onset of the episode. An EEG demonstrated right-sided frontal slowing without epileptiform discharges. However, she was administered a loading dose of intravenous phenytoin as she was suspected to have had a focal seizure followed by postictal paresis. A repeat brain MRI/MRA was performed and this did not demonstrate any new areas of cerebral infarction, or hemorrhagic conversion. The MRA demonstrated return of flow through the proximal MCA (M1) with residual stenosis at the site of prior occlusion. Conventional angiography confirmed stenosis and irregularity of the right A1 and M1. A lumbar puncture revealed a lymphocytic pleocytosis with 17×10^6 white cells. The cerebrospinal fluid (CSF) bacterial culture and polymerase chain reaction (PCR) for viral infections were negative. Her erythrocyte sedimentation rate (ESR) was elevated at 45 mm/h. Investigations for systemic inflammation and/or autoimmunity such as antinuclear antibody (ANA) were negative. A prothrombotic evaluation and transthoracic echocardiography did not demonstrate any abnormalities.

A diagnosis of transient cerebral arteriopathy (TCA) with a probable inflammatory basis was made. Due to the substantial risk of recurrent stroke or TIA in children with TCA, the initial treatment with unfractionated heparin was followed by transition to low molecular weight heparin. The decision was made to avoid immunosuppressive therapy agents despite the presumed inflammatory basis, due to the generally observed spontaneous resolution of arteriopathy in TCA despite conservative treatment. During follow-up no further events occurred and over the course of 6 months, MRA demonstrated significant improvement in the right MCA and ACA stenosis, prompting transition from anticoagulation therapy with low molecular weight heparin to antiplatelet therapy with aspirin. An MRA 4 years later demonstrated complete normalization of the right MCA and ACA (Figure 2.5).

Discussion

This case demonstrates the need to maintain a high index of suspicion for TIA and stroke in children. Despite having an episode of sudden onset hemiparesis, she was

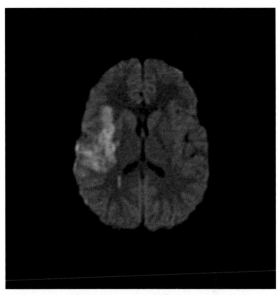

Figure 2.4 Diffusion-weighted imaging demonstrating diffusion restriction in the right middle cerebral artery territory.

(a)

(b)

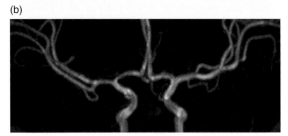

Figure 2.5 Magnetic resonance angiography (MRA): initial (a) and 6-month follow-up (b). The initial MRA shows complete occlusion of the proximal MCA (M1, thick arrow) and stenosis of the proximal ACA (A1, thin arrow) on the right. Follow-up imaging 6 months later shows near complete resolution with only mild reduction in caliber of the right A1 and M1.

discharged from the emergency department without a diagnosis. Hemiparesis is the most common symptom of cerebral ischemia and should prompt strong consideration of TIA or AIS regardless of patient age. Early identification would have allowed for timely investigations and management in this case, perhaps preventing irreversible cerebral injury. Characteristic features of TIA and its differential diagnoses are outlined in Table 2.3. The challenges and important factors to differentiate between TIA or AIS and postictal paresis are illustrated by this case. Postictal paresis can occur following a focal or apparent generalized seizure and identification of suspected seizure activity, such as the tonic posturing seen in this case, preceding the onset of weakness is crucial for diagnosis. However, seizures are a common presenting feature of childhood stroke [18] so a brain MRI is often required to rule out AIS, particularly in a first episode of postictal paresis. Clinical experience suggests that seizures do not occur as a feature of TIA in childhood; however, large studies of TIA in the pediatric population are lacking. Since rapid recovery and brief duration of hemiparesis are common in both TIA and postictal paresis these characteristics are not necessarily helpful in differentiating the two conditions [19]. A past history of epilepsy should be sought, as this is a supporting feature of postictal paresis.

The provisional diagnosis of transient cerebral arteriopathy was made in the context of vascular imaging demonstrating a unilateral stenosing arteriopathy involving the proximal portions of the right middle and anterior cerebral arteries. Given that this child had a varicella infection 2 months prior to her stroke, the most accurate diagnosis would be post-varicella angiopathy (PVA). Transient cerebral arteriopathy and post-varicella angiopathy are both terms for unilateral non-progressive arteriopathies of childhood [20]. Both are suspected to have an inflammatory basis and are major causes of childhood TIA and stroke. Due to the presumed inflammatory basis some centers may treat select patients with TCA and/or PVA with immunosuppressive therapy (typically corticosteroids), as for any other form of central nervous system vasculitis. Treatment with immunosuppressive agents remains controversial in these conditions, as there is a lack of evidence supporting benefit. For the majority of patients with TCA or PVA the arteriopathy spontaneously improves and is monophasic in nature [21]. If immunotherapy is used, the practice would likely include addition of acyclovir in cases of PVA.

Case 3

Case description

A 17-year-old female presented to the emergency department with left-sided weakness and sensory symptoms. After waking from a brief afternoon nap she noticed tingling of the left side of her face. Within a few minutes she developed a mild bilateral occipital headache. Over 5–10 minutes the tingling progressed to involve her left arm and leg. She got into her car to drive to work and noticed that her left arm and leg felt heavy and numb. When she arrived at work a colleague noticed drooping of the left side of her face and slurred speech. This was now 1 hour after initial symptom onset. On arrival in the emergency department her neurological examination demonstrated mild left arm and leg weakness. Her sensation was intact and there was no facial weakness or dysarthria. She made a full recovery within 2 hours of symptom onset. Brain MRI and intracranial and cervical time-of-flight MRA and magnetic resonance venography (MRV) were performed 6 hours after symptom onset and no abnormalities were demonstrated.

Her past history was significant for deep vein thrombosis (DVT) of the right lower limb 9 months prior to this presentation. The DVT was thought to be precipitated by trauma to the leg while playing hockey. She was also on the oral contraceptive pill (OCP) and prior prothrombotic testing had demonstrated heterozygosity for the factor V Leiden gene mutation. For the DVT she had been treated with an oral vitamin K antagonist and she remained on this at the time of presentation with hemiparesis. The international normalized ratio (INR) had been consistently within the target range of 2–3.

Her past medical history included intermittent mild "band-like" frontal headaches, most consistent with tension type headaches. There was no history of migraine in her immediate family. Doppler ultrasound of the right leg showed a persistent non-occlusive thrombus in the proximal superficial femoral vein. Transthoracic echocardiography and electrocardiography were normal. She was diagnosed with a probable spontaneous hemiplegic migraine and was discharged home the following day.

Discussion

The differential diagnosis of hemiparesis is broad and includes common stroke mimics such as hemiplegic migraine, postictal paresis, and functional disorders (Table 2.3). The two main differential diagnoses in this case were TIA or AIS and hemiplegic migraine (HM). A detailed history including mode of onset, symptom characteristics, and episode duration followed by careful analysis is critical for differentiating these two

Table 2.3 Characteristic features of TIA and the common differential diagnoses

	Onset	Symptoms	Duration
TIA	Sudden onset; deficit maximal at onset	Negative symptoms	Minutes to hours. The majority last <60 minutes
Hemiplegic migraine	Gradual progression of symptoms over 20–30 minutes	Motor aura occurs with at least one other aura symptom. Almost always accompanied by headache	Typically >20 minutes. Most resolve in <60 minutes but may last up to 72 hours
Migraine with aura	Gradual development of aura; symptoms evolve over 5–20 minutes	Positive and/or negative aura symptoms; visual aura most common Headache occurs following aura but can occur with aura or within 60 minutes of aura	Each individual aura symptom lasts 5–60 minutes
Post-ictal paresis/Todd's paresis	Weakness follows focal motor seizure and is maximal at onset	Weakness is usually mild to moderate. May have past history of focal seizures	Duration typically ranges from seconds up to 30 minutes, with some reported cases of up to 36 hours duration

disorders. Difficulty can, however, arise due to atypical presentations and overlap in clinical features.

In this case the mode of onset was gradual and progressive with spreading of symptoms from face, to arm and leg and from sensory to motor, over 30–60 minutes. This is typical of HM where the aura symptoms characteristically slowly evolve. Although rare, symptoms can rapidly evolve over less than 1 minute in HM [22]. Her sensory symptoms were initially positive (tingling) but then became negative (numbness) and this evolution from positive to negative symptoms is common in HM. Headache occurs in the majority of patients with HM and usually has the characteristics of a typical migraine headache (e.g., unilateral and pulsating in nature) but mild nonspecific headaches, as seen in this patient, can occur. Headaches also occur in up to 20–40% of patients with cerebral ischemia, so the differentiating value of headache alone is limited [23,24]. A past history of migraine with aura, particularly if there have been previous similar episodes, may be helpful; however, it is important to remember that migraine is common and a past history of migraine may also be present in young patients with stroke [25]. Hemiplegic migraine can be spontaneous or familial so it is important to seek a family history as this may assist in the diagnosis.

This case was also complicated by the history of deep vein thrombosis. Although a patent foramen ovale (PFO) was not demonstrated on transthoracic echocardiography, paradoxical embolism resulting in cerebral ischemia should still be considered due to

the possibility of a false negative echocardiogram and also because right-to-left shunting can occur at the pulmonary level. However, taking into account all of the clinical characteristics, the final diagnosis in this case was hemiplegic migraine. Regardless, investigations for TIA including MRI/MRA brain, echocardiography, and a prothrombotic work-up were performed before excluding this possible diagnosis. This is advisable in any first episode of suspected HM and also in subsequent episodes if the symptoms of an event are atypical for an individual.

Case 4. Young woman with sudden onset homonymous hemianopsia

Case description

A 28-year-old woman presented to the emergency department after having had two episodes of transient visual loss. In the first episode she had sudden onset of a severe headache associated with sudden complete right-sided visual field loss. From the patient's description, the visual loss was consistent with a right homonymous hemianopsia. She had confirmed the presence of binocular visual loss by opening and closing each eye in turn during the episode. Her visual symptoms resolved over 2 hours; however, the headache gradually resolved over the course of the day. The following day she had a similar episode of sudden visual loss but there was no associated headache on this occasion. Examination demonstrated normal visual fields and normal visual acuity, and the remainder of the ophthalmological, neurological, and systemic examinations were normal.

Her past medical history was significant for frequent headaches beginning in adolescence. These occurred up to 2–3 times per month and were typically unilateral (could be either side) and pulsating in nature. There had never been any visual, sensory, or other type of aura symptom associated with the headaches but there could be nausea and/or mild photophobia. The description of these headaches was consistent with migraine without aura. Her most recent migraine occurred 2 weeks prior to the first episode of visual loss. She was not taking any medications for migraine prophylaxis and for acute attacks she used ibuprofen only. The severe headache that occurred in association with her first episode of visual loss differed from her typical migraine headaches, in that it was bilateral and lacked a pulsating quality. Both her usual migraine headaches and the headache associated with her visual loss were frontotemporal in location. Of note, for 5 days leading up to the first episode of visual loss, she had been taking an OCP to delay her menstrual period for an important athletic event. She had never smoked and was not pregnant.

She was referred to the stroke prevention clinic on an urgent basis and a number of investigations were performed including brain MRI and MRA, a prothrombotic work-up, and a transthoracic echocardiogram with bubble study. The brain MRI/MRA was normal. Her echocardiogram demonstrated a small PFO and the prothrombotic work-up demonstrated a mildly low protein S. She was diagnosed with a probable TIA and was commenced on low dose aspirin. She was advised to avoid taking the OCP in future. No further similar events have occurred; however, she continues to have migraine without aura 2–3 times per month.

Discussion

The cause of transient isolated visual symptoms can be challenging to diagnose [26]. Homonymous hemianopsia is a common type of transient visual loss that localizes to the retrochiasmal optic pathway, and occipital lobe lesions or dysfunction are most commonly responsible. The main differential diagnoses in this case were TIA and migraine with aura. Occipital lobe seizures should also be considered as a differential diagnosis along with other less common possibilities including metabolic disorders such as MELAS

(mitochondrial encephalomyopathy with lactic acidosis and stroke like episodes) that may mimic occipital lobe TIA or stroke.

The same general principles apply as per Case 3 in differentiating TIA from migraine with aura. The diagnosis in this case was a probable TIA affecting the left posterior cerebral artery territory. A number of clinical features were helpful in reaching this diagnosis. Her visual symptoms were reported to come on suddenly with a maximal deficit at onset. This is consistent with TIA. However, it is important to carefully question patients about the tempo of symptom onset, as it is not uncommon for a patient to report sudden onset of symptoms when on further questioning it becomes clear that the symptoms actually developed over a number of minutes. She developed a complete right-sided homonymous visual field loss consistent with ischemia involving the left occipital cortex. In a visual migraine aura the symptoms are also typically homonymous, but they usually commence around fixation and spread outwards. Negative visual symptoms can occur in migraine aura and TIA but positive symptoms (e.g., spots, lines, scintillations, shapes, and flickering lights) are more characteristic of a migraine aura. The 2-hour duration of this young woman's visual field loss was also not typical for migraine aura, where symptom duration is usually 5–60 minutes, although rarely prolonged aura occurs [27]. The headache that occurred during the first episode was not characteristic for a migraine headache as it occurred concurrently with the visual symptoms, was bilateral, and lacked a pulsating quality. It is important to note, though, that headaches in migraine with aura can be atypical in nature or even absent.

As in this case, some diagnostic uncertainty frequently exists due to the overlap in clinical characteristics between migraine with aura and TIA. If there is uncertainty then it is imperative to comprehensively evaluate for cerebral ischemia as the findings may help to confirm the clinical suspicion of TIA and will guide management. No major risk factors or causes of TIA were found following further investigations in this young woman although a number of potential minor risk factors were identified including the OCP use, a history of migraine, mildly low protein S levels, and a patent foramen ovale. She had been taking the OCP preceding the event and in population studies the OCP has been associated with a small increased risk of stroke. Her past history of migraine may also have been a risk factor as it has been established that people who suffer from migraine with aura have an approximately twofold increased risk of ischemic stroke. However, it is less certain whether those with migraine without aura also carry an increased risk [25]. The combination of migraine with aura and the OCP may further increase the risk of stroke in young women, particularly in those who smoke. On prothrombotic testing, a mildly low protein S was found in this patient. This is another potential risk factor as an association between low protein S levels and stroke has been reported. However, her protein S level was only mildly low and repeat testing while off the OCP would be required.

It is common practice to evaluate for prothrombotic disorders in young patients with cryptogenic TIA or stroke, but some controversy exists around the utility of testing. In children, the presence of a prothrombotic disorder plays a role in initial and recurrent stroke [28,29] risk, albeit most commonly as an additive factor. A 2010 meta-analysis of observational studies looked at the impact of thrombophilia on the risk of first AIS in children. The highest odds ratios were seen for protein C deficiency (odds ratio [OR] 11, 95% confidence interval [CI] 5.13–23.59), antiphospholipid antibodies/lupus anticoagulant (OR 6.95, 95% CI 3.67–13.14), and lipoprotein (a) (OR 6.53, 95% CI 4.46–9.55) [30]. Modest associations were also seen for the factor V Leiden and prothrombin gene mutations. Despite the reported associations between these hematological disorders and first AIS, their true relevance as risk factors for recurrent TIA and stroke in young adults, particularly when atherosclerosis is becoming more prevalent, is uncertain. The clinical value, cost effectiveness, and psychological implications of testing should be considered in individual cases prior to testing.

The role of PFO in TIA and stroke is discussed in Case 6.

Case 5

Case description

A 5-year-old boy presented to the emergency department after having a 2-hour episode of nausea, dizziness, and gait unsteadiness. This was preceded by a 2–3 day history of upper respiratory tract symptoms. There was no history of recent head or neck trauma. When seen in the emergency department, his symptoms had fully resolved and his neurological and systemic examinations were normal. Four days later he returned with identical symptoms; however, on this occasion they persisted for 24 hours. Neurological examination demonstrated mild gait ataxia and dysmetria of the right arm. A brain CT was performed and this was reported as normal. Following this he had a brain MRI and this showed an area of diffusion restriction in the right cerebellar hemisphere, consistent with acute infarction. Intracranial and cervical time-of-flight MRA were reported as normal. He was diagnosed with posterior circulation arterial ischemic strokes, specifically involving the territory supplied by the right posterior inferior cerebellar artery (PICA). He was commenced on low dose daily aspirin for secondary stroke prevention. At discharge he had no residual neurological deficits. A follow-up brain MRI was performed 3 months later and this demonstrated the expected evolution of the right cerebellar hemisphere stroke, with no new areas of infarction seen.

Eighteen months later, he presented to the emergency department with ataxia, nausea, dizziness, slurred speech, and drowsiness. He had complained of headache for a few days leading up to this presentation. Brain MRI showed multifocal acute infarctions involving the cerebellar hemispheres bilaterally (right more than left) and the inferior temporal lobe on the right (Figure 2.6). Intracranial and cervical time-of-flight MRA showed reduced flow signal in the proximal right posterior cerebral artery, and moderate reduction in

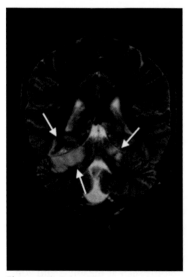

Figure 2.6 Coronal T2 sequence demonstrating multifocal high signal changes (see arrows) in the cerebellum and right inferior temporal lobe that conform to arterial territories.

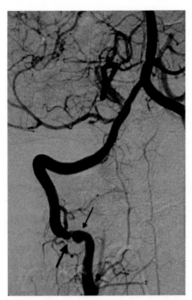

Figure 2.7 Conventional cerebral angiography of the right vertebral artery demonstrating an area of stenosis (thick arrow) and proximal to this, an area of dilatation (thin arrow) representative of a pseudoaneurysm.

the caliber of the right vertebral artery. Conventional angiography was subsequently performed and this demonstrated approximately 50% stenosis of the right vertebral artery at the level of the second cervical vertebral body (C2). Focal dilatation proximal to the stenosis (Figure 2.7) and narrowing of the proximal right PICA were also seen. These findings were consistent with previous vertebral artery dissection. Anticoagulation was commenced in addition to aspirin as stroke recurrence had occurred while on aspirin therapy alone. Follow-up vascular imaging over a 6–18 month period demonstrated resolution of the arterial abnormalities and only mild stenosis of the vertebral artery remained. For ongoing secondary stroke prophylaxis, clopidogrel was chosen over aspirin due to concern related to previous treatment failure while on aspirin.

Discussion

This case posed significant difficulties both with the initial recognition of posterior circulation ischemic symptoms and in the diagnosis of vertebral artery dissection (VAD). Posterior (vertebrobasilar) circulation TIAs can be very challenging to diagnose [31]. Non-localizing symptoms such as dizziness and vomiting may occur, young children may find it difficult or impossible to describe symptoms such as vertigo, and

the differential diagnosis is broad. The posterior circulation provides blood supply to the cerebellum, the brainstem, the occipital lobes, the inferior temporal lobes, and the thalami. Symptoms of posterior circulation ischemia depend on the area of brain affected but can include ataxia, vertigo, dizziness, visual field deficits, eye movement disorders, dysarthria, alterations in level of consciousness, unilateral or bilateral weakness, autonomic disturbance, confusion, disorientation, and memory loss. Some symptoms, such as hemiparesis, can occur in either anterior or posterior circulation ischemia, so in these cases it is important to look for other clinical signs referable to the posterior circulation such as those that localize to the brainstem. The differential diagnosis of posterior circulation TIA or stroke includes acute cerebellar ataxia, cerebellitis, posterior fossa tumors, vestibular disorders, migraine with aura (including brainstem aura), and demyelination, among others.

Vertebral artery dissection [32,33] is a major cause of posterior circulation ischemia in children and young adults [34,35]. The diagnosis is reliant on neuroimaging evidence of dissection but this can be challenging due to the limitations of current vascular imaging techniques and the lack of definitive neuroimaging criteria. Characteristic findings of dissection include an intimal flap, a double lumen sign or a wall hematoma; however, it is common to find only nonspecific signs such as arterial stenosis. Where nonspecific findings are seen, the location of the abnormality can be helpful diagnostically as vertebral artery dissection typically occurs at the C1–C2 vertebral level [36]. The first line of cerebral vascular imaging for suspected dissection is typically MRA or CT angiography (CTA) of the cervical and intracranial vessels. In many pediatric centers MRA is preferred due to the superior safety profile. The choice of anticoagulation or antiplatelet therapy in VAD is controversial. The treatment guidelines, as with much of the academic literature on dissection, combine VAD with internal carotid artery dissection and intracranial dissection under the term cervicocephalic artery dissection (CCAD). Pediatric guidelines generally recommend treatment with anticoagulation. However, the American Heart Association (AHA) scientific statement on the *Management of Stroke in Infants and Children 2008* states that antiplatelet therapy can be used as an alternative [13]. Anticoagulation is not recommended for patients with an intracranial dissection or for those with a subarachnoid hemorrhage resulting from CCAD. A Cochrane meta-analysis of anticoagulation versus antiplatelet therapy in adults with internal carotid artery dissection found no significant difference in initial or recurrent stroke rates; however, it was underpowered according to the authors [37]. Currently no adult or pediatric clinical trial data is available. Stroke recurrence is seen in up to 20% of children with CCAD so clinicians should have a high degree of suspicion for TIA or stroke if a child with a past history of dissection presents with acute onset of neurological symptoms. There are no pediatric guidelines for treatment of stroke recurrence in dissection, so decisions are made on a case-by-case basis. Long-term follow-up vascular imaging is important to assist in the prediction and prevention of stroke recurrence. Very late stroke recurrence as seen in this case, although relatively rare, has been reported in childhood [38].

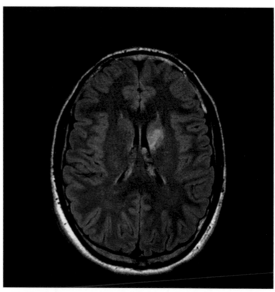

Figure 2.8 MRI brain axial FLAIR sequence demonstrating high signal change in the head of the caudate on the left.

Case 6

Case description

A previously healthy 16-year-old male woke up late one morning. He attempted to reach for his mobile phone with his right hand but was unable to do so. He also noticed that his right arm felt numb. When he got out of bed he immediately fell due to weakness of the right leg. He managed to stand up and walk to the bathroom at which time he noticed asymmetry of his lower face when looking in the mirror. The lower right side of his face also felt numb. His father drove him immediately to the nearest emergency department where right-sided hemiparesis and hemisensory loss were demonstrated on examination. Approximately 30 minutes after waking up, the numbness of his arm started to improve and 15 minutes later he was completely asymptomatic. He had participated in kick-boxing and wrestling in the weeks leading up to the event but he did not recall any significant trauma to the head or neck. Routine laboratory testing and ECG were performed and were normal. He was informed that he had most likely suffered a TIA. An outpatient brain MRI was requested and he was discharged from the emergency department.

A brain MRI was performed 2 weeks later and this showed evidence of a subacute arterial ischemic stroke in the left basal ganglia (see Figure 2.8). Following this, MRA of the head and neck arteries was performed but no abnormalities were found. Due to concern about possible CCAD, cerebral angiography was also performed but again no abnormalities were demonstrated. A transthoracic echocardiogram with contrast (bubble study) showed a PFO with limited passage of bubbles across the intra-atrial septum. Prothrombotic testing did not demonstrate any abnormalities. He was commenced on daily low dose aspirin for secondary stroke prevention and to date, he has had no recurrent events.

Discussion

This young man awoke from sleep with a right-sided hemiparesis. The differential diagnosis of hemiparesis has been discussed in previous cases. The sudden and concurrent onset of a complete left-sided motor and hemisensory deficit was very suggestive of cerebral ischemia. Although his symptoms were gradually recognized over the course of a few minutes, further questioning confirmed that sudden onset was probable. It is important to note that as he *awoke from sleep* with his symptoms and he was last seen well prior to going to bed the evening before, the precise symptom duration is unknown and may have been significantly longer than the 45 minutes reported. Although he was diagnosed with a transient ischemic attack, further investigations including neuroimaging were not performed acutely. A transient ischemic attack is considered a medical emergency and urgent neuroimaging should be performed to assess for diffusion-weighted changes, to investigate etiology, and to rule out certain differential diagnoses. Studies have shown that TIAs of incremental duration are more likely to demonstrate diffusion-weighted changes on brain MRI; up to 30% in TIAs lasting 0–3 hours, 50% in TIAs lasting >3–12 hours, and 70% in those over 12 hours [39]. The presence of diffusion-weighted changes increases the likelihood of recurrent stroke and further increases the importance of initiating secondary stroke prevention strategies early. The recurrence risk is also dependent on underlying etiology, again highlighting the need for urgent investigations so that specific management can be commenced.

Despite extensive, albeit delayed, investigations in this patient no definitive cause for his stroke was identified. Cervicocephalic artery dissection was strongly considered, particularly given his recent participation in contact sports; however, MRA of the intracranial and cervical vessels and conventional angiography did not demonstrate any abnormalities suggestive of dissection. Transthoracic echocardiography with contrast did demonstrate a PFO in this young man. Determining whether or not his PFO was incidental or pathogenic was not possible, as is often the case. Paradoxical embolism via a right-to-left shunt is a purported mechanism of stroke in the presence of a PFO, but the role of PFO in stroke remains controversial and further studies are required for clarification. The management of a child or adolescent with a PFO and TIA or AIS is also controversial. Observational studies in the adult population suggested a benefit for percutaneous PFO closure; however, recent randomized controlled trials did not demonstrate a benefit for PFO closure over medical therapy alone for prevention of recurrent cerebral ischemia [40]. The choice between antiplatelet and anticoagulant agents for medical therapy is also unclear, as clinical trials are lacking. Adult stroke guidelines generally recommend antiplatelet therapy over anticoagulation unless there is stroke recurrence while on aspirin, or there is a high-risk feature such as a DVT or a prothrombotic state. Pediatric stroke guidelines do not make specific recommendations regarding medical therapy for children with stroke and a PFO. In this case, the patient was commenced on aspirin. Had another risk factor, such as a DVT or prothrombotic state been identified, then anticoagulation would have been strongly considered.

References

1. Adil MM, Qureshi AI, Beslow LA, Jordan LC. Transient ischemic attack requiring hospitalization of children in the United States: kids' inpatient database 2003 to 2009. *Stroke* 2014;45(3):887–8.

2. Easton JD, Saver JL, Albers GW, Alberts MJ, Chaturvedi S, Feldmann E, et al. Definition and evaluation of transient ischemic attack: a scientific statement for healthcare professionals from the American Heart Association/American Stroke Association Stroke Council; Council on Cardiovascular Surgery and Anesthesia; Council on Cardiovascular Radiology and Intervention; Council on Cardiovascular Nursing; and the Interdisciplinary Council on Peripheral Vascular Disease. The American Academy of Neurology affirms the value of this statement as an educational tool for neurologists. *Stroke* 2009;40(6):2276–93.

3. Giles MF, Rothwell PM. Transient ischaemic attack: clinical relevance, risk prediction and urgency of secondary prevention. *Curr Opin Neurol* 2009;22(1):46–53.

4. Furie KL, Kasner SE, Adams RJ, Albers GW, Bush RL, Fagan SC, et al. Guidelines for the prevention of stroke in patients with stroke or transient ischemic attack: a guideline for healthcare professionals from the American Heart Association/American Stroke Association. *Stroke* 2011;42(1):227–76.

5. Rafay MF, Armstrong D, Deveber G, Domi T, Chan A, MacGregor DL. Craniocervical arterial dissection in children: clinical and radiographic presentation and outcome. *J Child Neurol* 2006;21(1):8–16.

6. Shellhaas RA, Smith SE, O'Tool E, Licht DJ, Ichord RN. Mimics of childhood stroke: characteristics of a prospective cohort. *Pediatrics* 2006;118(2):704–9.

7. Mackay MT, Chua ZK, Lee M, Yock-Corrales A, Churilov L, Monagle P, et al. Stroke and nonstroke brain attacks in children. *Neurology* 2014;82(16):1434–40.

8. Fujiwara H, Momoshima S, Kuribayashi S. Leptomeningeal high signal intensity (ivy sign) on fluid-attenuated inversion-recovery (FLAIR) MR images in moyamoya disease. *Eur J Radiol* 2005;55(2):224–30.

9. Weinberg DG, Rahme RJ, Aoun SG, Batjer HH, Bendok BR. Moyamoya disease: functional and neurocognitive outcomes in the pediatric and adult populations. *Neurosurg Focus* 2011;30(6):E21.

10. Srinivasan J, Miller SP, Phan TG, Mackay MT. Delayed recognition of initial stroke in children: need for increased awareness. *Pediatrics* 2009;124(2):e227–34.

11. McGlennan C, Ganesan V. Delays in investigation and management of acute arterial ischaemic stroke in children. *Dev Med Child Neurol* 2008;50(7):537–40.

12. Scott RM, Smith ER. Moyamoya disease and moyamoya syndrome. *N Engl J Med* 2009;360(12):1226–37.

13. Roach ES, Golomb MR, Adams R, Biller J, Daniels S, Deveber G, et al. Management of stroke in infants and children: a scientific statement from a Special Writing Group of the American Heart Association Stroke Council and the Council on Cardiovascular Disease in the Young. *Stroke* 2008;39(9):2644–91.

14. Monagle P, Chan AK, Goldenberg NA, Ichord RN, Journeycake JM, Nowak-Gottl U, et al. Antithrombotic therapy in neonates and children: Antithrombotic Therapy and Prevention of Thrombosis, 9th ed: American College of Chest Physicians Evidence-Based Clinical Practice Guidelines. *Chest* 2012;141(2 Suppl):e737S–801S.

15. Ganesan V. Moyamoya: to cut or not to cut is not the only question. A paediatric neurologist's perspective. *Dev Med Child Neurol* 2010;52(1):10–13.

16. Fung LW, Thompson D, Ganesan V. Revascularisation surgery for paediatric moyamoya: a review of the literature. *Childs Nerv Syst* 2005;21(5):358–64.

17. Smith ER, Scott RM. Spontaneous occlusion of the circle of Willis in children: pediatric moyamoya summary with proposed evidence-based practice guidelines. A review. *J Neurosurg Pediatr* 2012;9(4):353–60.

18. Abend NS, Beslow LA, Smith SE, Kessler SK, Vossough A, Mason S, et al. Seizures as a presenting symptom of acute arterial ischemic stroke in childhood. *J Pediatr* 2011;159(3):479–83.

19. Gallmetzer P, Leutmezer F, Serles W, Assem-Hilger E, Spatt J, Baumgartner C. Postictal paresis in focal epilepsies–incidence, duration, and causes: a video-EEG monitoring study. *Neurology* 2004;62(12):2160–4.

20. Elbers J, Benseler SM. Central nervous system vasculitis in children. *Curr Opin Rheumatol* 2008;20(1):47–54.

21. Lanthier S, Armstrong D, Domi T, deVeber G. Post-varicella arteriopathy of childhood: natural history of vascular stenosis. *Neurology* 2005;64(4):660–3.

22. Russell MB, Ducros A. Sporadic and familial hemiplegic migraine: pathophysiological mechanisms, clinical characteristics, diagnosis, and management. *Lancet Neurol* 2011;10(5):457–70.

23. Mallick AA, Ganesan V, Kirkham FJ, Fallon P, Hedderly T, McShane T, et al. Childhood arterial ischaemic stroke incidence, presenting features, and risk factors: a prospective population-based study. *Lancet Neurol* 2014;13(1):35–43.

24. Tentschert S, Wimmer R, Greisenegger S, Lang W, Lalouschek W. Headache at stroke onset in 2196 patients with ischemic stroke or transient ischemic attack. *Stroke* 2005;36(2):e1–3.

25. Kurth T, Diener HC. Migraine and stroke: perspectives for stroke physicians. *Stroke* 2012;43(12):3421–6.

26. Thurtell MJ, Rucker JC. Transient visual loss. *Int Ophthalmol Clin* 2009;49(3):147–66.

27. The International Classification of Headache Disorders, 3rd edition (beta version). *Cephalalgia* 2013;33(9):629–808.

28. Ganesan V, Prengler M, Wade A, Kirkham FJ. Clinical and radiological recurrence after childhood arterial ischemic stroke. *Circulation* 2006;114(20):2170–7.

29. Rodan L, McCrindle BW, Manlhiot C, MacGregor DL, Askalan R, Moharir M, et al. Stroke recurrence in children with congenital heart disease. *Ann Neurol* 2012;72(1):103–11.

30. Kenet G, Lutkhoff LK, Albisetti M, Bernard T, Bonduel M, Brandao L, et al. Impact of thrombophilia on risk of arterial ischemic stroke or cerebral sinovenous thrombosis in neonates and children: a systematic review and meta-analysis of observational studies. *Circulation* 2010;121(16):1838–47.

31. Markus HS, van der Worp HB, Rothwell PM. Posterior circulation ischaemic stroke and transient ischaemic attack: diagnosis, investigation, and secondary prevention. *Lancet Neurol* 2013;12(10):989–98.

32. Debette S, Leys D. Cervical-artery dissections: predisposing factors, diagnosis, and outcome. *Lancet Neurol* 2009;8(7):668–78.

33. Schievink WI. Spontaneous dissection of the carotid and vertebral arteries. *N Engl J Med* 2001;344(12):898–906.

34. Mackay MT, Prabhu SP, Coleman L. Childhood posterior circulation arterial ischemic stroke. *Stroke* 2010;41(10):2201–9.

35. Ganesan V, Cox TC, Gunny R. Abnormalities of cervical arteries in children with arterial ischemic stroke. *Neurology* 2011;76(2):166–71.

36. Fullerton HJ, Johnston SC, Smith WS. Arterial dissection and stroke in children. *Neurology* 2001;57(7):1155–60.

37. Lyrer P, Engelter S. Antithrombotic drugs for carotid artery dissection. *Cochrane Database Syst Rev* 2010(10):CD000255.

38. Tan MA, Armstrong D, MacGregor DL, Kirton A. Late complications of vertebral artery

dissection in children: pseudoaneurysm, thrombosis, and recurrent stroke. *J Child Neurol* 2009;24(3):354–60.

39. Kidwell CS, Alger JR, Di Salle F, Starkman S, Villablanca P, Bentson J, et al. Diffusion MRI in patients with transient ischemic attacks. *Stroke* 1999;30(6):1174–80.

40. Wolfrum M, Froehlich GM, Knapp G, Casaubon LK, DiNicolantonio JJ, Lansky AJ, et al. Stroke prevention by percutaneous closure of patent foramen ovale: a systematic review and meta-analysis. *Heart* 2014;100(5):389–95.

Chapter 3

Transient ischemic attacks (TIAs) – an underrecognized and undertreated disorder

Patrícia Canhão

Introduction

Transient ischemic attack (TIA) is clinically defined as "a sudden loss of focal cerebral or monocular function lasting less than 24 hours due to inadequate cerebral or ocular blood supply as a result of low blood flow, thrombosis or embolism associated with disease of the arteries, heart or blood" [1]. This classical definition has been a topic of debate and a tissue-based definition has been more recently proposed: "a transient episode of neurologic dysfunction caused by focal brain, spinal cord, or retinal ischemia, without acute infarction on MRI" [2]. Regardless of the definition used, TIA patients have a high risk of stroke and other cardiovascular events. Establishing the diagnosis of TIA offers an excellent opportunity to prevent a devastating stroke. However, these transient ischemic events are frequently underdiagnosed and undertreated.

Case 1. TIA is underrecognized – a potentially preventable stroke

Case description

A 72-year-old man, with diabetes and hypertension, was brought to the emergency department (ED) due to severe speech disturbance and loss of strength in the right limbs. His wife told that 2 days earlier he had a transient numbness of the right hand and some word-finding difficulties. Symptoms lasted about 30 minutes, and as he became completely normal, he did not seek medical attention. He thought the symptoms could have been due to diabetes. However, he did not test his blood glucose. He was usually treated with a calcium channel blocker, a diuretic, and an oral antidiabetic drug. On initial neurologic examination, he had a global aphasia, forced gaze deviation to the left side, right homonymous hemianopsia, right central facial paresis, and a flaccid right hemiplegia. A CT scan displayed early signs of ischemia in the left middle cerebral artery (MCA) territory and a hyperdense left MCA sign, suggestive of an occlusive thrombus (Figure 3.1).

Because the last time he was seen well was more than 5 hours earlier, he was not treated with thrombolytic therapy with recombinant tissue plasminogen activator (rtPA). Further etiological investigation with a neck vascular ultrasound showed an occlusion of the left internal carotid artery (ICA) due to a large atheromatous plaque. Transcranial Doppler (TCD) ultrasound confirmed the absence of flow in the left MCA compatible with occlusion of this vessel. The patient received conservative treatment aimed at preventing medical complications, correction of risk factors, and secondary prevention. Three weeks after admission he was discharged dependent to a rehabilitation clinic, scoring 5 on the modified Rankin scale (mRS).

Discussion

The first episode presented by this patient had characteristic symptoms of a TIA. Speech disorder and unilateral weakness are typical symptoms of TIA. Many stroke awareness campaigns include these symptoms as warning signs of stroke and educate the public to seek emergency assistance. Just because symptoms abate, it does not mean that the situation has become less urgent. Indeed, urgent evaluation of this patient at the time he had the initial TIA could have led to the institution of therapy to modify the natural history of the disease. Conversely, if the institution of preventive therapy was not enough to prevent stroke that occurred during hospitalization, the patient could have been treated with rtPA and might have suffered a less devastating consequence of his stroke.

Common Pitfalls in Cerebrovascular Disease: Case-Based Learning, ed. José Biller and José M. Ferro. Published by Cambridge University Press. © Cambridge University Press 2015.

(a)   (b)

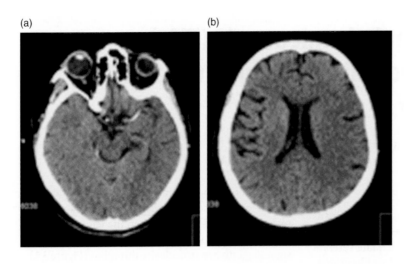

Figure 3.1 Unenhanced CT show signs of acute stroke of the left MCA territory. (a) Hyperdense left MCA sign, in which high attenuation thrombus is seen extending from the left internal carotid artery terminus through the distal left M1 segment. (b) Parenchymal early changes of ischemic stroke are seen, such as effaced sulci and cortical swelling on the left cerebral hemisphere.

Unfortunately, this is not a rare occurrence. About 15–20% of patients who suffered a stroke had previously experienced a TIA, 17% had a TIA on the same day as the stroke, 9% on the day before, and 43% within the previous 7 days [3]. Many of these patients had not sought medical assistance.

Although a TIA does not cause immediate sequelae, affected individuals have a high risk for future ischemic events. A recent systematic review of stroke risk following TIAs showed the pooled risk of recurrent stroke to be 5.2% at 7 days, 6.7% at 90 days, and 11.3% at >90 days [4].

Timely and appropriate treatment of TIAs can drastically reduce stroke risk. This is supported by at least two leading sources of evidence: (1) The EXPRESS (Early Use of Existing Preventive Strategies for Stroke) study examined the effect of immediate care compared with delayed care among 1278 TIA and stroke patients, and found that early care resulted in an 80% reduction in the 90-day risk of secondary stroke [5]. Management included assessment and referral for carotid endarterectomy if appropriate, warfarin for patients in atrial fibrillation, and immediate initiation or adjustment of antiplatelets, statins, and antihypertensive agents if the systolic blood pressure was >130 mmHg. (2) A French study showed the feasibility of assessing and treating TIA patients as soon as possible after the event in a TIA clinic providing 24-hour access (SOS-TIA). At the end of 2 years, the 90-day stroke risk in more than 1000 TIA patients was 1.24%, lower than could have been expected according to the potential risk of recurrence if these patients were not treated on an emergency basis [6].

It is of the utmost importance to treat these patients as soon as possible following the TIA. The risk of stroke is particularly high immediately after the TIA. In a prospective population-based incidence study of TIA and stroke (OXVASC), the risks of stroke at 6, 12, and 24 hours were 1.2%, 2.1%, and 5.1%, respectively [7]. Therefore, these transient events warrant complete evaluation and management in an acute setting. This setting should be defined according to local resources, and may be at emergency rooms, stroke units or TIA clinics. Most guidelines now recommend that patients with TIAs should be assessed within 24 hours of their event, but undoubtedly the feasibility of this depends on patients' behavior.

Tip

Increased awareness of symptoms and signs of TIA and stroke is needed among the population. Even if symptoms subside patients should be urgently evaluated. TIAs warrant complete evaluation and management in an acute setting, because the risk of stroke is particularly high in the first days following these transient events.

Case 2. TIA – can I go home while awaiting etiological investigation?

Case description

A 67-year-old woman went to the ED complaining of difficulties in moving her right limbs. Symptoms began suddenly when she was setting the table for lunch. She sat up, and the symptoms abated after 40 minutes. She did not have changes in her speech, sensation, or limb coordination. She had never had similar episodes or other diseases of the nervous system. Past medical history was remarkable for hypertension, dyslipidemia, and cigarette smoking. She was receiving atorvastatin 20 mg daily, and atenolol 50 mg daily. At the ED, blood pressure was 163/85 mmHg, and heart rate was 54 beats per minute and regular. She had a left cervical bruit. Otherwise, general physical and neurologic examinations were normal. An emergent brain CT scan was normal. Blood analyses were normal. Except for sinus bradycardia, the electrocardiogram was normal.

This index event occurred around Christmas, and her wishes were to go home rather than being hospitalized. However, she was told of the potential risks of stroke, and finally agreed to be hospitalized. The patient was immediately started on aspirin 250 mg daily and 80 mg of atorvastatin daily. Atenolol was replaced by an angiotensin-converting enzyme inhibitor (ACEI).

A carotid Doppler ultrasound displayed a high-grade (90%) atherosclerotic left internal carotid artery stenosis, and a moderate (50%) atherosclerotic right carotid stenosis. TCD ultrasound demonstrated diminished flow velocities on the left MCA, and collateral blood flow through the circle of Willis secondary to extracranial carotid stenosis. Diffusion-weighted MRI showed several small bright signals compatible with acute ischemia at the border zone between the MCA and anterior cerebral artery (ACA) vascular territories (Figure 3.2).

A left carotid endarterectomy (CEA) was performed the same week, and the patient was discharged home without neurologic deficits. She was encouraged to quit smoking, optimize risk factor control, increase her physical activity, and continue on antiplatelet drugs, high dose statins, and a combination of a diuretic and ACEI.

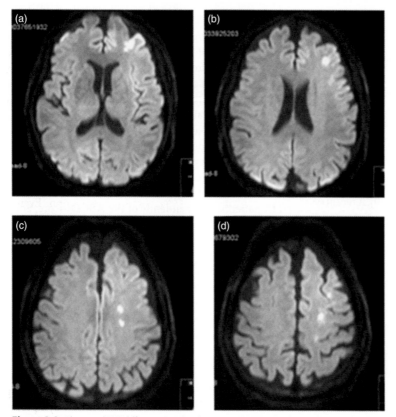

in successive brain slices associated with acute ischemia at the border zones between left MCA and ACA vascular territories.

Figure 3.2 Abnormal MRI diffusion-weighted imaging showing multiple hyperintense signals

Discussion

Given the presence of vascular risk factors and clinical presentation, her transient symptoms were easily attributed to TIA. There were no other neurologic conditions suspected as an alternative diagnosis. Furthermore, the cervical bruit raised suspicion of carotid artery stenosis as the possible cause of the event. All these characteristics were taken into consideration to estimate the immediate risk of stroke, and to decide whether she should be admitted to hospital immediately or discharged to complete the investigation and treatment in an outpatient clinic.

Several clinical risk prediction scores have been developed to identify patients at high risk of stroke and assist clinicians to decide how urgently those patients need to be evaluated. The $ABCD^2$ score has achieved particular relevance and has been adopted by many stroke services, emergency departments, and primary care physicians to guide triaging of patients with TIAs. The $ABCD^2$ score includes: age (>60 years, 1 point); blood pressure elevation on first assessment after TIA (systolic >140 mmHg or diastolic >90 mmHg, 1 point); clinical presentation (unilateral weakness (2 points), speech disturbance (1 point, if there is not motor weakness)); duration of symptoms (≥60 minutes, 2 points; 10–60 minutes, 1 point) and diabetes mellitus (1 point) as clinical variables [8].

The $ABCD^2$ score classifies TIA patients at low, moderate, or high risk using cutoff points of <4, 4–5, and >5. Some clinical guidelines advocate admission to hospital and early assessment/treatment for patients with an $ABCD^2$ score of ≥3, others recommend a specialist assessment and investigation within 24 hours of symptoms for patients with an $ABCD^2$ score of ≥4 and within 1 week for those patients with an $ABCD^2$ score of <4 [9]. A recent systematic review evaluated data on the performance of the $ABCD^2$ score to predict stroke recurrence among patients at high risk (score ≥4) and low risk (score of <4) of stroke [4]. The corresponding pooled risks of stroke for patients with $ABCD^2$ score of ≥4 and <4 at 7 days were 7.5% (95% CI 4.7–11.7) and 2.4 (95% CI 1.3–4.2), respectively.

Our patient had an $ABCD^2$ score of 5. Based on the score, we had enough data to recommend her to be admitted to hospital and start secondary prevention without delay. But we additionally suspected the patient might have left ICA stenosis which would further increase the risk of stroke [10]. Accordingly, we strongly recommended her to be hospitalized despite her wish not to spend Christmas in hospital. Doppler ultrasonography confirmed she had a severe symptomatic left ICA stenosis and thus, she was referred for urgent endarterectomy, the benefit of which is highest when performed within 2 weeks of the index ischemic event [11].

Thus, the addition of information obtained from etiological investigation and brain imaging may further improve the prediction of stroke among TIA patients. Although this was not the case in our patient because she already had a very high $ABCD^2$ score, an important pitfall of using the $ABCD^2$ score alone may be not identifying other established markers of high stroke risk, such as carotid stenosis or atrial fibrillation [12–16]. Adding carotid artery stenosis to the $ABCD^2$ score improves stroke risk prediction [17,18]. Refined versions of this score were proposed, including data based on imaging and vascular assessment, deriving a new score ($ABCD^3$-I) [17].

Approximately 10–15% of patients with an $ABCD^2$ score of <4 have carotid artery stenosis of >50% or even >70% and should therefore be referred for endarterectomy [12,15,16]. In a French cohort, patients with TIAs and $ABCD^2$ scores of <4 had similar 90-day risk of recurrent stroke (3.9%) as those with a score of ≥4 (3.4%) in the presence of internal carotid or intracranial artery stenosis of ≥50% estimated by North American Symptomatic Carotid Endarterectomy Trial (NASCET) criteria, or major cardiac source of embolism [15].

Another interesting finding in our patient concerns the results of brain MRI, because it displayed several acute ischemic lesions. Diffusion-weighted imaging (DWI) shows a definite acute ischemic lesion in about one-third of TIA patients, being negative in two-thirds [19]. The presence of an ischemic lesion on DWI MRI has been associated with an increased risk of stroke in TIA patients, independently of the $ABCD^2$ score, and these findings have been incorporated in the proposed $ABCD^3$-I score (I – lesion in the brain) [4,17].

Taking all these data into consideration, we can summarize that our patient had several characteristics that placed her at high risk of a stroke: high $ABCD^2$ score, severe degree of carotid artery stenosis, and an acute ischemic lesions on DWI MRI. Urgent evaluation was thus essential for the good outcome she had.

Tip

The $ABCD^2$ score is a useful tool to stratify the risk of stroke among patients with TIAs. If the $ABCD^2$ score is ≥4, patients need urgent evaluation and treatment. But a low ABCD² score cannot exclude other conditions that potentially increase stroke risk. Brain imaging and carotid vascular studies should be urgently performed aiming to further individualize the stroke risk and appropriate treatment of these patients.

Case 3. Repeated TIAs – does it change the patient's management?

Case description

A 58-year-old left-handed physician with a history of ischemic heart disease and heavy cigarette smoking was admitted because of sudden onset of slurred speech and weakness of his left limbs. Symptoms started upon awakening, and completely resolved after 2–3 minutes. He had had similar symptoms one month earlier; symptoms consisted of decreased strength on the left side of the body which lasted a minute or two. He was noncompliant with the medications proposed for control of ischemic heart disease, and only took aspirin on an irregular basis. On admission, blood pressure was 120/65 mmHg, and heart rate was 67 per minute and regular. General physical and neurologic examinations were normal. While waiting for the CT scan on the ED, he had another transient event consisting of left limb paresis. This episode was observed by the ED physician, confirming the weakness of both left limbs that transiently became hypotonic. The patient also had left facial paresis and dysarthria. During these episodes he never mentioned sensory or visual symptoms, lack of coordination, or clonic movements.

CT scan was normal. Blood analysis showed a high cholesterol of 223 mg/dL and a low-density lipoprotein (LDL) of 164 mg/dL. ECG was normal. Due to the repeated occurrence of the TIAs a carotid ultrasonography was performed at the ED, which showed small regular atheromatous plaques in both carotid bifurcations without stenosis. The patient was admitted to the stroke unit to be monitored and complete etiological investigation. Aspirin 250 mg daily and atorvastatin 80 mg daily were started.

TCD revealed a marked increase in flow velocities at the origin of the right MCA (systolic velocity 290 cm/s; diastolic velocity 200 cm/s). Brain MRI was normal. Cerebral angiography showed a focal stenosis of the proximal segment of the M1 portion of the right MCA (Figure 3.3). No other abnormalities were found in the other cerebral arteries. Testing for orthostatic hypotension was negative.

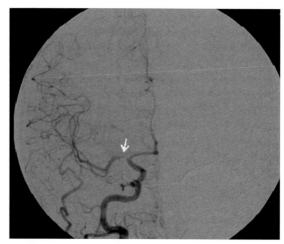

Figure 3.3 Cerebral angiography shows a severe right MCA (M1) stenosis (arrow).

During the first day of hospital stay, the patient had another transient event while lying down. Blood pressure was 137/78 mmHg and the episode resolved after one minute. At that time, clopidogrel 75 mg daily was added to aspirin. The patient was discharged 3 days after. No further TIAs were reported. The patient was seen at the TIA clinic one month later and he did not report further events. A TCD was repeated, and was similar to that performed during hospital admission. The patient did not completely quit smoking, but was otherwise compliant with his medications.

Discussion

This patient presented with repeated stereotyped negative symptoms, suggestive of a TIA. Once the diagnosis of TIA is established, one of the first steps is to determine which vascular territory is affected, as this may guide further etiological investigation and treatment. However, this may be difficult because of the paucity of neurologic abnormalities at the time of evaluation, and the need to rely on the patient's description. Moreover, similar symptoms can be produced by ischemia in different vascular territories. Such an example is the clinical presentation of our patient, which was characterized by unilateral motor deficits and slurred speech. In general, isolated unilateral symptoms are taken as suggestive evidence for anterior circulation ischemia, but ischemia involving the pons, the cerebral peduncles, or the medullary pyramids produce virtually indistinguishable symptoms. In our patient, the absence of cortical symptoms suggested a subcortical or brainstem location. Sometimes, MRI can help determine which is the vascular territory affected, but this was not the case with our patient as his MRI was normal.

The recurrent symptoms at the time he went to hospital, consisting of a burst of stereotyped TIAs with unilateral motor deficits involving at least two of three body parts (face, arm, or leg) without cortical symptoms, were evocative of the "capsular warning syndrome" [20] or "pontine warning syndrome" [21]. These syndromes have been closely linked to single penetrating artery disease, and have been associated with a high early risk of lacunar infarction. The pathophysiology is complex, and may involve hemodynamic mechanisms in penetrating arterial territories. Contrary to what is described in those warning syndromes, our patient reported a similar event about one month earlier. This argued against a small vessel etiology, and ultimately, the demonstration of a right MCA stenosis established the cause of his recurrent TIAs.

Our patient had an $ABCD^2$ score of 2, which portends a low recurrence risk, but this case highlights that we would have incurred a pitfall if our decision was based exclusively on this score. If we had decided against admitting him to hospital because of the low $ABCD^2$ score and normal ultrasound study of the extracranial vessels, we could have referred him for a less urgent evaluation, missing an important etiology and underestimating the true stroke risk.

The presence of two or more TIA symptoms within 7 days has been associated with a higher short-term risk of stroke. Indeed, the refined $ABCD^3$ score (the third "D" meaning dual TIA) is more accurate in identifying patients at high risk compared with the $ABCD^2$ score [17]. Moreover, recent studies have shown that intracranial arterial stenosis is associated with recurrent stroke after TIA [22].

Taking all these data into consideration – the clinical presentation, recurrence of TIAs, and the presence of intracranial stenosis – we concluded that the patient had a high stroke risk. Once he had a subsequent TIA while on aspirin, we added clopidogrel. Dual antiplatelet therapy is not a standard recommendation for secondary stroke prevention, but among selective high-risk patients, where conventional maximal therapy fails, it might be reasonable to prescribe dual antiplatelet therapy. The Clopidogrel in High-Risk Patients With Acute Non-disabling Cerebrovascular Events (CHANCE) trial, demonstrated a benefit of combination therapy (aspirin plus clopidogrel vs. aspirin alone) for patients with an acute minor ischemic stroke or TIA within 24 hours of their event [23]. This trial only enrolled Chinese patients, thus we should be prudent when generalizing its results.

Tip

The risk after TIA needs to be individualized. Even patients with low $ABCD^2$ may have other features that place them at high risk of stroke, such as those with large vessel stenosis or multiple TIAs in a short period of time.

Case 4. TIA is underrecognized

Case description

A 45-year-old woman, without known vascular risk factors, presented to the ED because of a transient visual blurring but she was uncertain if it afflicted her right eye or the right field of vision. She was also unable to recall if her visual impairment was progressive or sudden in appearance. She had no positive phenomena like scintillating scotomata. The visual symptom lasted less than 3–5 minutes, and was accompanied by headache, progressive in onset and of throbbing quality. A few minutes later, she experienced sensory loss on her right arm and face and felt anxious. Again, she was not able to describe if the symptoms had a progressive onset. Her colleagues at work became very worried and brought her to the ED. Past medical history was noteworthy for some episodes of headaches fulfilling diagnostic criteria of migraine, but without aura, and anxiety, occasionally taking benzodiazepines. She did not smoke or use illicit drugs.

In the ED, she was hyperventilating and appeared very anxious. General and neurologic examinations were normal. Blood pressure was 107/57 mmHg. Blood analysis and ECG did not show any abnormalities. The ED physician assumed her symptoms were due to anxiety and prescribed diazepam. However, because of the transient focal symptoms he requested a brain CT scan and a neurologic examination. The neurologist was uncertain about the diagnosis, hesitating between migraine with atypical aura versus anxiety with hyperventilation-related symptoms. After 6 hours of clinical monitoring she was discharged home to be re-evaluated in the TIA outpatient clinic. The next day she attended the TIA clinic. She was calm and gave a more detailed description of the symptoms. It was then clear that the first symptom was headache, followed by

(a)　　　　　　　　　　　　　(b)　　　　　　　　　　　　　(c)

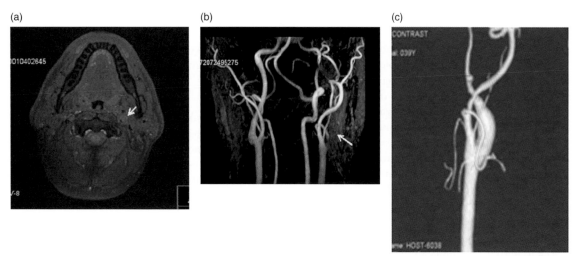

Figure 3.4 MRI and angio-CT scan of the patient with left ICA dissection. (a) T1-SPIR brain MRI shows intramural iso/hypersignal with crescent morphology in the wall of the left ICA, associated with diminished void arterial sign (arrow). (b) In the angio-MR the left ICA is not visualized between the carotid bifurcation and the base of the skull (arrow). (c) Angio-CT shows permeability of the carotid bulb despite a narrowing of the ICA in accordance with the diagnosis of cervical artery dissection.

visual blurring. Since the patient did not attempt alternating closure of either eye, it was still impossible to know if she had a right homonymous hemianopsia or decreased vision of the right eye. However, it became clear that her sensory symptoms affected simultaneously her right hand and right corner of her mouth, and it was also clear that those symptoms preceded anxiety and hyperventilation.

Thus, the stroke neurologist at the TIA clinic established TIA as the most likely diagnosis and a carotid ultrasound was immediately performed that showed a tight stenosis of the left ICA probably due to ICA dissection. This diagnosis was confirmed by T1-weighted axial cervical MRI scans with use of a fat-saturation technique that showed a crescent-shaped rim of hyperintense signal surrounding the lumen of the left ICA. This sign is indicative of a mural hematoma (Figure 3.4). Angio-CT scan was also performed, showing a filiform flow in the left ICA.

She was then admitted to the stroke unit, where she was monitored and treated with anticoagulation. She experienced no further events, and was discharged without neurologic deficits.

Discussion

This young woman presented with transient focal signs which were elusive to the physicians who first assessed her. The symptoms were not sufficiently detailed due their very short duration. The anxious mood induced

the ED physician to attribute her symptoms to anxiety. Indeed, hyperventilation can induce some visual disturbance and paresthesias. However, anxiety can also be the reaction to abnormal phenomena, such as those that this patient had.

Headache was another confusing symptom, which may have led the physician to the diagnosis of migraine, rather than TIAs. Headache is not a common symptom of TIA. So, considering the young age of our patient, the previous migraine history, and the apparent succession of symptom appearance (visual followed by sensory symptoms) the first neurologist who evaluated the patient in the ED considered migraine with aura as the most probable diagnosis. But the clinical description was not entirely typical for a first episode of aura: (1) symptoms were "negative" type, whereas auras more often have positive symptoms; (2) headache occurred at onset of focal symptoms, whereas it more typically appears when focal symptoms have subsided. Finally, the stroke neurologist at the TIA clinic obtained the data from the history without the confounding factor of anxiety, and considered that the most likely diagnosis was a TIA. When headache is a prominent symptom in patients with transient neurological symptoms, a cervical dissection should be suspected as a possible cause of the TIAs. Other conditions that need to be included in the differential diagnosis are the reversible vasoconstriction syndrome or, less commonly, cerebral venous thrombosis.

This case clearly illustrates the difficulties in the clinical diagnosis of TIAs, and also exemplifies the poor interobserver agreement in TIA diagnosis [24–27].

The following symptoms are typical of TIAs: (1) weakness, clumsiness, or sensory alteration in one or both limbs on the same side; speech or language disturbance; loss of vision in one eye or part of the eye, or homonymous hemianopsia for symptoms that relate to the carotid territory; (2) weakness or clumsiness (sometimes shifting from one side to another); sensory alteration; complete blindness or homonymous hemianopsia; ataxia, imbalance or unsteadiness not associated with vertigo; diplopia; dysphagia; dysarthria; or vertigo for symptoms related to the vertebrobasilar territory.

The following symptoms are nonspecific or atypical of TIA: disturbances of vision in one or both eyes consisting of flashes, distorted-view tunnel vision, or images moving on change of posture; tiredness or heavy sensation in one or more limbs, either unilateral or bilateral; gradual spread of sensory symptoms; isolated disorder of swallowing or articulation, double vision, vertigo, or dizziness; and accompanying symptoms including unconsciousness, limb jerking, tingling of the limbs or lips, disorientation, and amnesia [28].

Patients with TIAs initially seek healthcare from primary care practices and emergency departments. Accurate recognition of TIA at the first healthcare contact is crucial in reducing early stroke risk. But this is a difficult and complex task for primary care physicians. Around 50% of referrals to TIA clinics do not have a cerebrovascular diagnosis [29]. The most frequent diagnoses of such patients are migraine, seizure/epilepsy, syncope, vestibular disease, or psychiatric disorder. Less frequent diagnoses are peripheral nerve conditions, postural hypotension, transient global amnesia, toxic or metabolic causes (e.g., drugs, hypoglycemia), and brain tumors.

Diagnosis requires a thorough clinical assessment. Although MRI may be helpful, it can be normal in up to two-thirds of cases [4]. There are some tools or scales which assist physicians in triaging and easier identification of stroke patients. But there are no such tools in the triage of TIA patients. Dawson and colleagues reported a recognition tool for TIA which is based on the physical signs elicited from patients [30] and the ABCD^2 score was also evaluated in order to try to distinguish between TIA and mimics [31]. However, these tools do not have good accuracy to distinguish between TIA and non-vascular events, and they cannot replace patients' descriptions of their experience of TIA and the judgment of the physician. Moreover, they might help with the triage process, but they are insufficient to establish the diagnosis.

Tip

An accurate and detailed description of the symptoms by the patient or proxy may increase the accuracy of the diagnosis. Knowledge of the main conditions that can mimic TIAs can assist physicians in establishing a proper differential diagnosis. If symptoms are typical for TIAs, patients should be urgently evaluated and treated.

Case 5. Right middle cerebral artery TIA – a possibly underdiagnosed TIA

Case description

A 79-year-old man was evaluated in the ED due to transient paresthesias of the left upper limb. Symptoms were brief in duration (<1 hour), but the patient was not able to recall the circumstances in which they occurred, how symptoms had settled, or their duration. The proxy accompanying the patient described that he had some difficulty in telling what was happening. She also explained that he was sitting at the dinner table and that his left arm seemed a little odd, making some inappropriate movements. She told him several times to remove his left hand from the bowl of soup, but the patient did not seem to recognize what was happening. The patient had had a right CEA 4 years earlier, and had hypertension, dyslipidemia, and peripheral artery disease. He was on aspirin 150 mg daily, perindopril plus indapamide, and atorvastatin. At the ED, blood pressure was 137/69 mmHg and heart rate was 63 per minute. Physical and neurological examinations were normal; CT scan showed an old right parietal ischemic stroke. Carotid ultrasound did not show significant changes. The patient was discharged home and referred to the TIA clinic the next day. Because of atypical symptoms and lack of awareness of symptoms, the normal appearance of the right ICA, and the presence of an old parietal lesion, the ED physician considered that the transient neurologic event might have been a partial seizure or a TIA. The next day the patient presented to the TIA clinic and the neurologic examination now disclosed a left hemiparesis neglect, and anosognosia. MRI confirmed an acute ischemic infarction involving the right MCA territory, on the

(a)

(b)

(c)

(d)

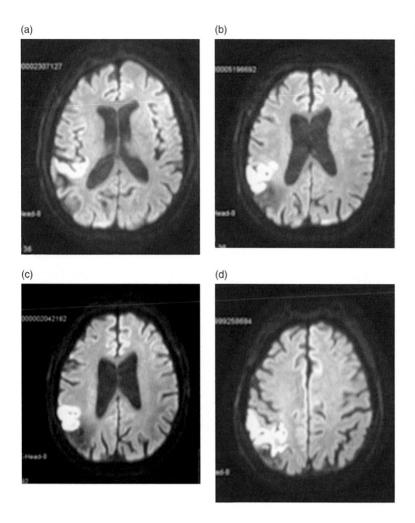

Figure 3.5 MRI diffusion-weighted imaging shows an acute ischemic lesion involving the right supramarginal and angular gyri and parietal convexity in the MCA territory. There is also adjacent parietal hypointensity corresponding to old parietal ischemia in the same vascular territory.

supramarginal and angular gyri and parietal convexity (Figure 3.5).

A 24-hour Holter recorded paroxysmal atrial fibrillation. Aspirin was switched to anticoagulation one week later.

Discussion

This case illustrates how difficult it is to diagnose transient cognitive dysfunction of the right carotid artery territory. Once the stroke had occurred, it was probably easier to recognize that the patient might have suffered a transient event related to ischemia of the right MCA territory. However, because the diagnosis relied on the description of the symptoms, the doctor at the ED was unable to establish that diagnosis. The detailed information given to the neurologist in the TIA clinic the following day immediately raised the hypothesis that

the patient had symptoms of the right MCA territory, underdiagnosed by the doctor at the ED. The main concern in the emergency room was whether the symptoms were due to a carotid restenosis. Once stenosis was ruled out, the patient was discharged home. The ABCD^2 score was 3 at the maximum. Unfortunately, he had a recurrence of symptoms before attendance at the TIA clinic, and during hospitalization paroxysmal atrial fibrillation was discovered. This case presents two potential pitfalls: (1) lack of recognition of symptoms of right cortical MCA territory; (2) scoring 3 or less on the ABCD^2 score does not necessarily identify the precise risk associated with the etiology of the TIA, in this particular case, atrial fibrillation.

This case reinforces that the ABCD^2 score is insufficient to decide when etiologic investigation may be deferred. Although patients with scores <4 had a lower stroke risk than patients with scores ≥4, the score is unable to identify if there is a potential underlying etiology that increases stroke risk. In the SOS-TIA study (SOS Transient Ischaemic Attack), which enrolled a total of 1176 TIAs, one-fifth of patients with an ABCD^2 score of <4 had a serious risk factor. Among 679 patients with ABCD^2 scores of <4, 9%, 6%, and 8% of patients, respectively, had carotid stenosis of >50%, atrial fibrillation, or some other high-risk factor requiring immediate attention [14].

Tip

Right cortical MCA territory TIAs represent diagnostic challenges that may be underdiagnosed. Suspicion of isolated cortical deficits should prompt a search for a cardioembolic source if no abnormal findings are demonstrated in large vessels. Patients with TIA should be evaluated without delay regardless of ABCD^2 score because some patients with lower scores have treatable causes associated with higher short-term risks of stroke.

Case 6. Did I have a new TIA because I stopped treatment?

Case description

A 79-year-old retired teacher decided to consult his family doctor because he had an episode he thought it was a TIA. Seven months earlier, he had suffered from a transient episode of slurred speech and weakness of the left limbs lasting less than one hour. After evaluation in the ED with a CT scan, ECG, and carotid artery ultrasound, he was told he had suffered a TIA, and medicated with aspirin, statins, and antihypertensive drugs. He had a past history of hypertension. After that TIA, he made same changes to his diet and increased his physical activity, taking frequent daily walks.

The current symptoms were quite different but also transient. While walking, he would suddenly lack strength in his right limbs, mostly in the leg in such a way that he was unable to walk and had to sit. The upper limb was not particularly weak, but the hand was clumsy so it was difficult for him to use the phone to request help from his son. Speech was not affected. About 10 minutes after symptoms cleared the first thing he thought was "This was a TIA" and he went home and took the medication he had stopped taking

regularly. Because he had a consultation with his primary care physician the following week, he decided to resume all medications and wait for that consultation. The primary care physician agreed with the presumed diagnosis made by the patient, and because the episode had occurred more than one week earlier, the patient was sent to a TIA clinic for further stroke specialist advice.

Discussion

The transient symptoms experienced by this patient correspond to a TIA. Etiological investigation did not disclose large vessel disease, and both clinical presentations may be related to lacunar syndromes, the first one a pure motor syndrome, and the second one ataxic hemiparesis. The main problem of this patient might have been that he abandoned his therapy, or at least, was not very compliant.

This case demonstrates that TIA patients continue to have a risk of further vascular events even after the first days. A recent systematic review showed that the pooled risk of stroke after TIA at 90 days is nearly 7%, and at >90 days is around 11% [4]. The risk for an individual patient is affected by specific characteristics of the event, event type and cause, risk factors, and adherence to preventive therapy. In this particular case, it was clear that, although the patient had made some changes to his lifestyle, he was not fully compliant with hypertension therapy, statin and antiplatelet drugs.

Medication adherence is important for optimal secondary stroke prevention. Several classes of medications are effective in modifying stroke risk factors and preventing stroke recurrence. However, up to one-third of stroke patients discontinue medications prescribed at the time of stroke or TIA [32]. Regimen compliance for secondary prevention decreases over time, and may affect medications differently. Sometimes, these changes are based on post-discharge healthcare provider recommendations. Other reasons may be associated with adverse effects, low access to medical consultations to reinforce and explain the need to be complaint, the multiplicity of drugs that need to be taken, and high cost.

It is possible that patients with TIAs do not recognize the severity of the disease because the symptoms disappear, and thus, might be less compliant with medications. Continuously educating the patient to

Table 3.1 Management of patients with transient ischemic attacks

Immediate evaluation (TIA clinic, emergent department, stroke unit)

Lab testing – full blood count, serum electrolytes and creatinine; fasting blood glucose and lipids

Electrocardiography

Brain imaging – CT or MRI

Vascular imaging – carotid imaging, CT or MR angiography, or TCD

Hospitalization (may be considered for patients with high risk of stroke)

$ABCD^2 \geq 4$

High-grade stenosis of intra- or extracranial vessel

Atrial fibrillation

Repeated TIAs

Immediate treatment

Antithrombotic therapy

Atherothrombotic TIA – antiplatelet therapy: combination extended-release dipyridamole plus aspirin, clopidogrel, or aspirin alone
Cardioembolic TIA – anticoagulation

Carotid endarterectomy (CEA)
TIA with ipsilateral severe (70–99%) carotid artery stenosis – CEA as soon as possible (within 2 weeks)
Ipsilateral moderate (50–69%) stenosis – CEA may be considered for certain patients and at centers with perioperative complication rate <6%

Hypertension – lower blood pressure to <140/90 mmHg, with an ACE inhibitor alone or in combination with a diuretic

Lipids – initiate a statin

Diabetes – screen for diabetes and treat

Smoking – initiate a cessation program

Nutritional assessment – look for signs of overnutrition or undernutrition

Motivate for increasing physical activity

maintain appropriate adherence to different measures of secondary prevention is crucial.

Tip

To prevent stroke recurrence, disability, and death, TIA patients should be compliant to measures controlling risk factors and maintain adherence to medications aimed at secondary prevention (Table 3.1). Primary care physicians, neurologists, or stroke specialists need to assess if patients are remaining compliant with all medications. Reasons limiting adherence need to be elucidated so patients continue to comply with all measures of secondary stroke prevention.

References

1. Hankey GJ. Redefining risks after TIA and minor ischaemic stroke. *Lancet* 2005;365:2065–6.

2. Easton JD, Saver JL, Albers GW, et al. Definition and evaluation of transient ischemic attack: a scientific statement for healthcare professionals from the American Heart Association/American Stroke Association Stroke Council; Council on Cardiovascular Surgery and Anesthesia; Council on Cardiovascular Radiology and Intervention; Council on Cardiovascular Nursing; and the Interdisciplinary Council on Peripheral Vascular Disease. The American Academy of Neurology affirms the value of this statement as an educational tool for neurologists. *Stroke* 2009;40:2276–93.

3. Rothwell PM, Warlow CP. Timing of TIAs preceding stroke: time window for prevention is very short. *Neurology* 2005;64:817–20.

4. Wardlaw J, Brazzelli M, Miranda H, et al. An assessment of the cost-effectiveness of magnetic resonance, including diffusion-weighted imaging, in patients with transient ischaemic attack and minor stroke: a systematic review, meta-analysis and economic evaluation. *Health Technol Assess* 2014;18(27):1–368.

5. Rothwell PM, Giles MF, Chandratheva A, et al. Effect of urgent treatment of transient ischaemic attack and minor stroke on early recurrent stroke (EXPRESS study): a prospective population-based sequential comparison. *Lancet* 2007;370:1432–42.

6. Lavallée PC, Meseguer E, Abboud H, et al. A transient ischaemic attack clinic with round-the-clock access (SOS-TIA): feasibility and effects. *Lancet Neurol* 2007;6:953–60.

7. Chandratheva A, Mehta Z, Geraghty OC, et al. Population-based study of risk and predictors of stroke in the first few hours after a TIA. *Neurology* 2009;72:1941–7.

8. Johnston SC, Rothwell PM, Nguyen-Huynh MN, et al. Validation and refinement of scores to predict very early stroke risk after transient ischaemic attack. *Lancet* 2007;369:283–92.

9. National Institute for Health and Care Excellence (NICE). *Stroke. The Diagnosis and Acute Management of Stroke and Transient Ischaemic Attacks*. London: NICE; 2008.

10. Eliasziw M, Kennedy J, Hill MD, et al. for the North American Symptomatic Carotid Endarterectomy (NASCET) Group. Early risk of stroke after a transient ischemic attack in patients with internal carotid artery disease. *CMAJ* 2004;170:1105–9.

11. Rothwell PM, Eliasziw M, Gutnikov SA, et al. for the Carotid Endarterectomy Trialists' Collaboration. Endarterectomy for symptomatic carotid stenosis in relation to clinical subgroup and timing of surgery. *Lancet* 2004;363:915–24.

12. Koton S, Rothwell PM. Performance of the ABCD and ABCD2 scores in TIA patients with carotid stenosis and atrial fibrillation. *Cerebrovasc Dis* 2007;24:231–5.

13. Purroy F, Montaner J, Molina CA, Delgado P, Ribo M, Alvarez-Sabin J. Patterns and predictors of early risk of recurrence after transient ischemic attack with respect to etiologic subtypes. *Stroke* 2007;38:3225–9.

14. Amarenco P, Labreuche J, Lavallée PC, et al. Does ABCD2 score below 4 allow more time to evaluate patients with a transient ischemic attack? *Stroke* 2009;40(9):3091–5.

15. Amarenco P, Labreuche J, Lavallée PC. Patients with transient ischemic attack with ABCD2 <4 can have similar 90-day stroke risk as patients with transient ischemic attack with ABCD2 ≥4. *Stroke* 2012;43:863–5.

16. Walker J, Isherwood J, Eveson D, Naylor AR. Triaging TIA/minor stroke patients using the ABCD2 score does not predict those with significant carotid disease. *Eur J Vasc Endovasc Surg* 2012;43:495–8.

17. Brazzelli M, Chappell FM, Miranda H, et al. Diffusion-weighted imaging and diagnosis of transient ischemic attack. *Ann Neurol* 2014;75(1):67–76.

18. Merwick A, Albers GW, Amarenco P, et al. Addition of brain and carotid imaging to the ABCD2 score to identify patients at early risk of stroke after transient ischaemic attack: a multicentre observational study. *Lancet Neurol* 2010;9:1060–9.

19. Giles MF, Albers GW, Amarenco P, et al. Addition of brain infarction to the ABCD2 Score (ABCD2I): a collaborative analysis of unpublished data on 4574 patients. *Stroke* 2010;41:1907–13.

20. Donnan GA, O'Malley HM, Quang L, et al. The capsular warning syndrome: pathogenesis and clinical features. *Neurology* 1993;43(5):957–62.

21. Muengtaweepongsa S, Singh NN, Cruz-Flores S. Pontine warning syndrome: case series and review of literature. *J Stroke Cerebrovasc Dis* 2010;19(5):353–6.

22. Coutts SB, Modi J, Patel SK, et al. Calgary Stroke Program. CT/CT angiography and MRI findings predict recurrent stroke after transient ischemic attack and minor stroke: results of the prospective CATCH study. *Stroke* 2012;43:1013–17.

23. Wang Y, Zhao X, Liu L, et al. CHANCE Investigators. Clopidogrel with aspirin in acute minor stroke or transient ischemic attack. *N Engl J Med* 2013;369:11–19.

24. Koudstaal PJ, van Gijn J, Staal A, Duivenvoorden HJ, Gerritsma JG, Kraaijeveld C. Diagnosis of transient ischemic attacks: improvement of interobserver agreement by a check-list in ordinary language. *Stroke* 1986;17:723–8.

25. Kraaijeveld CL, van Gijn J, Schouten HJ, Staal A. Interobserver agreement for the diagnosis of transient ischemic attacks. *Stroke* 1984;15:723–5.

26. Ferro JM, Falcao I, Rodrigues G, et al. Diagnosis of transient ischemic attack by the nonneurologist. A validation study. *Stroke* 1996;27:2225–9.

27. Castle J, Mlynash M, Lee K, et al. Agreement regarding diagnosis of transient ischemic attack fairly low among stroke-trained neurologists. *Stroke* 2010;41:1367–70.

28. Bots ML, van der Wilk EC, Koudstaal PJ, et al. Transient neurological attacks in the general population. Prevalence, risk factors, and clinical relevance. *Stroke* 1997;28(4):768–73.

29. Fonseca AC, Canhão P. Diagnostic difficulties in the classification of transient neurological attacks. *Eur J Neurol* 2011;18(4): 644–8.

30. Dawson J, Lamb KE, Quinn TJ, et al. A recognition tool for transient ischaemic attack. *QJM* 2009;102:43–9.

31. Quinn TJ, Cameron AC, Dawson J, et al. ABCD2 scores and prediction of noncerebrovascular diagnoses in an outpatient population. A case-control study. *Stroke* 2009;40:749–53.

32. Bushnell CD, Olson DM, Zhao X, et al. AVAIL Investigators. Secondary preventive medication persistence and adherence 1 year after stroke. *Neurology* 2011;77(12):1182–90.

When the diagnostic image is not diagnostic

David D. Pasquale and Jordan Rosenblum

This chapter provides a case-based review with imaging correlation to focus on the inherent limitations of imaging in the diagnosis of hemorrhagic and ischemic stroke. Diagnostic imaging studies are not created equal with regard to the stroke patient. Thus, an accurate history and physical examination are imperative in the selection of appropriate imaging to maximize sensitivity. Each case will provide the reader with the patient presentation, pertinent history, physical examination, and imaging findings followed by a discussion of why a particular imaging study was performed. The pitfalls of the particular imaging modality will be addressed as well as imaging alternatives and case relevant pearls.

Case 1. Acute subarachnoid hemorrhage (SAH)

Case description

A 35-year-old right-handed woman with a history of occasional mild headaches, presented with sudden onset of the "worst headache of her life" at 7 a.m. She was in her usual state of health when she experienced an acute, 9/10 bifrontal and periorbital headache that was pressure-like, non-radiating, and not relieved as usual with two "baby aspirins." She reported associated symptoms of nausea, photophobia and nuchal rigidity. On examination, blood pressure was 108/59 mmHg, pulse was 72 beats per minute, respiratory rate was 18 breaths per minute, and O_2 saturation was 100%. She was afebrile. Physical examination at presentation was otherwise normal. Toxicology screen was unremarkable. Emergent non-contrast computed tomography (NCCT) of the head was normal with the exception of punctate hyperdensity adjacent to or involving the basilar artery on a single axial image (Figure 4.1).

The clinical history and abnormal computed tomography (CT) findings prompted a magnetic resonance imaging (MRI) and MR angiogram (MRA) of the brain with and without contrast, which demonstrated single punctate foci of susceptibility within the occipital horns of the lateral ventricles consistent with hemorrhage or calcification but no aneurysm (Figure 4.2).

Ultimately, a diagnostic lumbar puncture (LP) was performed in the emergency department at approximately 5.5 hours post symptom onset because of the concern for subarachnoid hemorrhage (SAH). Cerebro spinal fluid (CSF) analysis showed 4 mL of blood-tinged CSF (reported as non-traumatic); red blood cells (RBCs) 48K on tube 1, 44K on tube 4; no xanthochromia; protein content 156 mg/dL (normal range 15–45 mg/dL). CSF was otherwise normal. The patient was admitted to the neurosciences intensive care unit (NICU) for aneurysmal SAH. The patient remained hemodynamically stable with a persistent 5/10 frontal headache. A diagnostic cervical and cerebral catheter angiogram was performed the next morning which demonstrated a 3 mm dorsal wall, blister-type aneurysm involving the ophthalmic/hypophyseal segment of the right internal carotid artery (Figure 4.3).

MRI of the entire spine with and without contrast and a repeat diagnostic LP was performed after the angiogram. The MRI of the spine was normal. The repeat LP was performed under fluoroscopy to yield the cleanest possible sample. CSF analysis of the second LP: opening pressure 12 cm H_2O; 10 mL of blood-tinged CSF; 5K RBCs on tube 1; 4K RBCs on tube 4; positive xanthochromia. Following a multidisciplinary discussion, the decision was made to treat the right internal carotid artery (ICA) blister-type aneurysm via an endovascular approach. The patient was loaded

Common Pitfalls in Cerebrovascular Disease: Case-Based Learning, ed. José Biller and José M. Ferro. Published by Cambridge University Press. © Cambridge University Press 2015.

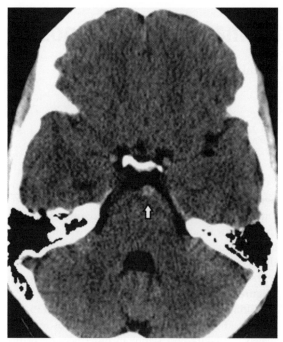

Figure 4.1 Non-contrast head CT axial image at the level of the basal cisterns demonstrates hyperdensity in the expected location of the basilar artery (arrow).

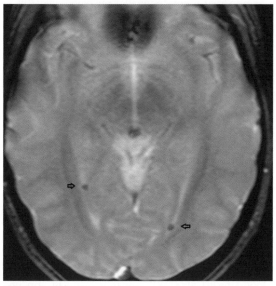

Figure 4.2 MRI brain; axial gradient-recalled echo (GRE) sequence demonstrates punctate foci of susceptibility within the occipital horns (arrows).

with aspirin and clopidogrel, as per protocol. The patient underwent uneventful treatment of the right ICA aneurysm with an endoluminal flow-diverting stent approximately 48 hours later.

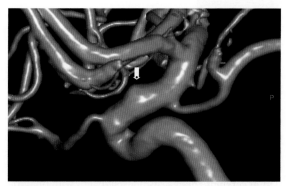

Figure 4.3 3D digital subtraction angiography (DSA) image of the right internal carotid artery, oblique lateral view, showing 3 mm dorsal wall, blister-type intracranial aneurysm (arrow).

Discussion

This patient presented with a "thunderclap" headache that is classic for SAH and 80% of the time secondary to aneurysm rupture. The diagnostic imaging in this patient was relatively unimpressive for a ruptured cerebral aneurysm. The sensitivity of an NCCT for acute SAH ranges from 97.5% to 93% but decreases with time to approximately 50% sensitivity at 7 days post ictus [1,2]. MRI of the brain begins to surpass the sensitivity of CT for the detection of SAH as the time from ictus increases. However, MRI is particularly fraught with susceptibility artifact near the skull base and aerated structures such as sinuses and mastoid air cells. In this particular case, the CT scan was essentially negative for SAH as there was lack of hemorrhage visible within the basal cisterns despite imaging at time interval less than 5 hours post ictus. Hemorrhage on MRI will have variable signal intensity (brightness or darkness) depending on the age of the intracranial blood breakdown products. Typically SAH hemorrhage will have increased signal or brightness on fluid-attenuated inversion recovery images (FLAIR) and decreased signal on gradient-recalled echo (GRE) or susceptibility-weighted imaging (SWI), which are generally the most sensitive sequences for the detection of SAH. Unfortunately, FLAIR and GRE/SWI images have a relatively low specificity secondary to pulsation and susceptibility artifact, respectively. The GRE images in this case did detect punctate foci of susceptibility within the occipital horns of the lateral ventricles; however, this could be hemorrhage, calcium, and/or mineralization. The lack of calcification on the prior NCCT confirms the MRI findings are secondary to heme. The initial diagnostic LP was suspicious for SAH given the persistently elevated RBC count in tubes 1 and 4 despite the lack of xanthochromia. Optimal timing of the LP is debatable but >6 hours and preferably at least 12 hours post ictus is recommended [3]. A sufficient time interval is necessary to allow hemoglobin breakdown and bilirubin formation within the CSF thus resulting in xanthochromia. Ultimately, our patient had a repeat LP with fluoroscopic guidance at approximately 20 hours post ictus which demonstrated persistent RBCs and xanthochromia. Digital subtraction cerebral angiography (DSA) remains the "gold standard" for the detection of cerebral aneurysms. However, the sensitivity of multidetector CT angiography (CTA) is near 99% and now approaches the sensitivity of DSA. A spinal MRI was performed in this patient to exclude a possible spinal vascular malformation or arteriovenous fistula as a cause of SAH. Although several studies have concluded that the addition of a spinal MRI in this setting is probably unnecessary [4].

Tip

The compelling force for decision-making and necessity to exclude aneurysmal SAH in this case hinged on the classic clinical presentation of "thunderclap and worst headache of life." The diagnostic imaging in this case was not particularly conclusive and possibly would have resulted in delayed diagnosis or non-treatment of a small (3 mm) ruptured cerebral aneurysm. Furthermore, one must exercise caution with regard to interpretation of ancillary laboratory data, particularly the CSF cell count and absence of xanthochromia, if the LP is performed within 0–12 hours post ictus. The differential diagnosis of SAH is broad and beyond the scope of this chapter but is most commonly associated with aneurysm rupture (80%) followed by perimesencephalic non-aneurysmal SAH and reversible cerebral vasoconstriction syndrome (RCVS). The inherent imaging pitfalls in the detection of subarachnoid blood are essentially identical regardless of the etiology. Pitfalls in the diagnosis of SAH are further discussed in Chapter 16.

Case 2. Cervicocerebral atherosclerotic disease and ischemic stroke

Case description

A 58-year-old right-handed woman with a history of hypertension, asthma, and 30 pack-years smoking presented with slurred speech and right-sided weakness

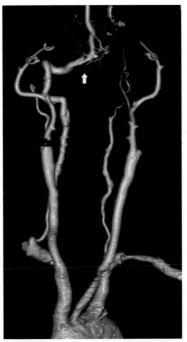

Figure 4.4 3D volume rendering, CTA of the head and neck demonstrating the right vertebral artery (arrow) as the single intracranial arterial supply. The bilateral internal carotid and left vertebral arteries are occluded.

which was worse and progressive relative to her baseline. The patient had been discharged approximately 2 weeks prior to admission after suffering left hemispheric watershed and embolic strokes. She was in her usual state of health with mild residual right-sided weakness, arm more involved than leg, intermittent spastic dysarthria and non-fluent aphasia when her symptoms worsened during an argument with her spouse. She had known bilateral ICA and left vertebral artery occlusion based on a prior cervicocerebral DSA and CTA (Figure 4.4).

She was previously discharged on a medical regimen of daily amlodipine 2.5 mg, lisinopril 2.5 mg, atorvastatin 80 mg, aspirin 81 mg, and clopidogrel 75 mg by mouth. On admission, she was afebrile, her blood pressure was 140/60 mmHg and pulse was 66 beats per minute. Respiratory rate was 18 breaths per minute, and O_2 saturation was 97%. Neurologic examination was notable for mild dysarthria and 4/5 right upper extremity grip strength. Laboratory data and transthoracic echocardiogram (TTE) were normal. MRI of the brain demonstrated two new foci of acute infarction within the left corona radiata (Figure 4.5), subacute anterior and posterior left border zone infarctions,

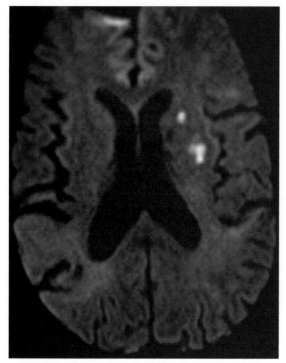

Figure 4.5 MRI brain; axial DWI demonstrating restricted diffusion within acute infarcts involving the left corona radiata.

left middle cerebral artery (MCA) territory embolic infarcts, chronic right MCA infarcts, and severe bilateral chronic border zone infarctions.

Antihypertensive medications were withheld and she was admitted to the NICU for observation and hemodynamic monitoring. She remained hemodynamically and neurologically stable and returned to her pre-admission baseline within 72 hours without the need for blood pressure augmentation. MR perfusion, CT perfusion, and CTA of the head and neck were performed prior to discharge. She was maintained on her initial medical regimen, remained asymptomatic, and was discharged to home.

Discussion

Given the patient's history of known cervical arterial vascular occlusion, intermittent, waxing and waning symptoms, the most appropriate and sensitive initial study for this new presentation was an MRI of the brain to determine areas of new infarction/ischemia. An NCCT scan would be appropriate if there was any indication of an acute hemorrhage; this was not the case here. The NCCT would have very low sensitivity

for an acute infarct in this setting, given her relatively low National Institutes of Health Stroke Scale (NIHSS) score and background of extensive chronic infarcts and ischemia. The favored diagnosis on admission was hypoperfusion syndrome and watershed/border zone infarcts which may be exacerbated by hyperventilation (following an argument with her spouse) resulting in decreased blood pCO_2 and cerebral vasoconstriction. However, the infarcts on the prior MRI where not entirely limited to a border zone territory but rather had an embolic component. Furthermore, the new and recent infarcts on MRI were primarily isolated to the left MCA territory. From where would such emboli originate and how could emboli get to the left MCA territory in the setting of bilateral ICA and left vertebral artery occlusion? The entire intracranial arterial vasculature in this patient was primarily supplied from the right vertebral artery through the posterior communicating arteries and pial/leptomeningeal collaterals. Embolic material traveling through the right innominate artery, right subclavian, and right vertebral artery to the intracranial arterial vasculature would inevitably result in embolic strokes within the posterior circulation and right anterior circulation rather than strokes isolated to the left MCA territory as in this patient. No additional vascular territory infarcts where demonstrated on three MRIs over the course of 3 weeks. An MR perfusion (MRP) examination was chosen to test the perfusion to the left MCA territory. Unfortunately, the MRP examination was extremely degraded by patient motion and was non-diagnostic (Figure 4.6).

The second available option was to try CT perfusion (CTP), which has rapid image acquisition and is less sensitive to motion. Drawbacks to CTP are necessity of iodinated contrast, radiation exposure, and questionable accuracy in defining core infarct volume and penumbral tissue [5]. A successful CTA and CTP examination was performed which demonstrated mildly prolonged (~2 s) mean transit time (MTT), preserved relative cerebral blood volume (rCBV), and relative cerebral blood flow (rCBF) within the left MCA territory (Figure 4.7).

At the time of the CTP examination the patient had returned to her baseline. Her symptoms remained unaffected by fluctuations in blood pressure, position, or ambulation. The embolic phenomenon was revisited with careful attention to the left internal carotid artery. Carotid ultrasonography/Doppler (not shown) demonstrated occlusion of both ICAs and left vertebral

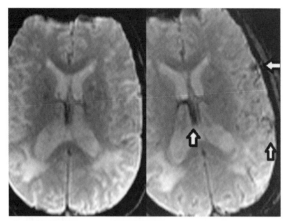

Figure 4.6 MR brain perfusion; axial contrast-enhanced susceptibility-weighted images demonstrating rotational head motion between the two scan intervals. Note the decreased signal intensity within the internal cerebral veins, left insula, and operculum secondary to the paramagnetic effects of gadolinium.

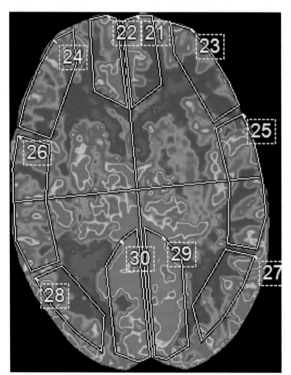

Figure 4.7 CT perfusion; axial map demonstrates relatively symmetric cerebral blood flow (rCBF).

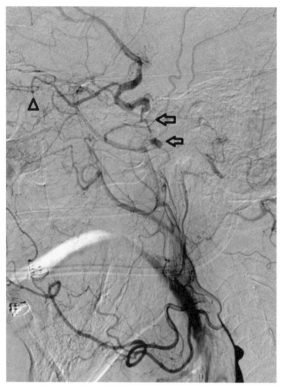

Figure 4.8 DSA; left common carotid injection, lateral projection demonstrates left internal carotid artery occlusion with intracranial reconstitution through the ophthalmic artery (arrowhead) and retrograde filling of the left cavernous and petrous carotid artery. Note the filling defects within the left petrous carotid (arrows).

artery. Carotid Doppler ultrasound is extremely operator dependent and not particularly specific in the evaluation of complete vessel occlusion or the acuity of the occlusion. With the exception of newborns and transcranial Doppler (TCD), ultrasound has a limited role for the evaluation of the intracranial vasculature because of the overlying cranium. The prior DSA demonstrated retrograde opacification of normal caliber left cavernous and petrous ICA and visualization of small geometric filling defects and a meniscus within the left petrous ICA consistent with thrombus (Figure 4.8).

Unfortunately, DSA can only image vessels and structures that fill with contrast. Vessel wall and surrounding tissue escapes detection with this modality. Fortunately, both MR and CT have the capability to image intra- and extraluminal structures as well as the vessel wall [6]. This patient's left ICA imaging findings – DSA, NCCT (hyperdense "clot" in the high left cervical ICA, not shown) and CTA (hypodense plaque and enhancing vessel wall) – indicated that the left carotid occlusion was a recent event and that she was probably experiencing "stump" emboli from the left ICA with or without hypoperfusion syndrome (Figure 4.9).

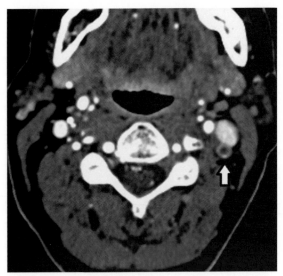

Figure 4.9 CTA; axial source image through the neck demonstrates peripheral enhancement of the left internal carotid artery wall and central non-enhancing plaque or thrombus (arrow).

Tip

The overwhelming majority of strokes that result from cervical carotid or vertebral artery occlusion or stenosis are secondary to thromboembolism rather than hypoperfusion. The ability of MR or CT perfusion imaging to identify at-risk ischemic penumbral tissue is debatable and continues to be investigated. MRI with diffusion-weighted imaging (DWI) is the best modality to assess acute cerebral infarct. The sensitivity and specificity of CTP to identify cerebral infarct core is debatable. Current available data does not support the routine use of perfusion imaging for the triage of acute stroke patients [7]. MRP is extremely vulnerable to motion and thus not always suitable for the acute stroke patient who might be aphasic. CT perfusion acquisition is rapid and less sensitive to patient motion at the expense of iodinated contrast and radiation exposure. CTA may be falsely positive for vessel occlusion in the setting of severe stenosis depending on the timing of contrast bolus. Research, mostly MRI, concerned with plaque imaging and composition to assess high or low stroke risk is ongoing.

Case 3. Non-contrast CT and ischemic stroke

Case description

A 60-year-old right-handed woman with a history of metastatic renal cell carcinoma presented to the

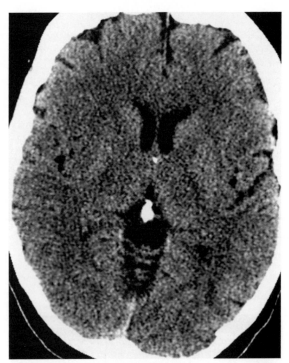

Figure 4.10 Axial NCCT head through the level of the lentiform nuclei and posterior insula demonstrates obscuration of the right putamen and insular cortex.

emergency department (ED) with acute onset of left hemiplegia, hemineglect, left facial droop, and dysarthria. She was in her usual state of health until her husband noticed that she acutely began slurring her words and could not move her left side. He immediately called the emergency services. Upon admission she had left hemiplegia, left hemineglect, left facial droop, and moderate dysarthria: NIHSS score 21. NCCT (spiral technique) was obtained at approximately 2 hours after symptom onset and read as negative (Figure 4.10).

Intravenous tissue plasminogen activator (IV tPA) was administered within 3 hours of symptom onset per protocol but her neurological examination failed to improve. MRI and MRA performed at approximately 10 hours following symptom onset demonstrated a large (>1/3) right MCA territory acute infarct, multiple acute left MCA territory infarcts, posterior circulation acute infarcts, and a distal right MCA occlusive thrombus. The patient was intubated for airway protection and transferred to the intensive care unit. Her neurological examination deteriorated in concordance with progressive brain swelling and subfalcine herniation. An emergent right hemicraniectomy was performed within 48 hours of stroke onset. Unfortunately her hospital course was complicated by pneumonia, atrial fibrillation (AF) with rapid ventricular response, acute renal insufficiency, and inability to wean from the ventilator. Per family request, she was terminally extubated.

Discussion

The patient's presentation is classic for an acute stroke, either ischemic or hemorrhagic. An NCCT of the brain is a necessity and usually the first imaging study obtained in the acute stroke setting. Advantages of an NCCT are: readily available, fast image acquisition, and 98% sensitivity for the detection of hemorrhage [8]. The exclusion of acute hemorrhage or hemorrhagic infarct is the most important use of the NCCT prior to the administration of IV tPA, which is the only FDA-approved treatment for acute ischemic stroke. But what about MRI in the setting of acute ischemic and/or hemorrhagic stroke? Yes it is true that MRI, specifically DWI, is the most sensitive imaging modality to detect acute ischemic infarct. An MRI, especially GRE and SWI, is especially sensitive for the detection of hemorrhage. But MRI is prone to false positives for the detection of hemorrhage when there is susceptibility artifact from air, bone, calcium, and/or metal. A focus of susceptibility on brain MRI should not prevent a patient from receiving appropriate treatment (IV tPA) as this finding is not necessarily hemorrhage. An NCCT must be reviewed or obtained to be sure that you are not looking at a false positive such as calcification on the MRI. The sensitivity of NCCT to detect an acute infarct within the first 3–6 hours is approximately 60%. Overall sensitivity and specificity of NCCT in the diagnosis of stroke is 64% and 85%, respectively. Sensitivity of NCCT approaches 100% at 24 hours or greater. The earliest signs of ischemia on NCCT are: decreased parenchymal attenuation; obscuration of the lentiform nucleus and/or insular ribbon; dense MCA sign and sulcal effacement. Ischemia is visualized on NCCT as hypodensity or hypoattenuation typically involving gray and white matter in an arterial vascular distribution because of the accumulation cytotoxic edema. Cytotoxic edema results from ischemia and depletion of ATP causing the failure of ion pumps and cellular swelling. Decreased density on NCCT is very specific for irreversibly damaged brain tissue if visualized in the first 6 hours

of symptom onset [8]. If one look carefully at this patient's NCCT, one can see early findings indicative of acute stroke: obscuration of the right lentiform nucleus and insular ribbon (see Figure 4.10).

If these findings had been made earlier, would this have changed the management in this case? Probably not. The patient was appropriately given IV tPA based on the clinical presentation and lack of hemorrhage on the NCCT. Whether or not this patient would have benefited from rapid or earlier advanced imaging such as MRI/MRA, CTA or perfusion studies and possible intra-arterial therapy is the basis of ongoing research and clinical trials. Endovascular stroke therapy will be discussed in Chapter 8.

Tip

Acute stroke diagnoses are made from the patient's history and physical examination. The primary role of the imaging study is to exclude hemorrhagic stroke prior to administration of IV tPA in appropriate selected patients. NCCT is the fastest, most readily available, and usually the most appropriate first diagnostic imaging study.

Case 4. Ischemic stroke secondary to carotid dissection

Case description

A 55-year-old right-handed man with no pertinent past medical history was transferred from an outside hospital for further management of bilateral anterior circulation hemispheric strokes secondary to bilateral cervical ICA dissections. One week prior to admission to the outside hospital he complained of having a headache, frequent cough, and sinusitis type symptoms. On the day of admission he experienced the sudden onset of transient visual disturbance more pronounced on the right while he was driving, at approximately 1 p.m. He then had two episodes of disequilibrium and falling after standing up to walk. Upon arrival at the ED, he had slurred speech and right facial droop but his symptoms resolved shortly thereafter. At approximately 6:30 p.m. he developed several minutes of transient dysarthria, right hemiparesis, and right facial droop. According to the provided records, he was treated for hypertensive emergency (systolic blood pressure was 180 mmHg and diastolic blood pressure 142 mmHg), with aspirin and blood pressure management. His symptoms prompted

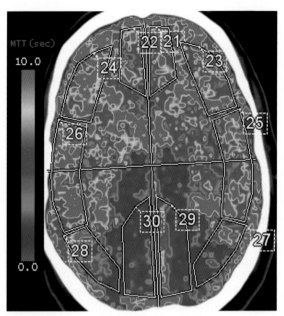

Figure 4.11 CT perfusion; axial MTT map demonstrating symmetric bilateral MTT (>5 seconds) within the anterior circulation (21–26) that is prolonged relative to the posterior circulation (2 seconds; 27–30).

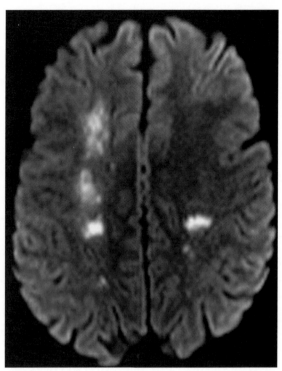

Figure 4.12 MRI brain; axial DWI demonstrates acute infarcts within the right greater than left watershed territory.

a CTA of the head and neck and MRI brain, which demonstrated bilateral cervical ICA dissections and small, scattered, left greater than right hemispheric, acute strokes. He was then started on intravenous unfractionated heparin due to the flow-limiting dissections, crescendo nature of the transient ischemic symptoms, and no clear indication for tPA. The patient remained symptom-free until 1 a.m. on the morning of transfer when he developed dysarthria and progressive left hemiparesis that progressed over the next several hours. Upon arrival at 8 a.m., his neurological examination was remarkable for global aphasia, left hemineglect, left homonymous hemianopsia, right gaze preference that was able to be overcome with Doll's eye maneuver, left central facial weakness, 0/5 left upper extremity plegia, 2/5 left lower extremity paresis, left lower extremity hyperreflexia, and bilateral extensor plantar responses; NIHSS score was 20. An emergent NCCT and CT perfusion study was performed. There was no acute hemorrhage. The CTP study was read as normal and demonstrated bilaterally symmetric perfusion and mean transit time (MTT) within the bilateral anterior circulation (Figure 4.11).

The on-call neuro-interventionalist was asked to evaluate the patient and was initially baffled by the

CT perfusion findings given the patient's profound neurologic deficits. The patient was rapidly transported to the MRI scanner for a single DWI sequence prior to an emergent catheter angiogram. The DWI sequence demonstrated new acute infarcts involving the right more than the left internal watershed territory (Figure 4.12).

The angiogram confirmed the presence of high cervical left ICA focal dissection resulting in near occlusion. The cervical right ICA was completely occluded just beyond the bifurcation. There was negligible angiographic collateral flow to the right MCA territory. The most important question was not whether to treat, but what to treat. The decision was made to recanalize the occluded right ICA with four self-expanding bare metal nitinol stents after initiating oral aspirin and clopidogrel. Even though severely narrowed, the left ICA dissection was left untouched. Fortunately, the patient made a rapid and full recovery. The 3-month follow-up CTA demonstrated a healed, near normal left ICA and patent right ICA stent construct.

Discussion

This patient developed bilateral cervical ICA dissections probably from repeated coughing episodes following an upper respiratory tract infection. Initial management with IV unfractionated heparin was probably appropriate for flow-limiting bilateral ICA dissections associated with small acute infarcts. Unfortunately, the neurological examination deteriorated which prompted transfer to a tertiary care center. After clinical deterioration, transfer and arrival the most appropriate imaging study was an NCCT to exclude hemorrhage given the prior aspirin and intravenous heparin administration in the setting of known infarcts. The CT perfusion study was performed immediately following the NCCT to assess at-risk or ischemic penumbra brain tissue. The new NCCT head was essentially unchanged from the previous NCCT and the CT perfusion study was read as symmetric. What explained his drastic deterioration and NIHSS score of 20? The patient's neurological deterioration probably corresponded to the onset of complete right ICA occlusion around 1 a.m. on the morning of transfer. This patient had insufficient collaterals from the posterior communicating arteries and a compromised contralateral anterior circulation. Although the anterior circulation was symmetric bilaterally on the CT perfusion study, there was a profound (>5 s) prolongation of MTT in the bilateral anterior circulation relative to the normal bilateral posterior circulation. In retrospect, the CT perfusion findings were not surprising given the bilateral ICA dissections and normal bilateral vertebral arteries. To save time he was taken emergently to MRI for a DWI sequence only (<10 min). The DWI sequence showed new acute infarcts in the internal border zones, right greater than left. This case is particularly illustrative of the potential pitfall of perfusion imaging when both of the compared vascular territories are abnormal such as bilateral ICA stenosis, carotid artery occlusion, or moyamoya disease. Fortunately, the single DWI sequence demonstrated primarily new watershed infarcts and a relatively small infarct core. Given an NIHSS score of 20 and a small infarct core on DWI, this patient had a large ischemic penumbra by definition and was likely to benefit from revascularization. Some investigators, including us, believe that this is much more valuable information than perfusion imaging to assess penumbra [9].

Tip

Perfusion imaging must be interpreted with respect to the known pitfalls as in this case [5]. DWI is the single best modality to define infarct core. Whether or not CT or MR perfusion imaging will prove beneficial for stroke patient triage or patient selection requires additional research. The natural history and prognosis of ICA dissection is usually quite favorable in the absence of large ischemic infarcts. The overwhelming majority of cerebral ischemia from ICA dissection is related to thromboembolism, NOT hypoperfusion as in this patient. Treatment with antiplatelet therapy alone is usually sufficient unless there is profound vessel narrowing or visible intraluminal thrombus which necessitates systemic anticoagulation.

Case 5. Venous ischemic and hemorrhagic stroke secondary to dural arteriovenous fistula

Case description

A 74-year-old right-handed man with a history of coronary artery disease, congestive heart failure, hypertension, hyperlipidemia, and diabetes presented to the emergency department with approximately 2 weeks of progressive altered mental status and one day of fluent aphasia. Upon admission he was normotensive, afebrile, and normoglycemic. He was alert and oriented to person and place (with cues). Neurological examination demonstrated naming and repetition errors, perseveration, and fluent aphasia. Strength, sensation, and cranial nerve examination was normal. Onset of aphasia was approximately 5 hours prior to presentation to the emergency department. Immediate NCCT head demonstrated punctate foci of acute hemorrhage within the left temporal lobe and obscuration of left temporal lobe sulci and gray-white differentiation consistent with edema, mostly cytotoxic (not shown). The primary concern was an acute infarct and MRI of the brain and MRA of the head and neck were performed with and without contrast. The MRI of the brain demonstrated left temporal lobe edema, primarily cytotoxic, and small foci of restricted diffusion confined to the left temporal and occipital lobes. The vascular distribution involved the left MCA and left posterior cerebral artery (PCA) territories. Post contrast MRI images demonstrated abnormal pachymeningeal, leptomeningeal, perivascular, and venous enhancement (see Figures 4.13 and 4.14).

3D time-of-flight (TOF) MRA of the brain demonstrated flow-related (arterialized) signal within the left transverse sinus and an enlarged left occipital artery

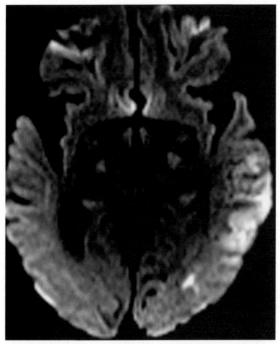

Figure 4.13 MRI brain; axial DWI demonstrates restricted diffusion within the left temporal cortex and left occipital juxtacortical white matter.

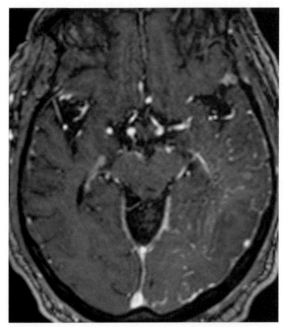

Figure 4.14 MRI brain; post contrast axial T1 image demonstrates abnormal left temporal and occipital lobe pachymeningeal, leptomeningeal, perivascular, and venous enhancement.

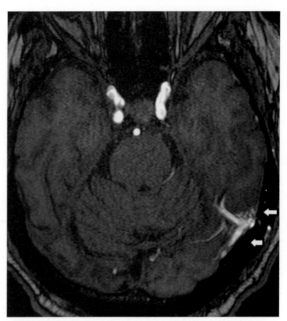

Figure 4.15 3D-TOF MRA; axial source image demonstrates flow-related, arterialized signal within the left transverse sinus.

(not shown). The arterialized signal within the left transverse sinus and enlarged left occipital artery were not recognized earlier and the initial conclusion from the MRI/MRA report was arterial ischemia or encephalitis (Figure 4.15).

The patient was admitted to the NICU for treatment of acute stroke and intracranial hemorrhage. An LP was performed to begin the encephalitis work-up, which was normal. EEG demonstrated slowing over the left temporal cortex without epileptiform activity. TTE was negative for thrombus or arteriovenous shunt. Additional, retrospective review of the available cerebral imaging suggested the presence of a left transverse sinus dural arteriovenous fistula (dAVF) from the abnormal MRA findings. A catheter cerebral angiogram was performed to confirm the presence of a dAVF and initiate treatment with endovascular embolization (Figure 4.16).

There was clinical and imaging improvement following the first session of embolization and the patient was discharged to an acute rehabilitation facility. The patient was scheduled for additional elective embolization of the dAVF.

Discussion

Given the presentation of acute onset of fluent aphasia in an elderly man with multiple cardiovascular risk

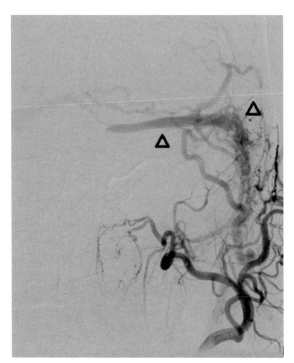

Figure 4.16 DSA; left external carotid artery injection, frontal projection. There is rapid arteriovenous shunting and visualization of the left transverse sinus (arrowheads) in the arterial phase consistent with a dAVF.

factors, the most likely diagnosis is ischemic stroke. The important variation in this case is the underlying pathophysiology of venous hypertension or occlusion resulting in ischemia and hemorrhage rather than the typical arterial event. Venous hypertension of any cause such as venous thrombosis, occlusion, or arteriovenous fistula may be symptomatic. Increased venous pressure results in increased capillary hydrostatic pressure and consequently decreased arterial perfusion. Decreased arterial perfusion may result in cytotoxic edema (infarct), blood–brain barrier breakdown (vasogenic edema), or capillary rupture and hemorrhage. The edema pattern in venous ischemia can be cytotoxic, vasogenic, or both. Areas of restricted diffusion which typically denote irreversibly damaged brain in acute arterial occlusion can and are often reversible in the setting of venous pathology. Hemorrhage is more often present on initial imaging of cerebral venous ischemia compared to hemorrhagic transformation of arterial ischemia, which is typically not present on initial imaging. Taking DSA as the gold standard for the diagnosis of dAVF, the reported sensitivity of 3D-TOF MRA and time resolved 3D contrast-enhanced MRA is

marginal at best and ranges from 47% to 100% and 72% to 100%, respectively. Thus a normal MRI and MRA does not exclude a dAVF [10].

Tip

The most important point of this case is to remember the existence and possibility of cerebral venous pathology as a cause of stroke and hemorrhage [11]. Cerebral venous ischemia will have a similar clinical and imaging presentation as arterial ischemia. However, the area of ischemia can and often does involve more than one arterial vascular territory such as in this case (left MCA and PCA). Involvement of more than one vascular territory is unusual for acute arterial ischemia. dAVFs are often missed with MRI and MRA. One must have a high index of suspicion to diagnose a dAVF. Catheter cerebral angiography remains the gold standard for diagnosis and embolization can be curative.

Case 6. Symptomatic left middle cerebral artery stenosis with normal MR perfusion imaging

Case description

A 37-year-old right-handed man presented to the ED with a 2-week history of progressive, intermittent right hemiparesis and aphasia. Symptoms were worse in the morning and during changes in position from sitting or recumbent to standing. He stated that symptoms occurred three to four times per day and lasted approximately one minute. There was no aura preceding the symptoms, nor did he experience post-ictal confusion or fatigue. He volunteered that approximately 2 days prior to symptom onset he experienced head trauma while hunting followed by 3 days of headache. Past medical history was unremarkable with the exception of a 10 pack-year history of cigarette smoking. He was currently not taking any medications with the exception of occasional acetaminophen (paracetamol) for headache. Upon admission to the emergency department he was asymptomatic and afebrile. Blood pressure was 163/76 mmHg and pulse was 78 breaths per minute. Neurologic examination was unremarkable with the exception of a trace right pronator drift. The patient did not report dizziness, vertigo, chest pain, or shortness of breath. NCCT performed in the ED was normal. Because the patient experienced an event just prior to arrival at the hospital, he was admitted for

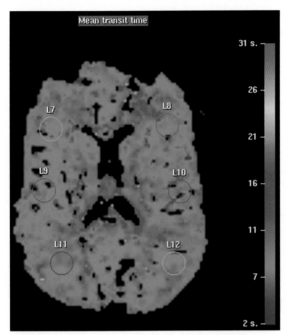

Figure 4.17 MR perfusion image; axial map demonstrating symmetric bilateral mean transit time (MTT).

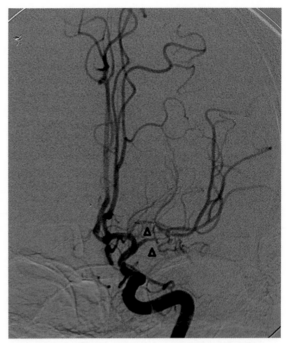

Figure 4.18 DSA; left internal carotid artery injection, frontal projection. There is severe, flow-limiting stenosis (arrowheads) within the M1 segment of the left middle cerebral artery.

observation and an MRI/MRA was performed. The brain MRI was normal. The MRA (not shown) demonstrated segmental occlusion of the M1 segment of the left MCA but visualization of the left M2, M3, and M4 segments. During an episode of relative hypotension, systolic blood pressure 128 mmHg, the patient experienced transient symptoms of right hemiparesis and aphasia on morning rounds, which prompted an MRI and MR perfusion imaging. The MRI and MR perfusion was normal; rCBV, rCBF, and MTT were symmetric. Not surprisingly, the patient was neurologically at baseline during MR imaging (Figure 4.17).

However, despite the MR perfusion findings there was continued fear of a large left MCA perfusion deficit, possible penumbra and potential M1 thrombus that might necessitate intra-arterial therapy should the patient deteriorate or develop a fixed neurological deficit. The patient continued to experience a transient left MCA syndrome which was responsive to hemodynamics and positional changes; therefore, a catheter cerebral angiogram was performed. The cervical and cerebral catheter angiogram demonstrated severe mid and distal left M1 segment stenosis without thrombus, distal occlusive disease, or embolism. Cervical and intracranial arterial vasculature was otherwise normal (Figure 4.18).

The patient underwent two additional studies: acetazolamide challenge with Tc99m cerebral spectroscopy and oxygen-15 positron emission tomography (^{15}O-PET). Both exams demonstrated abnormal perfusion within the left MCA territory while the patient was at rest and asymptomatic. The patient ultimately had an uneventful ECA–ICA bypass and experienced complete resolution of symptoms.

Discussion

The underlying disease affecting the left M1 segment could be atherosclerotic, thromboembolic, inflammatory, reactive (spasm), or traumatic (dissection). The most common cause of an M1 lesion is thromboembolic disease or intracranial atherosclerotic disease (ICAD). The MCA is most commonly affected in the setting of cerebral thromboembolism and ICAD. Although this patient did have a smoking history and possibly undiagnosed hypertension, he had no additional risk factors for thromboembolic disease or ICAD after completion of his inpatient stroke evaluation. He was hypertensive upon admission; however, the majority of the inpatient vital signs showed that he was normotensive. Perhaps some of the hypertensive episodes were compensatory in the setting of the severe left M1 stenosis. Furthermore, the entire imaged arterial vasculature was normal with the exception of the left M1 stenosis. Thus, thromboembolism and ICAD was less likely. An exhaustive search for inflammatory markers was also negative. Vasospasm or cerebral vasoconstriction syndrome was also thought unlikely given the atypical imaging appearance, isolated vessel involvement, and lack of identifiable risk factors. Although he did experience an acute onset of headache, which is typical of cerebral vasoconstriction syndrome, his symptom onset was associated with trauma. A diagnosis of left MCA stenosis secondary to arterial dissection was concluded. Dissection affecting the extracranial carotid and vertebral arteries is relatively common; however, dissection affecting the intracranial ICA is rare. Dissection of the MCA is rarer still. Given the patient's history of ipsilateral head trauma and angiographic appearance of the left M1 segment, dissection was the most likely diagnosis. He remained symptomatic despite maximum medical therapy, antiplatelet regimen, and vasopressor agents. After a multidisciplinary management discussion, he had an uneventful extracranial to intracranial (EC–IC) bypass surgery with complete symptom relief.

Tip

Symptoms related to left MCA stenosis may be secondary to hemodynamic compromise or thromboembolism [12]. The use of EC–IC bypass in the treatment of intracranial arterial stenosis or occlusion is highly debatable and beyond the scope of this chapter. Catheter cerebral angiography remains the gold standard for imaging intracranial arterial stenosis. TOF MRA often overestimates the degree of stenosis or occlusion, particularly within the M1 segment which is usually parallel to the axial source image acquisition. The role of CT or MR perfusion imaging in the triage of stroke patients requires further investigation. Although not as readily available, imaging of cerebral perfusion with spectroscopy or PET provides greater sensitivity than either CT or MR perfusion [13,14].

References

1. Edlow JA, Wyer PC. Evidence-based emergency medicine/clinical question. How good is a negative cranial computed tomographic scan result in excluding subarachnoid hemorrhage? *Ann Emerg Med* 2000;36:507–16.

2. Bambakidis N, Selman W. Subarachnoid hemorrhage. In: Suarez JI, ed. *Critical Care Neurology and Neurosurgery*. Totowa, NJ: Humana Press; 2004:365–77.

3. Vermeulen M, van Gijn J. The diagnosis of subarachnoid haemorrhage. *J Neurol Neurosurg Psychiatry* 1990;53:365–72.

4. Woodfield J, Rane N, Cudlip S, Byrne JV. Value of delayed MRI in angiogram-negative subarachnoid haemorrhage. *Clin Radiol* 2014; 69:350–6.

5. Lui YW, Tang ER, Allmendinger AM, Spektor V. Evaluation of CT perfusion in the setting of cerebral ischemia: patterns and pitfalls. *AJNR Am J Neuroradiol* 2010;31:1552–63.

6. Kim JJ, Wintermark M. Intracranial vascular imaging: pearls and pitfalls. *Appl Radiol* 2010;April:28–34.

7. Kidwell CS, Jahan R, Gornbein J, Alger JR, et al. A trial of imaging selection and endovascular treatment for ischemic stroke. *N Engl J Med* 2013;368:914–23.

8. Srinivasan A, Goyal M, Azri FA, Lum C. State of the art imaging of acute stroke. *Radiographics* 2006;26:S75–S95.

9. González RG. Low signal, high noise and large uncertainty make CT perfusion unsuitable for acute ischemic stroke patient selection for endovascular therapy. *J NeuroInterv Surg* 2012;4:242–5.

10. Meckel S, Maier M, Ruiz DS, et al. MR angiography of dural arteriovenous fistulas: diagnosis and follow-up after treatment using a time-resolved 3D contrast-enhanced technique. *AJNR Am J Neuroradiol* 2007;28:877–84.

11. Saposnik G, Barinagarrementeria F, Brown RD, et al. Diagnosis and management of cerebral venous thrombosis: a statement for healthcare professionals from the American Heart Association/American Stroke Association. *Stroke* 2011;42:1158–92.

12. Derdeyn CP, Powers WJ, Grubb RL. Hemodynamic effects of middle cerebral artery stenosis and occlusion. *AJNR Am J Neuroradiol* 1998;19:1463–9.

13. Grüner JM, Paamand R, Højgaard L, Law I. Brain perfusion CT compared with 15O-H2O-PET in healthy subjects. *EJNMMI Res* 2011;1:28.

14. Vagal AS, Leach JL, Fernandez-Ulloa M, Zuccarello M. The acetazolamide challenge: techniques and applications in the evaluation of chronic cerebral ischemia. *AJNR Am J Neuroradiol* 2009;30:876–84.

Further reading

Albers GW, Thijs VN, Wechsler L, et al. Magnetic resonance imaging profiles predict clinical response to early reperfusion: the diffusion and perfusion imaging evaluation for understanding stroke evolution (DEFUSE) study. *Ann Neurology*. 2006;60:508–517.

Davis SM, Donnan GA, Parsons MW, et al. Effects of alteplase beyond 3 h after stroke in the Echoplanar Imaging Thrombolytic Evaluation Trial (EPITHET): a placebo-controlled randomized trial. *Lancet Neurol*. 2008;7:299–309.

Essig M, Shiroishi MS, Nguyen TB, et al. Perfusion MRI: the five most frequently asked technical questions. *AJR Am J Roentgenol* 2013;200:24–34.

Heasley DC, Mohamed MA, Yousem DM. Clearing of red blood cells in lumbar puncture does not rule out ruptured aneurysm in patients with suspected subarachnoid hemorrhage but negative head CT findings. *AJNR Am J Neuroradiol* 2005;26:820–4.

Latchaw RE, Yonas H, Hunter GJ, et al. Guidelines and recommendations for perfusion imaging in cerebral ischemia: a scientific statement for healthcare professionals by the writing group on perfusion imaging, from the Council on Cardiovascular Radiology of the American Heart Association. *Stroke* 2003;34:1084–104.

Mohamed M, Heasely DC, Yagmurlu B, Yousem DM. Fluid-attenuated inversion recovery MR imaging and subarachnoid hemorrhage: not a panacea. *AJNR Am J Neuroradiol*. 2004;25:545–550.

Schellinger PD, Bryan RN, Caplan LR, et al. Evidence-based guideline: the role of diffusion and perfusion MRI for the diagnosis of acute ischemic stroke: report of the Therapeutics and Technology Assessment Subcommittee of the American Academy of Neurology. *Neurology* 2010;75:177–85.

Takasawa M, Jones PS, Guadagno JV, et al. How reliable is perfusion MR in acute stroke?: validation and determination of the penumbra threshold against quantitative PET. *Stroke* 2008:39:870–7.

Chapter

5

Choosing appropriate patients for anticoagulation

Sarkis Morales-Vidal and Alejandro Hornik

Introduction

Anticoagulants play a major role in stroke prevention. Warfarin is effective in reducing stroke risk in patients with non-valvular atrial fibrillation (NVAF). Most recently, novel oral anticoagulants (NOACs) have been shown to be a good alternative for stroke prevention in these patients. Appropriate antithrombotic agent selection is paramount to provide optimal stroke risk reduction and minimize bleeding risks among these patients. This chapter reviews some challenging cases for the appropriate selection of anticoagulant agents in stroke prevention.

Case 1. Stroke prevention in patients with mechanical prosthetic heart valves

Case description

A 67-year-old woman with history of atrial fibrillation (AF) and prosthetic mechanical mitral valve replacement was admitted to hospital following sudden onset of left hemiparesis, left hemisensory loss, and left hemineglect. She was not a candidate for intravenous recombinant tissue plasminogen activator (tPA) due to recent use of dabigatran. MRI of the brain showed a right middle cerebral artery (MCA) territory acute ischemic infarction (Figure 5.1). Symptoms steadily improved throughout her hospital stay. Transesophageal echocardiography (TEE) showed no intracavity thrombi. She was switched to warfarin with a target INR of 2.5 (range 2.0–3.0) for recurrent stroke prevention, and she was discharged to a rehabilitation facility.

Discussion

Prosthetic heart valve replacement is performed annually in thousands of patients worldwide [1]. Management of patients with prosthetic heart valves requires lifelong anticoagulant therapy. Patients requiring prosthetic heart valve replacement are faced with a choice of a longer lasting mechanical heart valve that is associated with decreased quality of life due to coagulation monitoring and treatment-associated dietary restrictions, or a bioprosthetic heart valve that has a higher risk of failure and replacement surgery, but which is associated with improved quality of life.

Dabigatran etexilate (dabigatran) is an orally administered thrombin inhibitor used for the prevention of embolism and stroke in patients with non-valvular atrial fibrillation (NVAF). In the Randomized Evaluation of Long-Term Anticoagulation Therapy (RE-LY) study, dabigatran was shown to be effective in the treatment of patients with NVAF. The subsequent RE-ALIGN study failed to demonstrate the ability of dabigatran to prevent thromboembolic complications in patients with mechanical heart valves [1]. Patients in the RE-ALIGN study were randomized to receive either dabigatran or warfarin. The trial was terminated prematurely due to an excess of thromboembolic and bleeding events in patients treated with dabigatran. Dose adjustment or discontinuation was required in 52 of 162 dabigatran-treated patients (32%). Ischemic or unspecified stroke occurred in 5% (9/162) of patients treated with dabigatran and in none of those treated with warfarin. Major bleeding occurred in 4% (7/162) of patients treated with dabigatran, and in 2% (2/81) of patients treated with warfarin. Pericardial bleeding was found in all patients with major bleeding. Excessive bleeding with dabigatran occurred in patients started on treatment within 7 days of heart valve surgery

---

Common Pitfalls in Cerebrovascular Disease: Case-Based Learning, ed. José Biller and José M. Ferro. Published by Cambridge University Press. © Cambridge University Press 2015.

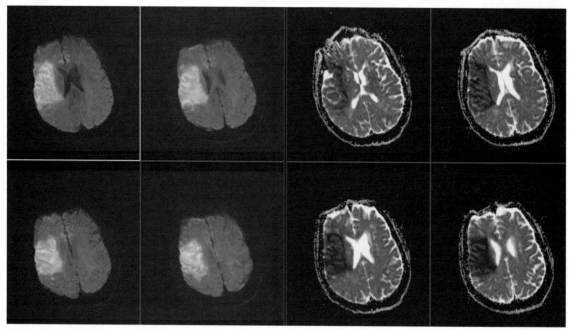

Figure 5.1 Axial diffusion-weighted (right) and apparent diffusion coefficient (left) images show evidence of restricted diffusion in the right MCA distribution consistent with an acute cerebral infarction.

and in patients who had had valve implantation for more than 3 months previously.

Patients with mechanical prosthetic heart valves have coagulation cascade and thrombin generation activated by the release of tissue factors from damaged tissues associated with valve placement. The artificial surface of the valve leaflets and sewing ring are also thrombogenic. Warfarin is thought to be more effective in these patients, as it has a broader effect on the coagulation system. Warfarin inhibits activation of tissue-induced coagulation (factor VII inhibition), contact-induced coagulation (inhibition of factor IX production), and common pathway factors (factor X and thrombin production). Dabigatran is effective in patients with NVAF where thrombus formation is believed to be triggered by blood stasis and endothelial dysfunction.

Tip

Warfarin is superior to dabigatran for stroke prevention in patients with prosthetic mechanical heart valves. Clinical trials of other novel oral anticoagulant agents (e.g., apixaban and rivaroxaban) in patients with AF excluded patients with prosthetic mechanical heart valves. Warfarin is the preferred anticoagulant agent for thromboembolic risk reduction in patients with prosthetic mechanical heart valve.

Case 2. Pitfalls in anticoagulation for stroke prevention in patients with low cardiac ejection fraction (EF) or severe cardiomyopathy

Case description

A 50-year-old man with history of coronary artery disease, non-ST elevation myocardial infarction (NSTEMI), ischemic cardiomyopathy, hypertension, and systolic chronic heart failure was admitted to hospital after sudden onset of word-finding difficulties, slurred speech, and right-sided weakness. MRI of the brain showed a cerebral infarction in the arterial distribution of the left anterior cerebral artery (ACA) and inferior division of the left MCA (Figure 5.2). Troponin levels were initially elevated. Transthoracic echocardiogram (TTE) and TEE reported a systolic ejection fraction (EF) of 20%. There were no intracavitary thrombi. He had no evidence of AF, and remained in sinus rhythm during his hospital stay. A 30-day event monitor recorded occasional premature ventricular complexes (PVCs). He was initially treated with warfarin, but approximately 6 months later he was switched to clopidogrel monotherapy. Follow-up TTE 6 months later showed persistent low EF (25%). He

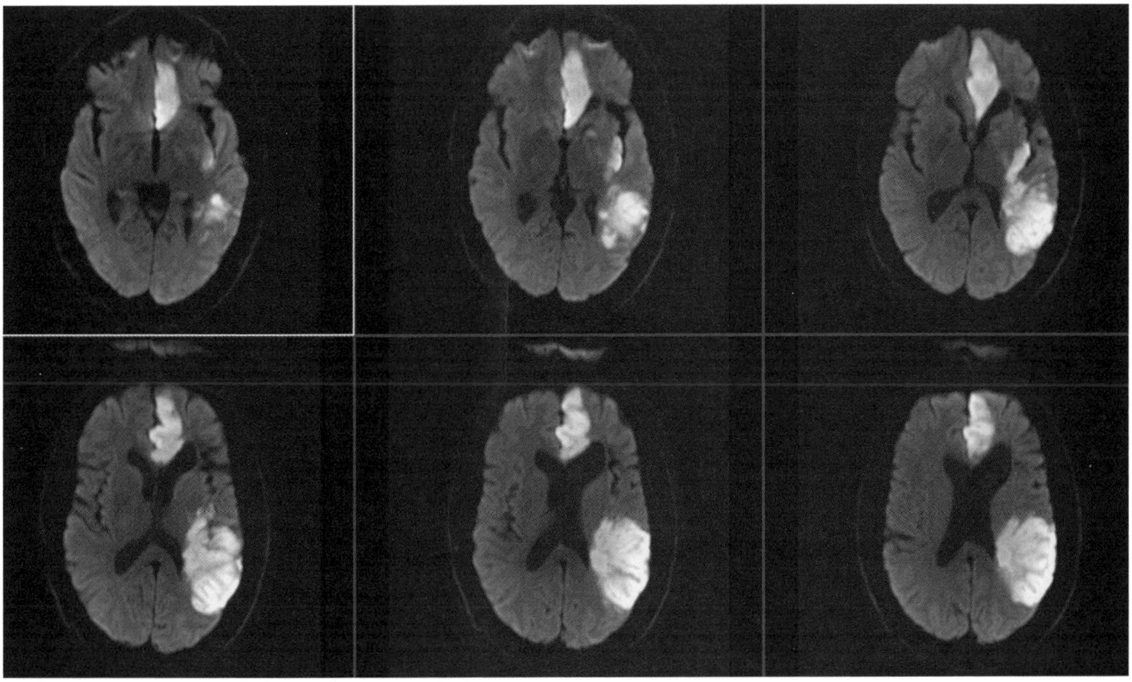

Figure 5.2 Axial diffusion-weighted imaging shows increased signal change in the left ACA and left MCA distribution consistent with acute cerebral infarction.

had no recurrent strokes or transient ischemic attacks (TIAs) while on warfarin or clopidogrel monotherapy.

Discussion

While the benefit of anticoagulation in patients with NVAF is robust and well established, its use in patients with normal sinus rhythm is controversial [2]. Individuals with a decreased EF <35% in sinus rhythm have an estimated 4% rate of embolic events, including stroke, pulmonary embolism, and peripheral artery embolization. Left ventricular thrombus (LVT) have been detected in 13%, and left atrial appendage (LAA) thrombus in 68% of these patients. These rates are decreased to 1.2% among patients treated with warfarin. Studies evaluating this benefit have not shown statistical significance by treatment type, including treatment with placebo. The modest benefit reported in the Warfarin and Antiplatelet Therapy in Heart Failure (WATCH) trial was associated with an increased risk of major hemorrhage [3].

The Warfarin versus Aspirin in Reduced Cardiac Ejection Fraction (WARCEF) trial evaluated patients with low cardiac EF and sinus rhythm [4]. No difference was noted in the rate of stroke, intracerebral hemorrhage or death between the two groups. Nevertheless, a subgroup analysis demonstrated a 48% relative risk reduction (RRR; $P = 0.005$) of ischemic stroke with warfarin use.

A further subgroup analysis defined ischemic stroke patients as definite, possible, or non-cardioembolic [4]. Warfarin treatment was associated with reduced rate of definite cardioembolic ischemic strokes compared to aspirin treatment (0.22 vs. 0.55 per 100 patient-years, $P = 0.012$), as well as a tendency for reduced rate of possible cardioembolic ischemic strokes (0.37 vs. 0.67 per 100 patient-years, $P = 0.063$). There was no difference in the rate of non-cardioembolic ischemic strokes by treatment.

Tip

Anticoagulation for recurrent stroke prevention in patients with EF <35% and sinus rhythm has not been established (2014 American Heart Association practice guidelines) [4]. Consider anticoagulation over antiplatelet therapy in patients with low EF (<35%) following a careful assessment of potential thromboembolic risk. Patients with history of strokes or TIAs have a high risk of recurrent thromboembolic events as compared to patients without history of cardioembolic events. In addition, anticoagulation may reduce cardiac mortality among these patients.

Case 3. Management of patients with atrial fibrillation with high thromboembolic risk (e.g., CHA2DS2-VASc score >1) not candidates for full anticoagulation due to high bleeding risk

Case description

A 90-year-old woman with a history of frequent falls, NVAF, arterial hypertension, coronary artery disease status post coronary artery cardiac stents, history of gastrointestinal bleeding attributed to gastric ulcers, and congestive heart failure was admitted to the neurology service after a left vertebral artery occlusion thrombosis with infarction in the distribution of the posterior inferior cerebellar artery (PICA) (Figure 5.3). Her HAS-BLED score was 4. Her CHA2DS2-VASc score was 7. Initial deficits included dysarthria, left upper and lower limb dysmetria, left Horner's syndrome, right hemibody sensory loss, and left facial sensory loss. The mechanism of ischemic stroke was presumed to be cardioembolic from AF and she was started on apixaban 2.5 mg twice daily, and subsequently she was discharged to an acute rehabilitation facility.

Discussion

NVAF is associated with a fivefold increased risk of stroke [5]. Vitamin K antagonists (VKAs) are commonly prescribed for patients with NVAF. Several risk factors, such as recurrent falls or trauma, can increase this risk of bleeding. About a third of patients who are candidates for VKA therapy either choose not to start, or rather discontinue therapy [6].

Aspirin, while better tolerated, is not as efficacious as warfarin, reducing stroke risk by only 20% [6]. Thus, aspirin use is reserved for NVAF patients who are not candidates for VKA therapy. Clopidogrel has been used in combination with aspirin to further reduce the risk of stroke in these patients, but with the drawback of an increased risk of major hemorrhage.

Apixaban is a direct and competitive inhibitor of factor Xa activity. The AVERROES study evaluated the efficacy of apixaban (2.5 or 5.0 mg by mouth, twice a day) in preventing stroke in AF patients who had failed or were unsuitable for VKA therapy [6]. Patients receiving 2.5 mg apixaban doses were older than 80 years of age, had a body weight of 60 kg or less, or a serum creatinine level of 1.5 mg/dL or higher.

The study was terminated prematurely due to a reduced efficacy in the aspirin (81–324 mg by mouth, every day) control group [6]. There were fewer strokes and peripheral artery embolism in the apixaban-treated

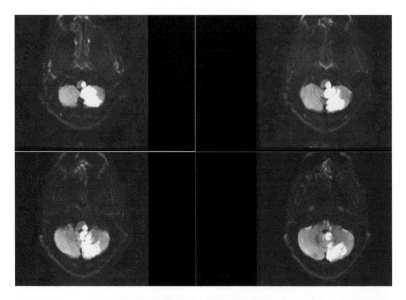

Figure 5.3 Axial diffusion-weighted imaging showing evidence of restricted diffusion in the left medial PICA distribution.

group than in the aspirin-treated group (1.6% per year vs. 3.7% per year, P < 0.001). Hospitalization for cardiovascular causes occurred less frequently in the apixaban group than in the aspirin group (12.6% per year vs. 15.9% per year, P < 0.001). Fewer patients taking apixaban chose to discontinue their medications (17.9% per year vs. 20.5% per year, P = 0.03). Major bleeding occurred with similar frequency in the two groups. The benefit of apixaban extended to both treatment doses. Outcomes of each apixaban dose group were not compared.

The ARTESiA study (Apixaban for the Reduction of Thrombo-Embolism in patients with device-detected Sub-clinical atrial Fibrillation) is currently enrolling patients to compare the relative efficacy of these same agents in patients with pacemakers and subclinical AF [7].

Tip

Consider novel oral anticoagulants (NOACs; e.g., apixaban) in patients with AF and high thrombo-embolic risk who are not candidates for full anticoagulation therapy with warfarin therapy.

Case 4. Pitfalls in choosing anticoagulant agents for stroke prevention in patients with AF

Case description

A 59-year-old man with history of hypertension, diabetes mellitus, and osteoarthritis was admitted to hospital after sudden onset of a left visual blurring. He arrived at the hospital 6 hours after onset of symptoms.

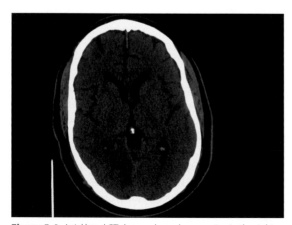

Figure 5.4 Axial head CT shows a hypodense region in the right medial PCA consistent with subacute cerebral infarction.

TTE showed an EF of 45%, mild diastolic dysfunction, and no intracardiac thrombi. He was unable to have an MRI due to claustrophobia. CT head showed a subacute right posterior cerebral artery (PCA) distribution infarction (Figure 5.4). CT angiogram (CTA) of the extracranial and intracranial circulation showed no significant stenosis of the vertebrobasilar system. ECG showed evidence of AF. CHA2DS2-VASc score was 4. HAS-BLED score was 2. The patient remained clinically stable during his hospital stay, he was educated about lifestyle modification for recurrent stroke prevention, and atorvastatin was started. In addition, apixaban 5 mg twice daily was chosen as the antithrombotic agent for recurrent stroke prevention.

Discussion

Anticoagulation is of proven benefit in patients with AF. Warfarin reduces the risk of stroke in these patients by about two-thirds. A new generation of drugs, factor Xa inhibitors, are currently available for the prevention of thromboembolism. At present, NOACs lack reversible antidotes and, as yet, have no reliable assays to accurately measure drug activity.

Apixaban is an orally administered inhibitor of factor Xa with predictable anticoagulant activity. The activity of apixaban was compared to that of warfarin in the Apixaban for Reduction in Stroke and Other Thromboembolic Events in AF (ARISTOTLE) study [8]. Over 18 200 patients were treated who had at least one additional risk factor for stroke. Apixaban-treated patients had a similar frequency of ischemic or hemorrhagic stroke or peripheral artery embolic events as warfarin-treated patients (1.27% per year vs. 1.60% per year). Fewer major bleeding events (2.13% per year vs. 3.09% per year, P < 0.001), deaths from any cause (3.52% per year vs. 3.94% per year, P = 0.047), and hemorrhagic strokes (0.24% per year vs. 0.47% per year, P < 0.001) were seen in the apixaban-treated group.

Dabigatran is a competitive inhibitor of thrombin that is renally excreted and does not require frequent monitoring for dose adjustments [9]. Over 18 000 patients with NVAF were randomized to receive either dabigatran or warfarin in the RE-LY trial. In this trial, patients on dabigatran 150 mg twice daily were less likely to experience strokes than patients on warfarin. The event rate (stroke or systemic embolism), per year, was 1.11% for those patients administered dabigatran 150 mg twice daily. The event rate was 1.53% for those patients administered dabigatran 110 mg twice daily.

By comparison, the event rate was 1.69% for those treated with warfarin [9].

The yearly rate of major bleeding in the warfarin-treated group was 3.36%, in the 110 mg dabigatran-treated group was 2.71% ($P = 0.003$ compared to warfarin), and in the 150 mg dabigatran-treated group was 3.11%. The yearly rate of hemorrhagic stroke in the warfarin-treated group was 0.38%, in the 110 mg dabigatran-treated group was 0.12% ($P < 0.0001$ compared to warfarin), and in the 150 mg dabigatran-treated group was 0.10% ($P < 0.0001$ compared to warfarin). The mortality rate of the three groups was not different.

The US Food and Drug Administration evaluated the outcome of dabigatran use among 134 000 Medicare patients aged 65 years or older with AF [10]. Dabigatran use was associated with a lower risk of stroke, cerebral hemorrhage, and death, than warfarin. Dabigatran use was associated with a higher risk of major gastrointestinal bleeding compared to warfarin. There was no difference in the risk of myocardial infarction (MI) between the two treatment groups.

Edoxaban is an orally administered factor Xa inhibitor with predictable anticoagulant activity [11]. The activity of edoxaban (60 mg by mouth, every day or 30 mg by mouth, every day) was compared to that of warfarin in over 21 100 patients with AF who were at moderate to high risk of stroke. The two treatments had similar rates of stroke or peripheral artery embolism (higher dose edoxaban, 1.18% per year; low dose edoxaban, 1.61% per year; warfarin, 1.5% per year). Warfarin was associated with a higher rate of major bleeding compared to high dose edoxaban (3.43% per year vs. 2.75% per year, $P < 0.001$) and low dose edoxaban (3.43% per year vs. 1.61% per year, $P < 0.001$). Less bleeding was seen in patients who had their dose of edoxaban further reduced, without loss of anti-thromboembolic activity.

Rivaroxaban is an oral factor Xa inhibitor with a consistent and predictable anticoagulant profile that does not require frequent monitoring [12]. Over 14 000 patients with chronic AF were randomized to either rivaroxaban or warfarin [12]. In the rivaroxaban group, the primary event rate (composite of ischemic and hemorrhagic stroke and systemic embolism) was 1.7% per year (188/6958). In the warfarin group the primary event rate was 2.2% per year (241/7004). Clinically relevant bleeding occurred to a similar extent in both groups (14.9% per year vs. 14.5% per year). Intracranial hemorrhage (0.5% vs. 0.7%, $P = 0.02$) and

fatal bleeding (0.2% vs. 0.5%, $P = 0.003$) was seen less frequently in the rivaroxaban-treated group.

No studies have compared the relative efficacy and safety of factor Xa inhibitors and dabigatran.

Examination of these trials suggests there is no difference in the efficacy, mortality rate, myocardial infarction rate, or major bleeding rate of high doses of edoxaban and apixaban. Apixaban appeared to be associated with reduced rates of non-major bleeding. Dabigatran 110 mg by mouth, twice daily, and high dose edoxaban had similar efficacy and safety profiles. Dabigatran 150 mg by mouth, twice daily, was associated with fewer strokes and peripheral artery embolic events [13].

Tip

1. Apixaban 5 mg twice daily in patients with NVAF, as compared to warfarin with target INR 2.0–3.0, is associated with a lower rate of stroke, lower rate of hemorrhage, and lower mortality.
2. Dabigatran 150 mg twice daily in patients with NVAF, as compared to warfarin with target INR 2.0–3.0, is associated with a lower rate of strokes but similar hemorrhage rates.
3. Rivaroxaban 20 mg daily in patients with NVAF, as compared to warfarin (INR 2.0–3.0), is associated with similar rates of strokes and major bleeding.
4. Edoxaban (low dose and high dose) in patients with NVAF, as compared to warfarin with target INR 2.0–3.0, is associated with similar rates of strokes and major bleeding.

Case 5. Pitfalls in stroke prevention with anticoagulation following an anterior STEMI

Case description

A 75-year-old man admitted for an acute anterolateral ST elevation myocardial infarction (STEMI) (Figure 5.5) treated with coronary angioplasty and stenting, had sudden onset of right hemiparesis, right hemisensory loss, and aphasia attributed to inferior division of left MCA ischemic stroke, 3 days after acute coronary intervention. ECG showed normal sinus rhythm. TEE showed no evidence of anteroapical aneurysm or intracardiac thrombi. He was started on warfarin for stroke prevention. However, warfarin was discontinued following an episode of gastrointestinal bleeding. He

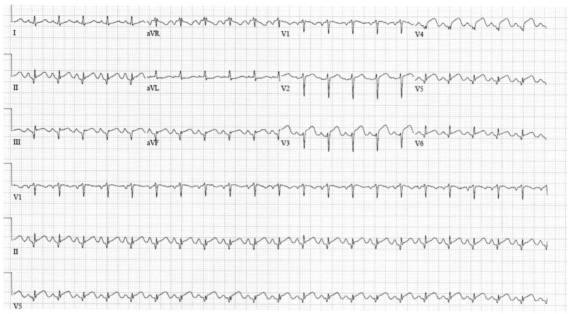

Figure 5.5 ECG shows evidence of ST segment elevation in anterolateral leads.

Discussion

was continued on aspirin alone. A 30 days event monitor showed no evidence of AF. Follow-up visit 7 months after ischemic stroke diagnosis showed mild to moderate improvement of residual neurologic deficits.

STEMI accounts for 25–40% of MIs. Patients with large anterior STEMI and anteroapical aneurysm formation are at highest risk for developing a left ventricular thrombus. Left ventricular aneurysm occurs in 2–15% of these patients. These findings have led to many patients being treated with warfarin therapy in order to decrease the risk of left ventricular thrombus formation and decrease the associated stroke risk. Some sources still consider left ventricular thrombus as a common complication of MI and recommend anticoagulation for at least 3 months [14].

Patients treated with rapidly available, percutaneous coronary revascularization techniques appear to have a reduced risk of aneurysm formation, thrombus formation, and stroke. A left ventricular mural thrombus was reported in 4–18% of a modern cohort of patients with STEMI [15]. The risk of stroke in these patients treated with anticoagulation is not clear, while the risk of bleeding requiring rehospitalization is well defined. ACC/AHA guidelines for the use of vitamin K antagonists following anterior STEMI provide only Class IIA, B level type of evidence to support its use.

Patients at high risk for left ventricular thrombus formation following STEMI treated with modern revascularization techniques were retrospectively evaluated for all-cause mortality, ischemic stroke, and clinically relevant bleeding [16]. High risk was considered a post-MI, left ventricular EF <40%. Patients were treated with or without VKA therapy.

The development of stroke was uncommon in these patients, occurring in only 1.9% of patients during the first 6 months of follow-up after MI. These findings are similar to previous reports. All-cause mortality, ischemic stroke, and clinically relevant bleeding occurred in 24.7% of treated patients and 20.5% of patients not receiving VKA therapy (adjusted hazard ratio [HR], 1.30). Ischemic stroke occurred in 2.5% and 0.9%, respectively, of treated patients (adjusted HR, 2.81). There was no difference in the rate of bleeding or mortality between the two treatment groups. Patients treated with the addition of low-molecular-weight heparin (LMWH) had an increased risk of bleeding (adjusted HR, 2.55). This lack of benefit suggests that further studies are needed to support the use of VKA therapy in these patients.

Tip

No data support the use of anticoagulation for stroke prevention during the first 6 months following an anterior STEMI, including those with low ejection fraction, without evidence of intracardiac thrombi. Consider monitoring patients for development of arrhythmias or cardiac thrombus which may require anticoagulation.

Case 6. Use of anticoagulant agents in patients with multiple asymptomatic cerebral microhemorrhages on brain MRI

Case description

A 72-year-old man with history of hypertension, diabetes mellitus, and dyslipidemia was admitted with a transient episode of word-finding difficulties, which resolved within 2 hours. ECG showed AF. MRI of the brain showed no evidence of restricted diffusion. However, there were multiple microhemorrhages (Figure 5.6). CTA of the head and neck showed no significant stenosis or atherosclerotic changes. TTE showed no intracardiac thrombi. Clinical impression was a TIA secondary to AF. His CHA2DS2-VASc score was 5. He had no prior history of head trauma, falls, gastrointestinal hemorrhage, or other potential contraindications for long-term anticoagulation. Apixaban 2.5 mg twice daily was used as antithrombotic agent.

Discussion

The development and increased use of anticoagulant agents to prevent stroke in an aging population of patients with AF has been associated with a fivefold increase in the rate of treatment-related intracerebral hemorrhages [17]. NOACs have been associated with a lower rate of intracerebral hemorrhage (~40–70% RRR) [17].

Hypertension, abnormal renal and liver function, history of stroke, bleeding tendency, labile INRs if on warfarin, age >65 years, and drug or alcohol use are associated with increased risk of intracerebral hemorrhage in patients on oral anticoagulants (HAS-BLED score). Some of these risk factors for bleeding are also risk factors for the presence of microangiopathy.

More than 75% of spontaneous intracerebral hemorrhages in the elderly are associated with small vessel hypertensive arteriopathy or cerebral amyloid

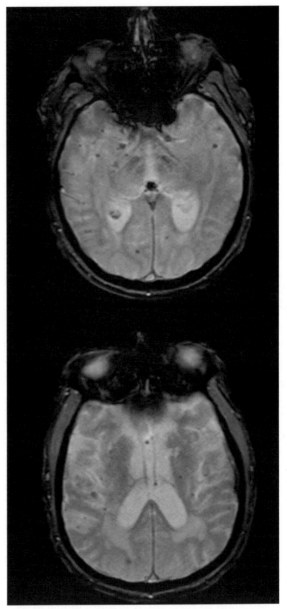

Figure 5.6 Axial gradient echo image shows multiple hypointense regions consistent with cerebral microhemorrhages.

angiopathy (CAA). Cerebral microbleeds (CMBs) occur from small cerebral vessels, increase in number over time, and are common in individuals at risk for treatment with anticoagulant drugs. While CMBs are usually asymptomatic, they can progress into symptomatic intracerebral hemorrhage. Prospective studies have suggested an increased risk of symptomatic intracerebral hemorrhage after ischemic stroke in patients with CMBs [17]. An excess of CMBs has been reported in patients treated with warfarin compared to ischemic stroke cohorts not taking warfarin. There are no large prospective studies of the use of MRI to screen patients for CMBs in patients with AF treated with anticoagulants.

Tip

Extensive CMBs appear to be a risk factor for intracerebral hemorrhage in patients with atrial fibrillation treated with anticoagulants. Consider avoiding full dose anticoagulation in patients with extensive CMBs or known diagnosis of CAA.

References

1. Eikelboom JW, Connolly SJ, Brueckmann M, et al. Dabigatran versus warfarin in patients with mechanical heart valves. *N Engl J Med* 2013;369:1206–14.

2. Mischie AN, Chioncel V, Droc I, Sinescu C. Anticoagulation in patients with dilated cardiomyopathy, low ejection fraction, and sinus rhythm: back to the drawing board. *Cardiovasc Ther* 2013;31(5):298–302.

3. Massie BM, Krol WF, Ammon SE. The Warfarin and Antiplatelet Therapy in Heart Failure trial (WATCH): rationale, design, and baseline patient characteristics. *J Card Fail* 2004;10(2):101–12.

4. Pullicino PM, Thompson JL, Sacco RL, et al. Stroke in heart failure in sinus rhythm: the Warfarin versus Aspirin in Reduced Cardiac Ejection Fraction trial. *Cerebrovasc. Dis. Basel Switz* 2013; 36:74–8.

5. January CT, Wann LS, Alpert JS, et al. 2014 AHA/ACC/HRS Guideline for the Management of Patients With Atrial Fibrillation: A Report of the American College of Cardiology/American Heart Association Task Force on Practice Guidelines and the Heart Rhythm Society. *Circulation*; published online March 28, 2014.

6. Diener HC, Eikelboom J, Connolly SJ, et al. AVERROES Steering Committee and Investigators. Apixaban versus aspirin in patients with atrial fibrillation and previous stroke or transient ischaemic attack: a predefined subgroup analysis from AVERROES, a randomised trial. *Lancet Neurol* 2012;11(3):225–31.

7. Healey, J. A Comparison of Apixaban Versus Aspirin for Preventing Stroke in Patients With Pacemakers (ARTESiA). NCT01938248. (2013). At http://clinicaltrials.gov/show/NCT01938248.

8. Granger CB et al. Apixaban in patients with atrial fibrillation. *N Engl J Med* 2011;364:806–17.

9. Connolly SJ, Ezekowitz MD, Yusuf S. Dabigatran versus warfarin in patients with atrial fibrillation. *N Engl J Med*. 2009;361:1139–51.

10. US FDA. FDA Drug Safety Communication: FDA study of Medicare patients finds risks lower for stroke and death but higher for gastrointestinal bleeding with Pradaxa (dabigatran) compared to warfarin. (2014). At www.fda.gov/Drugs/DrugSafety/ucm396470.htm.

11. Giugliano RP, Ruff CT, Braunwald E, et al. Edoxaban versus warfarin in patients with atrial fibrillation. *N Engl J Med* 2013;369:2093–104.

12. Patel MR, Mahaffey KW, Garg J, et al. Rivaroxaban versus warfarin in nonvalvular atrial fibrillation. *N Engl J Med* 2011;365:883–91.

13. Skjoth F, Larsen, TB, Rasmussen LH, Lip GYH. Efficacy and safety of edoxaban in comparison with dabigatran, rivaroxaban and apixaban for stroke prevention in atrial fibrillation. An indirect comparison analysis. *Thromb Haemost* 2014;111:981–8.

14. Lip GY, Manning WJ, Weissman NJ. Left ventricular thrombus after acute myocardial infarction. (2014). At www.uptodate.com/contents/left-ventricular-thrombus-after-acute-myocardial-infarction.

15. Shacham Y, Leshem-Rubinow E, Ben Assa E, et al. Frequency and correlates of early left ventricular thrombus formation following anterior wall acute myocardial infarction treated with primary percutaneous coronary intervention. *Am J Cardiol* 2013;111:667–70.

16. Buss NI, Friedman SE, Andrus BW, DeVries JT. Warfarin for stroke prevention following anterior ST-elevation myocardial infarction. *Coron Artery Dis* 2013;24:636–641.

17. Charidimo, A, Shakeshaft C, Werring DJ. Cerebral microbleeds on magnetic resonance imaging and anticoagulant-associated intracerebral hemorrhage risk. *Front Neurol* 2012;3:133. eCollection 2012.

Chapter 6

Antithrombotic management of recurrent atherothrombotic cerebrovascular disease

Murray Flaster

Introduction

When considering pitfalls or failure to prevent recurrent stroke there are several things to think about first. We must consider time – do we mean stroke later that day, that week, or at some distant time point? Do we mean stroke from the same etiology, known or surmised or some other etiology? Perhaps as importantly, we must humbly acknowledge the weakness of our remedies. For instance, consider the unimpressive performance of aspirin, probably the single most widely used agent for the prevention of recurrent ischemic stroke, which in extensive meta-analyses reduced recurrent stroke rate by 20%. In other words, there is an expected failure rate of 80%. With this caveat in mind we will consider a few pitfalls in the recognition and prevention of recurrent stroke.

Case 1. Carotid disease

A 57-year-old man with a past medical history that included arterial hypertension, cigarette smoking, chronic low back pain, and occasional analgesic overuse developed sudden weakness and numbness of the left upper and lower extremity while driving a vehicle with a manual transmission on a dirt road. He became understandably alarmed, managed to stop the vehicle, and called his wife on his cell phone. She noticed slurred speech. While speaking to his wife, his motor function began to improve enough to allow him to resume driving from his remote location. His condition continued to improve and he believed himself to be back to normal when he reached home almost 2 hours later. Still, he and his wife went immediately to the local, rural emergency department (ED) where the ED physician found him without deficit 2 hours and 45 minutes after the onset of his symptoms. Blood

pressure in the ED was recorded as 150/90 mmHg. The patient appeared anxious. He was treated first with intravenous fluids and was placed on oxygen by nasal cannula. Complete blood count, complete metabolic panel, and troponins were obtained with all values returning normal. An ECG showed evidence of old inferior wall ischemia which had not been, to the patient's knowledge, previously noted. The patient remained anxious and complained that he simply did not feel well. He then complained that his left side again seemed numb. Three hours after arrival at the ED, he received an anxiolytic. Almost immediately thereafter, he complained of marked weakness of the left upper extremity and a lesser degree of weakness of the left lower extremity. His speech was again slurred. A CT scan of the head was ordered but this was unavailable for technical reasons and the patient was moved by air transport to an urban hospital stroke center.

Clinically, the initial event should be considered a transient ischemic attack (TIA), at least by the classic clinical definition [1]. Neither anxiety nor the past history of chronic pain including the use of narcotic analgesics should deter the evaluating physician from considering the neurologic complaint to be primary. If the primary complaint may be ischemic, it is disadvantageous to give anxiolytic unless absolutely necessary. The event may have been an ischemic stroke with resolution of symptoms but we could not know this without obtaining a diffusion-weighted image (DWI) had a brain magnetic resonance imaging (MRI) scanner been available. That being said, if this was an ischemic event, what is the risk of a recurrent ischemic event? The ABCD^2 score [2] is a simple, validated way of estimating risk. This score has a maximum of 7 points, 1 for age greater than 60, 1 point for systolic blood pressure greater than 140 mm Hg or diastolic blood

Common Pitfalls in Cerebrovascular Disease: Case-Based Learning, ed. José Biller and José M. Ferro. Published by Cambridge University Press. © Cambridge University Press 2015.

pressure greater than 90 mm Hg, 2 points for lateralized weakness reported or present on examination, one point for abnormal speech if lateralized weakness is not present, one point for the duration greater than 10 minutes but less than 1 hour and 2 points for duration greater than 1 hour, and finally a single point for a history of diabetes. This man's score is 4. A score of 0–3 indicates mild stroke risk, a score of 4–5 moderate stroke risk, and scores of 6 or 7 a severe stroke risk. Cigarette smoking presents an added risk, harder to quantify but which should never be ignored when evaluating patients with possible cerebral ischemia. An ECG suggesting old cardiac ischemia is a further cause of concern in this case.

The patient arrived at the stroke center roughly 12 hours after the initial ictus and about 6.5 hours after definitive clinical worsening, the flight having been delayed for non-medical reasons. The patient's examination demonstrated mild left facial weakness, severe paresis but not plegia of the left upper extremity, mild weakness (drift) of the left lower extremity, and mild dysarthria. The NIH Stroke Scale (NIHSS) score was 6 points. CT scan of the head showed no hemorrhage but multiple subtle, probably ischemic changes in the left middle cerebral artery (MCA) territory and boundary zone. These findings were subsequently substantiated by MRI (Figure 6.1). Aspirin was administered and computed tomography angiograms (CTA) of the head and neck were obtained. This showed a widely patent right MCA, bilateral carotid artery bifurcation atherosclerotic plaque, worse on the right than on the left, but with stenosis of less than 50% (Figure 6.2). Additionally an intraluminal filling defect in the intracranial, horizontal petrous segment of the internal carotid artery (ICA) on the right was detected (Figure 6.3).

These findings when taken together strongly imply that the patient experienced recurrent embolization from the highly irregular, ruptured plaque at the origin of the right ICA. The presence of irregular plaque is a well-established risk factor associated with increased risk of ischemic stroke recurrence [3]. This case also illustrates the very important relationship between TIAs or minor strokes and ischemic recurrence. Classically defined TIA has been known to predict stroke in about 10% of cases in the next 90 days, half of them within the next 48 hours [4]. A more recent effort to better define the fine structure of stroke recurrence following an initial minor ischemia demonstrated that 42% of strokes which would occur in the following 30 days occurred within the first 24 hours as our

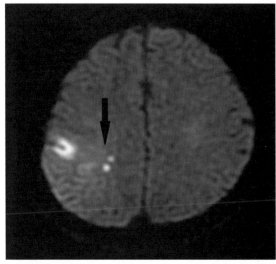

Figure 6.1 MRI diffusion-weighted imaging shows acute ischemia in the primary motor cortex and in neighboring white matter along the MCA–anterior cerebral artery (ACA) boundary zone (arrow).

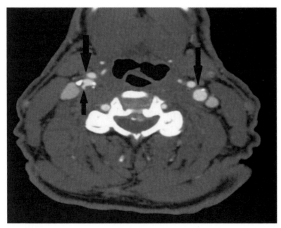

Figure 6.2 CTA source image at the origin of the ICAs (down arrows) shows an extremely irregular plaque on the right with peripheral calcification (up arrow).

case clearly illustrates. Furthermore, these early recurrences frequently involve extracranial or intracranial large artery stroke [5,6].

Case 2. More carotid disease

A 67-year-old right-handed man was seen in neurologic outpatient consultation for recurrent spells. The first spell took place 2 months before the patient's visit. Hospital reports indicated that there was an episode of near syncope followed by confusion. These records further indicated that the patient was transiently aphasic

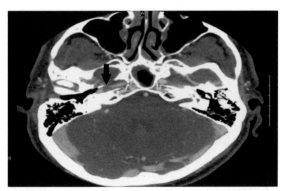

Figure 6.3 CTA source image at the level of the horizontal petrous segment of the intracranial carotid artery shows intraluminal filling defect consistent with embolus (arrow).

with aberrant behavior. The patient recalled only that he had been looking for his dog outdoors only to have neighbors discover and explain that his dog was in his trailer home. He also remembered failing to cover for his son at work as he had previously agreed to do. His recollection of the episode was limited and his recollection of the hospitalization was vague. MRI reportedly showed bilateral deep white matter changes. It was not clear if DWI was available at that site at that time. Carotid ultrasound study found left ICA stenosis estimated at between 50% and 79% with the detailed velocity data in the lower part of the velocity range. A transthoracic echocardiogram showed only mild mitral regurgitation and a normal ejection fraction. A 24-hour video EEG obtained during that hospitalization failed to show any epileptiform activity. The hospital discharge summary indicated that the patient had suffered either a TIA or mild stroke or possibly a seizure. The only medication added at discharge was clopidogrel.

His next medical encounter was initiated by a State policeman on a highway 2 months and 2000 miles distant from the initial event. The patient was detained after he was noted to be driving erratically on a highway. He was confused and initially thought to be intoxicated. He was brought to a local ED where he was evaluated and hospitalized. The ED staff as well as an evaluating neurologist initially thought the patient was intoxicated. He was confused but some aphasic features were noted by the examining neurologist. No blood alcohol was present. MRI of the brain again demonstrated bilateral deep white matter changes; however, DWI showed no restriction. An MR angiogram (MRA) of the head did suggest an asymmetry of flow, with less

flow evident in the distal branches of the left MCA but the quality was such as to make that finding uncertain. The patient was maintained in the intensive care unit and monitored for 2 days. No arrhythmias were noted. A routine EEG did not show epileptiform activity. The patient enjoyed a good cognitive recovery and was discharged after 2 days of close observation. Clopidogrel was discontinued and warfarin added instead. The patient was discharged from the hospital and an outpatient consultation for our stroke clinic was arranged. When the patient was evaluated in the stroke clinic 2 weeks later, he was found to have no evidence of aphasia, normal mentation as well as a normal neurologic examination. The only abnormality noted was an occasional aberrant heartbeat not consistent with atrial fibrillation (AF). There were no cervical bruits. We noted that the patient was a retired commercial chemist who lived alone, had a motor home, and enjoyed traveling. His past medical history was significant for treated hypothyroidism, well-controlled hypertension treated with sustained release verapamil, cigarette smoking discontinued 25 years prior, and significant alcohol use discontinued 20 years prior. At the completion of that evaluation, 81 mg of aspirin daily was added. A 24-hour Holter monitor was requested with the understanding that should that monitor fail to demonstrate AF, warfarin would be discontinued. A repeat MRI brain and MRA of the head was also requested.

Several weeks later, the patient again experienced an aphasic or confusional episode. He telephoned the stroke clinic and was instructed to come to the clinic emergently. Examination at that time found the patient unable to perform complex tasks when verbally instructed to do so. He had difficulty with anything more than simple calculations. Mild word-finding difficulties, scattered neologisms, and some perseveration were noted. Speech production was slowed. A mild right hemi-apraxia was noted. Immediate recall was impaired. The patient was able to give a partial history. He realized he was having difficulties but could not define them precisely. He did recall having a great deal of difficulty dialing the number to the stroke clinic but he drove there uneventfully. The patient was immediately admitted to hospital. There, he was evaluated by a neurology resident who found his speech was slurred. The patient was mistaken as to the year and when asked to name the current president, he erroneously named the prior president instead. There was no weakness and no sensory deficit. The Neurology Resident felt the patient was perhaps intoxicated with

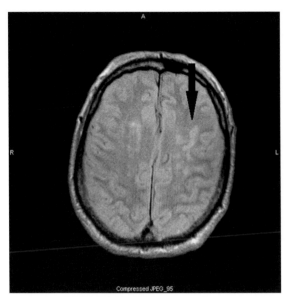

Figure 6.4 MR T2 FLAIR image demonstrating a large asymmetry in juxtacortical and corona radiata T2 bright signal which is considerably greater on the left (arrow).

something other than alcohol; however, a toxicology screen was negative. Within several hours, the patient's primarily left hemispheric deficits fully resolved. An EEG was obtained that day. Cerebral activity was described as diffusely slow, with 5–6 Hz predominance and an excess of bifrontal delta activity but again no epileptiform activity was noted. MRI of the brain again showed no diffusion restriction. MR T2 FLAIR sequences showed bilateral periventricular and juxtacortical white matter changes, more pronounced on the left than on the right (Figure 6.4). MRA of the head showed no definite abnormalities. MRA of the neck showed only minor changes suggestive of carotid bifurcation atherosclerosis with minimal stenosis on the left (Figure 6.5). Cardiac monitoring failed to show any evidence of AF. A catheter angiogram was proposed to the patient but he declined. The patient was discharged on aspirin and lamotrigine and warfarin was discontinued. The patient reported another confusional episode several weeks later, he was evaluated in the ED, and lamotrigine dose was increased. Subsequently, he agreed to a catheter cerebral angiogram (Figure 6.6). The biplane cerebral angiogram demonstrated a very large, severely ulcerated plaque at the left ICA origin with about 60% stenosis measured in the most affected plane. After some debate between stroke specialists and an epileptologist, a left carotid endarterectomy (CEA)

was recommended. Following uneventful CEA, lamotrigine was weaned over 3 months and the patient was event free for at least 7 months. He was lost to follow-up after he resumed his highway travels.

Lessons to be learned in this case are many. The most elementary are to be very circumspect about placing a patient on therapy for tentative diagnoses. The patient was placed on warfarin for a time although AF or other adequate indication had not been demonstrated. It is worthwhile noting that prolonged highly portable ECG recording (for example a 30-day event monitor) was not available at the time of this case presentation. Although epilepsy can be an elusive diagnosis, this patient had repeated normal EEG recordings including a full day of video continuous EEG monitoring, so making that diagnosis could be at best only tentative. Conventional ultrasound and conventional cervical MRA will on occasion fail to find significant atherosclerotic disease at the carotid bifurcations as this case strikingly demonstrated. Advanced multi-detector CTA, high resolution ultrasonography, or as in this case catheter angiography are remedies. Repeated carotid embolism would reasonably be expected to demonstrate MR diffusion restriction if timely images, within 1 week, are obtained but this is not always the case. Rigorous clinically defined TIA may fail to show diffusion restriction at least 50% of the time. Atherosclerotic carotid plaque with ulceration is notably associated with high risk of recurrent ischemic events [7,8]. Although recurrent carotid ischemia can be devastating as in Case 1, on some occasions it can be somewhat subtle, as in this case. This patient's lesion had a very unusual appearance which may correlate with the unusually elusive clinical presentation. In general, symptomatic ICA disease carries a very high risk of early recurrence and should be treated promptly [9].

Case 3. Intracranial atherosclerosis

A 94-year-old man was doing relatively well, living alone and managing most of his own affairs successfully, when he developed abrupt weakness which he described as a "ball and chain" suddenly fastened to his right leg. He also felt shortness of breath and thought that he might have some bilateral lower extremity weakness as well. He had two such episodes. The first lasted 1 hour, resolved completely and about which he chose to do nothing. The second episode the following morning he found sufficiently alarming that he called for

(a) (b)

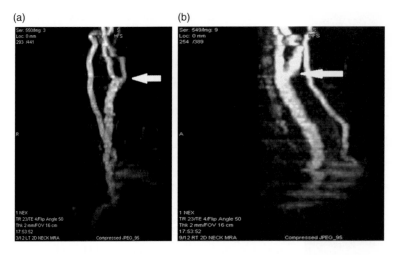

Figure 6.5 Rotational projection 2D time-of-flight MRA of the cervical left carotid artery. Images a and b are approximately 90° apart. Arrows indicate the carotid bifurcation. Only mild atherosclerotic disease is demonstrated.

(a) (b)

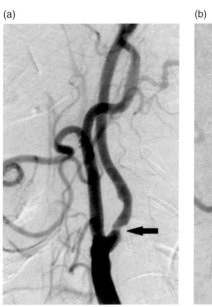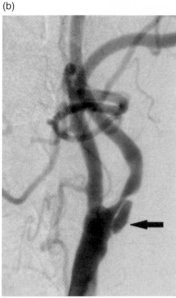

Figure 6.6 Catheter angiogram left common carotid artery injection with two orthogonal views. Arrows indicate the carotid bifurcation. A deep, elongated unusually large ulceration is well seen in image b (arrow) but is not even suspected in image a, which only shows what appears to be smooth plaque and at most moderate stenosis.

emergent medical assistance. His weakness completely resolved by the time he reached the ED of our hospital.

Past medical history included arterial hypertension, hypothyroidism, chronic mild macrocytic anemia, benign prostate hypertrophy, and peripheral vascular disease. His peripheral vascular disease never progressed to the point of requiring intervention. Similarly, he had known, mild to moderate asymptomatic cervical carotid and subclavian atherosclerotic disease which had been followed by ultrasound studies for the prior 7 years and had not required intervention.

Examination in the ED demonstrated no neurologic deficits. CT scan of the brain showed bilateral periventricular white matter changes but no discrete infarcts. The patient was diagnosed with either TIA or transient orthostatic hypotension. He received intravenous (IV) fluids and mild systolic hypotension was soon replaced by isolated systolic hypertension with relatively wide pulse pressure. The neurologic consultant

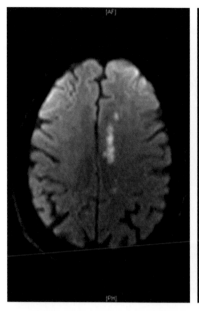
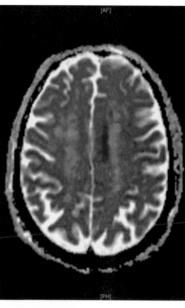

Figure 6.7 Echo-planar MR DWI consistent with acute ischemia in the left ACA territory (left) and apparent diffusion coefficient (ADC) map confirming restricted diffusion (right).

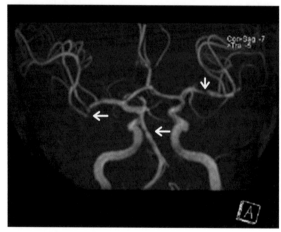

Figure 6.8 MRA (circle of Willis maximum intensity projection [MIP]) consistent with intracranial stenoses involving left mid-MCA (vertical arrow), right MCA bifurcation (horizontal arrow to left), and basilar artery (horizontal arrow center). Abnormalities of the ACA are inapparent.

recommended an MRI of the brain, which showed no acute diffusion restrictions. That study did demonstrate bilateral periventricular and juxtacortical white matter changes as well as changes in the pons consistent with small vessel vasculopathy. Carotid ultrasound studies were repeated and were read out as showing bilaterally 50–69% ICA stenosis with heterogeneous plaque. These ultrasound results were little changed

from studies performed 2 and 7 years prior. The patient had subjective orthostatic symptoms which resolved spontaneously. Lipid profile demonstrated a total cholesterol of 121 mg/dL, an HDL of 57 mg/dL and a calculated LDL of 60 mg/dL. Repeated ECGs showed sinus rhythm or mild sinus bradycardia with few premature atrial complexes. He was discharged home the following morning on his previous medications which included 325 mg of aspirin daily, lisinopril with hydrochlorothiazide, levothyroxine, and tamsulosin.

Five days later the patient was readmitted to hospital after experiencing transient right lower extremity weakness again. He had fallen twice while at home but without significant injury. Mild, transient systolic hypertension was again noted in the ED. Fluids were again given. The patient's neurologic examination was considered normal, unchanged. He was admitted for further investigation and physical therapy. The ED physician and internists expected placement would be necessary at discharge as it was doubted that the man could continue to live independently. Peripheral vascular studies were repeated which showed no significant change. A plain radiograph of the knee showed a subacute to chronic fracture of the medial femoral condyle on the right. Echocardiography demonstrated a left ventricular ejection fraction of 60% and mild diastolic dysfunction. On the third hospital day the patient was transferred to the rehabilitation service.

(a)   (b)   (c)   (d)

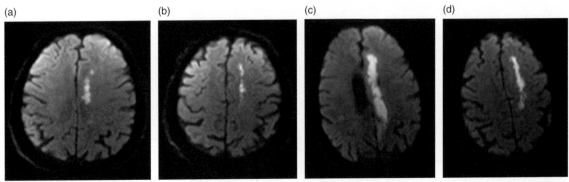

Figure 6.9 MR DWI showing ACA territory and ACA/MCA boundary zone ischemia of the initial stroke (a and b) and new, larger DWI lesions in the same distribution exactly 2 weeks later (c and d).

The following day, in mid-afternoon, the patient was noted to be less responsive, with right-sided weakness and language difficulties. An acute stroke code was initiated. Examination demonstrated mild aphasia and significant right-sided weakness as well as right gaze preference with an NIHSS score of 11. CT scan demonstrated no other bleeding or signs of acute infarction. The patient did not receive acute thrombolytic therapy because time of onset was uncertain. He was last seen well 3½ hours before his deficits were recognized. The patient was subsequently transferred to the neurology service. MRI of the brain demonstrated ischemic changes involving the territory of the anterior cerebral artery (ACA) on the left (Figure 6.7). MRA of the head was obtained and this was read out as showing minor intracranial atherosclerosis and otherwise unremarkable (Figure 6.8). The patient was judged to have moderate symptomatic stenosis of the left ICA origin, carotid artery endarterectomy was tentatively offered but the patient and family declined. The patient was placed on atorvastatin. Aspirin was substituted with clopidogrel. The patient made a good recovery with respect to language and right upper extremity function, but his right lower extremity remained weak. He was discharged to a skilled nursing facility for further rehabilitation 2 days after his acute stroke.

Twelve days later, the patient was readmitted to hospital. Over the prior 10 days he had developed increasing confusion, difficulties with speech, and increased right-sided weakness. A urinary tract infection was diagnosed and treated. The patient was relatively hypotensive with significant pre-renal azotemia and hypernatremia. Dehydration was diagnosed and treated. A repeat MRI of the brain demonstrated new ischemia (Figure 6.9). MRA of the head was repeated (Figure 6.10) and MRA of the

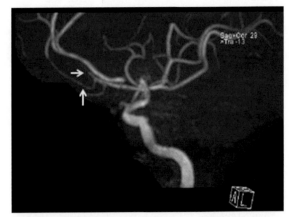

Figure 6.10 MRA MIP projection left intracranial ICA shows cutoff of the pericallosal branch of left ACA (horizontal arrow) and diminished flow in the proximal segment of the neighboring fronto-polar branch (vertical arrow). The right ACA (immediately above left ACA) appears artifactually discontinuous in this projection.

neck was obtained. Neurologically, the patient was arousable but unable to speak clearly. He could follow simple commands with effort. He was noted to have increased motor tone throughout with significant right-sided weakness. Fluid resuscitation reversed the patient's renal failure and hyponatremia. There were no further signs of infection. Despite these treatments, his cognitive status further declined. After discussion with family, comfort care was elected. The patient was transferred to a skilled nursing facility for hospice care and died several days later.

The pitfalls in this case are many. Evaluating the very elderly patient clinically is complex and involves consideration of many comorbidities and competing possibilities. When our patient was initially admitted with TIA considered likely, vascular imaging other than repeated carotid ultrasound studies was not obtained. Carotid ultrasound studies alone are often obtained with the idea that should symptomatic and sufficiently severe stenosis be demonstrated, effective intervention is possible or at least should not be overlooked. The value of this approach in a nonagenarian is far from clear. In general and regardless of age, comprehensive vascular imaging should be obtained in any TIA patient in the hopes of elucidating the likely origin of the patient's ischemic symptoms and in selecting the most appropriate care.

This patient's primary problem was multiple intracranial atherosclerotic stenoses. Long recognized as an important cause of ischemic stroke in patients of non-European origin with a prevalence as high as 50% in stroke patients from China or Japan, symptomatic intracranial atherosclerotic stenosis with a prevalence as high as 10–20% is now recognized in stroke patients of European origin [10,11]. Like other stroke etiologies, the frequency of intracranial atherosclerosis increases significantly with age. When MRA of the head is obtained, it is important to personally review the projection images and source images carefully while bearing in mind MR diffusion and T2 FLAIR imaging results and correlate them. In this instance, these considerations would have led to the discovery of subtle but clear-cut evidence of the absence of a major branch of the A2 segment of the left ACA (Figure 6.10) as well as clinically important distal left MCA stenosis (Figure 6.8). These findings best explain the recurrent left ACA stroke and MCA/ACA border zone infarct pattern.

A reduction in antihypertensive medications, the early addition of a statin, and an understanding of the critical importance of good hydration might have altered outcome in this patient, at least in the short run. It is common clinical practice to augment or alter antiplatelet therapy in the setting of recurrent TIA or recurrent stroke. Although this practice may not be well supported by evidence-based reasoning in many instances, the brief use of dual antiplatelet therapy may arguably have been helpful in this case. It is important to exercise considerable caution when assigning stroke etiology based on carotid ultrasound data alone. In this case, careful review of serial carotid ultrasound studies showed that peak proximal and mid internal carotid artery velocities were variable between studies and did not show progression overall. An analysis of cervical MR angiography which in this case was marred by movement demonstrates marked tortuosity of the

left internal carotid artery origin and fails to confirm the ultrasound estimate of stenosis. Discordant results with respect to degree of carotid artery stenosis when different imaging modalities are compared is not uncommon [12]. Surgical treatment of symptomatic, mild carotid artery origin disease may not be appropriate for all patients, particularly where life expectancy is limited [13]. In this instance, carotid disease contributed little to overall ischemic risk. Good decision-making requires consideration of all the data, cognizance of applicable treatment guidelines, and most importantly, consideration of the characteristics of the individual patient.

Recurrent stroke due to intracranial atherosclerosis in the same arterial distribution is common, noted in over 12% of patients radiologically and in 4% of patients clinically within 7 months of the index stroke in one recent prospective study including 353 patients participating in a randomized therapy trial [14]. Recurrent ischemic stroke in the same arterial distribution should influence the treating physician to consider intracranial atherosclerosis as a possible etiology that must be considered.

Case 4. More intracranial atherosclerosis

A 74-year-old woman with a history of previous stroke and previous TIA was referred to our stroke clinic regarding stroke etiology and further management. The patient suffered an ischemic stroke 13 months prior and a TIA 2 months prior to her office visit with us. Her stroke took place during a hospitalization for community-acquired pneumonia. MRI diffusion demonstrated multiple acute diffusion restrictions, all small and all in the distribution of the right MCA territory. None were at the cortical surface; most approximated the MCA boundary zone (Figure 6.11). The patient recalled experiencing left-sided numbness and tingling and some left-sided weakness as well. She was very frightened by the event. However, she regained good motor function within 1 to 2 weeks and her sensory symptoms also subsided. Records from that hospitalization indicated no unusual findings on cardiac telemetry or ECG, an echocardiogram showed mild left ventricular hypertrophy only, and a carotid ultrasound study reportedly showed mild calcific plaque in the left carotid bulb but no atherosclerotic disease on the right. She was placed on aspirin 81 mg and clopidogrel at hospital discharge but left without a defined

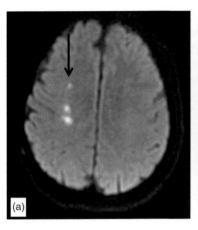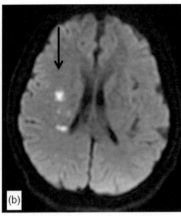

Figure 6.11 MR echo planar DWI demonstrating relatively linear cluster of small areas of restricted diffusion not extending to the cortical surface (arrow in a) and deeper not quite as linear areas of diffusion restriction approaching the lateral ventricle (b). This deeper MCA boundary zone pattern suggests artery to artery embolism associated with limited flow, more likely due to MCA than cervical ICA disease.

stroke etiology. Her past medical history was significant for hypertension and hypercholesterolemia, mild renal impairment, and gastroesophageal reflux. She also had a history of recurrent headache with migrainous features and recurrent depression with occasional manic features. She had been a heavy cigarette smoker at one time but stopped smoking 20 years before her visit to our clinic. Alcohol use was minimal. Family history included both coronary artery disease and hypertension in both parents. She had a sister with migraine headache.

The patient did well for 11 months but then developed new left-sided paresthesias which were accompanied by headache and an elevated blood pressure. MRI of the brain was again performed but this time there were no acute diffuse restrictions. Carotid ultrasound studies and echocardiography were repeated with results similar to the earlier studies. An LDL of 130 mg/dL was reported. Her symptoms resolved and she was discharged with additional antihypertensive medication, low dose rosuvastatin, and aspirin increased from 81 to 325 mg daily. She subsequently reported muscle aches associated with rosuvastatin and was placed on 20 mg of simvastatin which she tolerated better. At some point, fenofibrate was also added.

Her examination at her visit to our clinic demonstrated mild left-sided pronator drift and slightly abnormal gait with mild circumduction of the left lower extremity and slowed toe tapping on the left as well. There were no sensory findings and no reflex asymmetries. Blood pressure seemed well-controlled. Simvastatin dosage was doubled, fenofibrate was discontinued, and aspirin dosage was reduced to 81 mg daily. CTA was considered but because of the patient's chronic renal insufficiency and the chronicity of her symptoms, MRA of the head and neck were requested instead. Prior to her return visit she telephoned us complaining of renewed myalgias. Pravastatin was substituted for simvastatin and this proved to be well tolerated. MRA of the head and neck demonstrated little if any cervical disease; however, considerable intracranial atherosclerosis was uncovered (Figure 6.12). Pravastatin was increased to 80 mg daily. Aspirin was subsequently eliminated but clopidogrel was continued. Six months later the patient experienced some transient left facial numbness after she noticed a small conjunctival hemorrhage during physical exercise. The facial numbness resolved within an hour and a repeat MRI demonstrated no new diffusion abnormalities. Six months later, the patient developed abrupt language difficulties and was treated with tissue plasminogen activator at an outside hospital. Her language difficulties, lasting about 2 hours, total subsided during treatment. She was transferred to our hospital that evening where MR diffusion studies demonstrated no deficits. CT angiography was obtained, reconfirming widespread intracranial atherosclerosis and perhaps suggesting an increase in distal left middle cerebral artery disease (Figure 6.13). At that time, high dose atorvastatin was substituted for pravastatin and that medication has been well tolerated since. LDL has gradually declined from a historic high of 160 mg/dL to 112 mg/dL most recently. In subsequent follow-up visits, the patient complained of transient "dizzy spells." Her blood pressure regime was slightly relaxed and these symptoms disappeared. At this time, the patient has been stroke free for nearly 4 years.

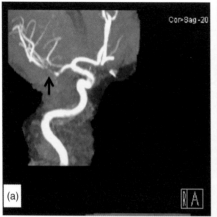

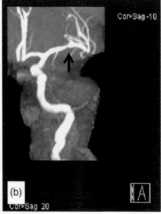

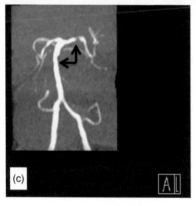

Figure 6.12 MRA of intracranial vessels (2D time-of-flight) MIP images showing severe distal M1 and M2 stenosis of the right MCA (arrow in a), mild distal stenosis of the left MCA (arrow in b), and marked stenosis of the left PCA (vertical arrow in c) and atherosclerotic plaque in the distal basilar artery (horizontal arrow in c).

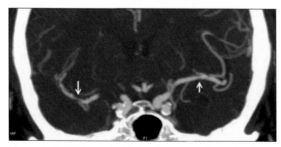

Figure 6.13 CTA (coronal MIP) showing severe atherosclerotic stenosis of proximal M2 branch of right MCA (down arrow) and milder stenosis of the distal left M1 segment (up arrow).

This case and the previous case illustrate the importance of considering intracranial atherosclerosis in ischemic stroke diagnosis and in subsequent management. In both instances, the patients were of European origin, which may help explain why intracranial disease was initially overlooked. Intracranial atherosclerotic disease is well recognized in Asian, Hispanic, African, and African-American populations but has only recently been recognized as common in white populations as well [11]. Worldwide, it may be the most frequent of all ischemic stroke subtypes [15]. In the past, definitive diagnosis required catheter cerebral angiogram whereas today, diagnosis can be reliably confirmed with either CTA or MRA while CTA may have slightly better sensitivity and specificity than MR methods [16]. Stroke recurrence rates can be high. Invasive management with intra-arterial stenting is not currently recommended. Best medical management is recommended including high dose statin, aggressive blood pressure management after the acute period, lifestyle alteration, and probably dual antiplatelet therapy for at least 1–2 months acutely [17].

Case 5. Aortic arch atheroma

A 77-year-old woman came to the ED at the urging of a friend because of left-sided headache and feeling "something is not right." The headache was gradual in onset, left frontal in location, and accompanied by a sense of not feeling well. There was a sudden sense of

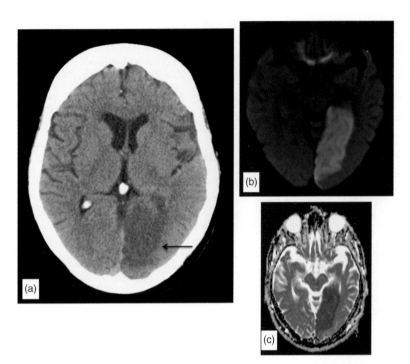

Figure 6.14 CT head obtained in the ED shows hypodensity consistent with acute left PCA territory infarction (a, arrow). MR DWI image (b) and ADC map (c) confirms same.

dysphoria which the patient attributed to feelings associated with recent illness and death amongst family members and friends. The friend who accompanied her felt that the patient had noticeably changed in recent days with slowed movement and speech. Physical examination in the ED was remarkable for a blood pressure of 163/75 mmHg and moderate obesity. A CT scan of the brain (Figure 6.14a) demonstrated an acute cerebral infarction involving the left posterior cerebral artery (PCA) territory. Neurologic examination in the ED demonstrated a dense right homonymous hemianopsia. Speech was mildly slowed. The patient had difficulty accepting the visual field loss even after it was demonstrated to her although she did not have anosognosia. Comprehension was intact. However, the examiner did feel that there was evidence for cognitive slowing which subsequently improved. MR imaging of the brain confirmed an acute left PCA infarction (Figure 6.14b and c) while MRA of the head demonstrated a flow gap involving the P3 segment of the posterior cerebral artery on the left (Figure 6.15). No other evidence of intracranial vessel abnormalities was noted while the circle of Willis was unexceptional other than a fetally derived right PCA (Figure 6.15). MRA of the neck including 2D time-of-flight and dynamic MR imaging demonstrated mild stenosis involving the left

ICA origin and what was interpreted as minor, likely calcific plaque involving the aortic arch and the origin of the left subclavian artery.

Past medical history was remarkable for arterial hypertension, hyperlipidemia, and hypothyroidism. There was no personal history of tobacco or alcohol use. Family history included a sister and two brothers with strokes. Additionally, the patient's mother had two strokes in her 80s, the second of which was fatal. The neurology team felt that the patient probably had artery to artery embolism but without a defined source. A lipid profile demonstrated a cholesterol of 149 mg/dL, HDL of 58 mg/dL, and LDL of 80 mg/dL. Hemoglobin A_{1c} was not elevated. Thyroid-stimulating hormone was within normal limits. Pravastatin was increased from 40 mg to 80 mg daily. (The patient had a previously demonstrated intolerance to atorvastatin.) Clopidogrel was begun and aspirin discontinued at hospital discharge. The patient improved uneventfully. Her headache diminished. Blood pressures seemed well-controlled. To further exclude a cardiac source of embolism, a 30-day event monitor was arranged as an outpatient and this failed to show significant arrhythmia. The patient was discharged with strict instructions not to drive. Outpatient physical therapy and speech therapy for cognition were also arranged.

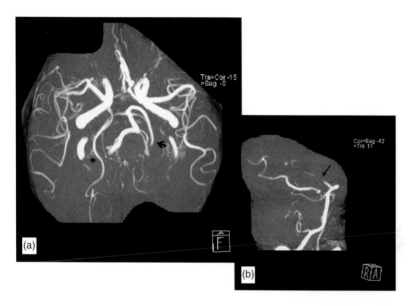

Figure 6.15 MRA head, maximum intensity projections (MIPs). (a) Slightly rotated top down view showing a fetally derived right PCA (finer arrow) and a left PCA derived from the basilar artery with what appears to be an abrupt cutoff (larger arrow).(b). A right anterior view of the basilar system clarifying the left PCA pathology, a severe flow gap (arrow) with a distal branch of left PCA faintly continuing. No other flow abnormalities are apparent intracranially.

Exactly 7 weeks after discharge the patient developed sudden numbness and pain in her right upper extremity. She hurried to the ED where she was found to have a cool, pale limb. Stat ultrasound of the right upper extremity showed reduced arterial flow in several vessels suggesting acute thrombosis. Emergent right brachial arteriotomy was performed with a successful embolectomy of the brachial artery, and also the right ulnar and radial arteries. Post-procedure CTA demonstrated widely patent vessels. Perioperatively, the patient was placed on a heparin drip and warfarin was begun postoperatively. Pain resolved and the limb returned to normal. The patient was discharged on warfarin. A thorough hypercoagulable work-up disclosed only a minimally elevated anticardiolipin IgM of uncertain significance.

The patient subsequently followed up in our neurology outpatient clinic where we became aware of the peripheral vascular event. A CTA of the head and neck was obtained and this demonstrated severe atherosclerotic disease of the aortic arch including widespread lipid-laden plaque of 3–4 mm thickness and an area of irregular and ulcerated plaque of 8 mm thickness which likely represents ruptured plaque remnant (Figure 6.16). Irregular atherosclerotic plaque was also present at the origins of both of the left common carotid artery and the left subclavian artery, the latter appearing more severe (Figure 6.17). A retrospective review of the CTA of the aorta obtained hours after the peripheral thrombectomy shows severe aortic arch plaque

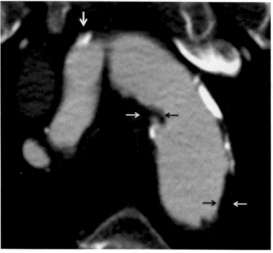

Figure 6.16 CTA of the aortic arch showing partially calcified plaque at the origin of the innominate artery (vertical arrow), smooth lipemic plaque of more than 4 mm thickness (lower paired arrows), and mixed, ulcerated plaque protruding into the aortic lumen with greater than 8 mm thickness (upper paired arrows).

which was not appreciated at that time (Figure 6.18). Retrospective analysis of the MRA of the neck at the time of the PCA infarction shows very subtle changes which failed to capture the significance of the lesions (Figure 6.19).

This patient suffered not recurrent stroke but recurrent systemic embolism from severe aortic atherosclerosis. This condition was not recognized at the time of the patient's embolic PCA stroke. Neither was it

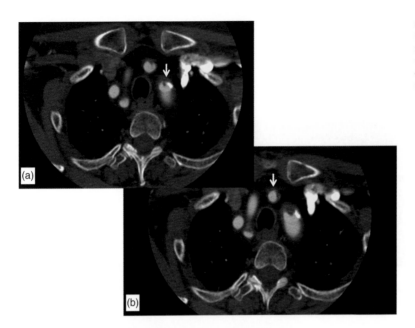

Figure 6.17 Successive CTA source images at the roof of the aortic arch showing the origins of the left subclavian (arrow in a) and left common carotid artery (arrow in b). Severe atherosclerotic plaque is present in abundance.

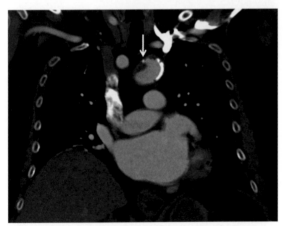

Figure 6.18 CTA of thorax obtained immediately after brachial arteriotomy. Coronal section shows large irregular plaque at the apex of the aortic arch measuring 8 mm in this slice (arrow).

specifically recognized by the surgical team or the radiologist following systemic embolization. First we will review the-related pitfalls to diagnosis. We will then review the importance of identifying aortic arch disease as a significant cause of ischemic stroke. Finally, we will discuss what is known regarding therapy for aortic atheromatous disease, an area that still contains much uncertainty.

The importance of disease of the aortic arch was not well recognized until the 1990s. Postmortem pathological studies demonstrated that severe atherosclerotic disease was commonly present in patients who had suffered major ischemic strokes but failed to demonstrate convincing disease elsewhere. Transesophageal echocardiography (TEE) provided a less invasive, reliable means of detecting aortic atherosclerosis and studies relying on TEE demonstrated that severe atherosclerosis with measured plaque thickness of 4 mm or more was associated with a high rate of stroke recurrence, almost 12% annually. A combined vascular event rate (ischemic stroke, myocardial infarction, peripheral vascular occlusions, or vascular death of 26% annually in these patients was particularly alarming [18]. An exact estimate of the contribution of aortic atherosclerosis to the burden of ischemic heart disease remains uncertain; however, some estimates place it at levels nearly equal to either cardioembolism or other large artery embolism. Approximately one-third of all ischemic strokes are of uncertain etiology, and about one-third of these, 10% of the total ischemic stroke burden, may be accounted for by severe aortic atherosclerosis [198].

The traditional gold standard for demonstrating aortic arch atherosclerosis is TEE. TEE does, however, have limitations as it is invasive, operator-dependent, and has a modestly limited field of view due to tracheal shadowing. CTA appears to be an excellent screening tool [20] and as methodology advances, may become in some ways superior to TEE [21]. As our case

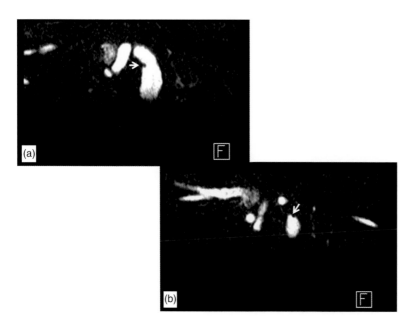

Figure 6.19 2D time-of-flight MRA source images showing small defects in the mid- aortic arch (a) and near the left subclavian origin (b). These small luminal abnormalities closely match the well-seen aortic wall abnormalities in Figures 6.16 and 6.17b.

demonstrates, severe arch disease can easily be overlooked by standardly available MRA technique.

It would be tempting to conclude that our patient's second ischemic event, embolism to the branches of the right subclavian artery, could have been prevented by "correct therapy." Unfortunately, this would be overstating the current state of our knowledge. Traditionally, most experts have chosen warfarin for secondary prevention in cases of aortic arch atheroma. A recently completed randomized trial comparing warfarin to the combination of aspirin and clopidogrel failed to reach conclusive results [22]. A decrease in vascular death was seen with dual antiplatelet therapy, but the primary endpoint of decreased vascular events combined suggested that dual antiplatelet might be more effective as a trend but was not statistically significant. Of great interest in this recently completed trial was the fact that the expected event rates of 12% annually, which was thought to be a conservative estimate when the trial was initiated, proved to be a large overestimate. Instead, expected ischemic stroke rates were decreased to 3.5% per year. This finding is similar to those of other recent stroke trials, where smaller than expected event rates were recorded when compared with event rates in comparable trials 15 to 20 years previously [23]. Better blood pressure control and the use of statins may have contributed significantly to these observed improvements. Statin therapy for aortic atherosclerosis is well established [24] and aggressive therapy is now a

guideline recommendation [25]. For the moment, dual antiplatelet therapy and high dose statin may be the preferred modality while trials including novel anticoagulants are being considered.

As a final point, this patient suffered subtle but important cognitive dysfunction as a consequence of her left PCA territory infarction. Severe impairment of both cognition and arousal are a well-known consequence of PCA infarction when the ipsilateral thalamus is involved. Involvement of the basal and mesial temporal lobe is associated with significant cognitive deficits which are too often overlooked. These patients almost always have more than just a visual field deficit. Cognitive impairments include visual memory, visual recognition, and verbal memory deficits that are important to recognize and are amenable to therapy [26,27].

Case 6. More aortic arch atheroma

A 66-year-old man developed sudden onset of chest pain during his habitual morning walk. He described a pressure-like sensation in the middle of his chest. The pain lasted about 20 minutes. He was not short of breath or diaphoretic. He experienced transient numbness in his left hand at that time and also headache. His symptoms were largely resolved by the time he arrived at our ED. There, the patient received a single injection of intravenous morphine which relieved his chest pain

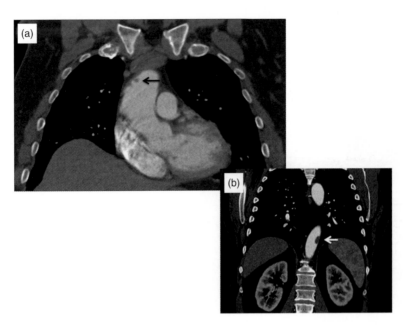

Figure 6.20 Coronal reconstructions of CTA of chest showing frond-like intraluminal thrombi in ascending aorta (a, black arrow) and elliptical thrombus in thoracic aorta (b, white arrow).

completely. He was minimally hypertensive but he rapidly became normotensive with relief of his pain. He was afebrile. Because of a history of ascending aortic aneurysm (dilatation) the ED physician obtained a CTA of the chest. This showed no change in ascending aortic diameter. However, there were multiple mural thrombi projecting into the aortic lumen at the top of the aortic arch and an ellipsoid thrombus in the descending thoracic aorta (Figure 6.20). Troponins were not elevated, and the patient was admitted to the General Medicine Service. Also noted at that time was a platelet count of 1 150 000 (K/µL) and a white blood cell count of 23 800 (K/µL). The patient was continued on 81 mg of aspirin daily and 40 mg of simvastatin daily. He had a complaint of ear pain and it was thought that he had an incompletely treated otitis media. He was placed on oral amoxicillin/clavulanic acid as well. Cardiovascular surgery and hematology consultations were placed and a transesophageal echocardiogram was scheduled for the following morning.

In addition to the history of a modest, 4.2 cm ascending aortic aneurysm, the patient had a history of arterial hypertension and hyperlipidemia. The patient had undergone a procedure for arthritis of the knee months earlier, which continued to cause him pain and had been intermittently infected. There was a history of thrombocytosis for which he was followed by observation only. He also had periodic headaches with migrainous features. He had a prior history of incompletely

explained paroxysmal chest pain. Coronary angiography had been performed 6 months prior to this admission and was reportedly without notable disease ("clean coronaries"). The second scheduled troponin measurement demonstrated an elevation to 2.71, he was diagnosed with a non-ST elevation myocardial infarction (NSTEMI), and a heparin drip was initiated.

Shortly after 5 p.m. that same day, the patient developed sudden numbness of his left hand, left facial droop, and dysarthria. A stroke emergency was called. Neurology noted mild left facial weakness and dysarthria as well as subjective paresthesias of the left hand. NIHSS score was 2. He again had a mild headache. Emergent head CT was felt to be unremarkable, without evidence of bleeding. The patient's symptoms resolved after about 20 minutes, and he was transferred to the neuroscience intensive care unit with a presumptive clinical diagnosis of TIA. Intravenous fluids were increased. Additional aspirin was given, simvastatin was continued, and after discussion with Hematology, hydroxyurea which had been initiated when the elevated troponins returned, was increased in dose, allopurinol was added, and MRI of the brain was urgently obtained. MRI brain demonstrated a number of small mostly punctate restrictions consistent with embolism. Some of these were scattered along the right MCA territory boundary zone and some nearer to the cortical surface including one punctate diffusion restriction just posterior to the primary sensory cortex at a

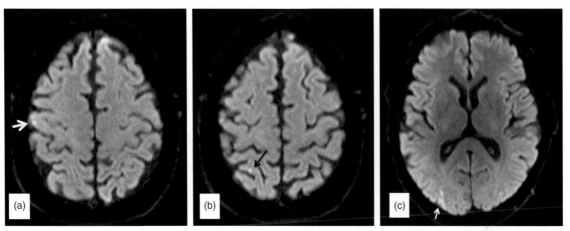

Figure 6.21 Arrows indicate punctate DWI lesions at the cortical rim (a), immediately posterior to the sensory strip (b), and a band extending along the posterior MCA border zone (c).

location in the sensory homunculus approximating the left hand (Figure 6.21). The patient was maintained on a heparin drip for the next several days. Troponin values rapidly returned to baseline, platelet count descended to 760 000, headache resolved, and intermittent left hand paresthesias ceased. TEE demonstrated a mobile mass in the descending aorta but visualized no disease in the aortic arch. Devoted cardiac CTA confirmed thrombus in the aortic arch, reconfirmed a thrombus in the ascending aorta but noted no disease in the coronary vessels. A bone marrow biopsy was obtained and demonstrated a myeloproliferative disorder consistent with essential thrombocytosis (ET) and myelofibrosis. The JAK-2 mutation was absent. The patient was discharged on enoxaparin 1 mg/kg twice daily and clopidogrel in place of aspirin. Two weeks later, a platelet count of 250 000 was measured. The patient had no paresthesias, headache, or chest pain. Enoxaparin was discontinued, aspirin 81 mg resumed and clopidogrel continued. Three months later, CTA of the chest demonstrated complete resolution of the aortic arch and thoracic aorta thrombi although small and splenic infarcts were noted. The patient has been followed for an additional 2 years without recurrence of chest pain or new neurologic symptoms other than a rare, mild headache. Hydroxyurea has been continued in moderating doses, platelet counts have remained well within normal limits, and dual antiplatelet therapy has been continued according to acute coronary syndrome guidelines.

A review of prior medical records disclosed that the patient had been admitted to this hospital 16 months earlier for an episode of sudden lightheadedness and diffuse weakness on arising from a chair. He did not lose consciousness but did need to hold onto a wall to allow himself to slide to the floor without injury. He had transient nausea and persistent chest tightness. In the ED, troponin was not elevated and ECG showed evidence of acute ischemia and no changes otherwise. CTA of the chest was obtained and showed no change in the ascending aortic aneurysm which by that time had been followed for over 4 years. CT did show a spherical mass within the aorta (Figure 6.22). Differential diagnosis for this mass ranged from thrombus to neoplasm. The interpreting radiologist was particularly concerned by "fat stranding" in the mediastinum immediately adjoining the intra-aortic mass. The patient's symptoms resolved completely. A follow-up TEE failed to demonstrate a mass. The patient was discharged after he declined to undergo gated cardiac MRI. Platelet count at that time was 846 000. In retrospect, it is abundantly apparent that this was a thrombus very similar in appearance to the thoracic aortic thrombus seen at a different location 14 months later.

Lessons to be learned from this case are many. Vascular problems can be both cerebral and systemic and so a patient's problems must be considered in their entirety. Our attention should never be limited to a single system. This patient presented with chest pain, headache, and focal paresthesias and just a few hours later developed more easily recognized cerebral ischemia. Both coronary ischemia and cerebral ischemia were in turn secondary to ET. Interestingly, the most common cause of coronary ischemia is disease of the coronary

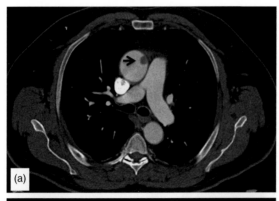

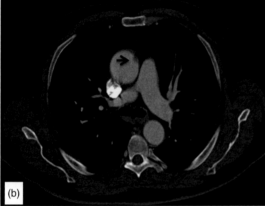

Figure 6.22 CTA of chest axial views showing intraluminal ascending aortic arch thrombus (arrow) present 14 months prior to stroke and MI (a) and likely remnant of the same thrombus on the day of stroke and NSTEMI (b).

arteries. In this instance, however, coronary ischemia was due to embolism. The most common cause of cerebral ischemia is embolism when large artery embolism and cardiac embolism are taken together.

We generally and appropriately do not consider unusual causes of stroke (i.e., "stroke in the young") in patients in their 60s, especially those with traditional stroke risk factors such as hypertension and hyperlipidemia. In this instance, however, cerebral embolism was due to an uncommon cause, ET. Although most patients with ET are asymptomatic at diagnosis, ET is associated with both arterial and venous thromboembolism, with arterial embolism being nearly twice as frequent. ET can present with ischemic stroke as a first manifestation [28]. Thrombosis is the major immediate cause of morbidity and mortality in ET while age greater than 60 and prior thrombotic events remain the best predictors of thrombotic events [29] and prompts definitive treatment [30]. Additionally, thrombotic

events in ET may be either macro- or microvascular. Included among the latter are headache, chest pain, and syncope, which we recognize in retrospect were the presenting symptoms in our patient 14 months before MI and ischemic stroke co-occurred.

As discussed in Case 5, cerebral embolism from the aortic arch may be underrecognized. In this fortunate case, the dangers of aortic arch intraluminal thrombus were recognized 14 months after thrombus was initially demonstrated on CTA. TEE is the traditionally accepted gold standard in detecting aortic arch atherosclerosis and intraluminal thrombus. CTA is only now being recognized as an important means of detection [21]. This is probably the case because of significant technical refinements over the past decade. As this case vividly demonstrates, TEE can repeatedly miss proximal aortic arch disease with its associated large stroke risk, probably because of tracheal air column interference [31].

References

1. Johnston SC, Nguyen-Huynh MN, Schwarz ME, et al. National Stroke Association guidelines for the management of transient ischemic attacks. *Ann Neurol* 2006;60(3):301–13.

2. Johnston S, Rothwell PM, Nguyen-Huynh MN, et al. Validation and refinement of scores to predict very early stroke risk after transient ischaemic attack. *Lancet* 2007;369(9558):283–92.

3. Lovett JK, Gallagher PJ, Hands LJ, et al. Histological correlates of carotid plaque surface morphology on lumen contrast imaging. *Circulation* 2004;110(15):2190–7.

4. Johnston SC, Gress DR, Browner WS, Sidney S. Short-term prognosis after emergency department diagnosis of TIA. *JAMA* 2000;284(22):2901–6.

5. Lovett JK, Coull AJ, Rothwell PM. Early risk of recurrence by subtype of ischemic stroke in population-based incidence studies. *Neurology* 2004;62(4):569–73.

6. Ois A, Gomis M, Rodríguez-Campello A, et al. Factors associated with a high risk of recurrence in patients with transient ischemic attack or minor stroke. *Stroke* 2008;39(6):1717–21.

7. Eliasziw M, Streifler JY, Fox AJ, et al. Significance of plaque ulceration in symptomatic patients with high-grade carotid stenosis. North American Symptomatic Carotid Endarterectomy Trial. *Stroke* 1994;25(2):304–8.

8. Coutts SB, Modi J, Patel SK, et al. CT/CT angiography and MRI findings predict recurrent stroke after transient

ischemic attack and minor stroke. Results of the Prospective CATCH Study. *Stroke* 2012;43(4):1013–17.

9. Rothwell PM, Eliasziw M, Gutnikov SA, et al. Analysis of pooled data from the randomised controlled trials of endarterectomy for symptomatic carotid stenosis. *Lancet* 2003;361(9352):107–16.

10. Suri MFK, Johnston SC Epidemiology of intracranial stenosis. *J Neuroimaging* 2009;19(S1):11S–16S.

11. Lau AY, Wong KSL, Lev M, et al. Burden of intracranial steno-occlusive lesions on initial computed tomography angiography predicts poor outcome in patients with acute stroke. *Stroke* 2013;44(5):1310–16.

12. Back MR, Wilson JS, Rushing G, et al. Magnetic resonance angiography is an accurate imaging adjunct to duplex ultrasound scan in patient selection for carotid endarterectomy. *J Vasc Surg* 2000;32(3):429–40.

13. Chaturvedi S, Bruno A, Feasby T, et al. Carotid endarterectomy – an evidence-based review. Report of the Therapeutics and Technology Assessment Subcommittee of the American Academy of Neurology. *Neurology* 2005;65(6): 794–801.

14. Jung JM, Kang DW, Yu KH, et al. Predictors of recurrent stroke in patients with symptomatic intracranial arterial stenosis. *Stroke* 2012;43(10):2785–7.

15. Gorelick PB, Wong KS, Bae HJ, Pandey DK. Large artery intracranial occlusive disease a large worldwide burden but a relatively neglected frontier. *Stroke* 2008;39(8):2396–9.

16. Degnan AJ, Gallagher G, Teng Z, et al. MR angiography and imaging for the evaluation of middle cerebral artery atherosclerotic disease. *Am J Neuroradiol* 2012;3(8):1427–35.

17. Chimowitz MI, Lynn MJ, Derdeyn CP, et al. Stenting versus aggressive medical therapy for intracranial arterial stenosis. *N Engl J Med* 2011;365(11):993–1003.

18. The French Study of Aortic Plaques in Stroke Group. Atherosclerotic disease of the aortic arch as a risk factor for recurrent ischemic stroke. *N Engl J Med* 1996;334:1216–21.

19. Di Tullio MR, Sacco RL, Homma S. Atherosclerotic disease of the aortic arch as a risk factor for recurrent ischemic stroke. *N Engl J Med* 1996;335(1464):1464–5.

20. Barazangi N, Wintermark M, Lease K, et al. Comparison of computed tomography angiography and transesophageal echocardiography for evaluating aortic arch disease. *J Stroke Cerebrovasc Dis* 2011;20 (5):436–42.

21. Ko Y, Park JH, Yang MH, et al. Significance of aortic atherosclerotic disease in possibly embolic stroke: 64-multidetector row computed tomography study. *J Neurol* 2010;257(5):699–705.

22. Amarenco P, Davis S, Jones EF, et al. Clopidogrel plus aspirin versus warfarin in patients with stroke and aortic arch plaques. *Stroke* 2014;45(5):1248–57.

23. George PM, Albers GW. Aortic Arch Atheroma A Plaque of a Different Color or More of the Same?. *Stroke* 2014;45(5):1239–40.

24. Tunick PA, Nayar AC, Goodkin GM, et al. Effect of treatment on the incidence of stroke and other emboli in 519 patients with severe thoracic aortic plaque. *Am J Cardiol* 2002;90(12):1320–5.

25. Hiratzka LF, Bakris GL, Beckman, JA, et al. 2010 ACCF/AHA/AATS/ACR/ASA/SCA/SCAI/SIR/STS/SVM Guidelines for the diagnosis and management of patients with thoracic aortic disease. *J Am Coll Cardiol* 2010;55(14):e27–e129.

26. Brandt T, Steinke W, Thie A, et al. Posterior cerebral artery territory infarcts: clinical features, infarct topography, causes and outcome 1. *Cerebrovasc Dis* 2000;10(3):170–82.

27. Park KC, Yoon SS, Rhee HY. Executive dysfunction associated with stroke in the posterior cerebral artery territory. *J Clin Neurosci* 2011;18(2):203–8.

28. Arboix A, Besses C, Acín P, et al. Ischemic stroke as first manifestation of essential thrombocythemia. Report of six cases. *Stroke* 1995;26(8):1463–6.

29. Bleeker JS, Hogan WJ. Thrombocytosis: diagnostic evaluation, thrombotic risk stratification, and risk-based management strategies. *Thrombosis* 2011, Article ID 536062.

30. Cortelazzo S, Finazzi G, Ruggeri M, et al. Hydroxyurea for patients with essential thrombocythemia and a high risk of thrombosis. *N Engl J Med* 1995;332(17):1132–7.

31. Krinsky GA, Freedberg R, Lee VS, et al. Innominate artery atheroma: a lesion seen with gadolinium-enhanced MR angiography and often missed by transesophageal echocardiography. *Clin Imaging* 2001;25(4):251–7.

Common pitfalls in intravenous thrombolysis for acute ischemic stroke

Shyam Prabhakaran

Introduction

Acute ischemic stroke is a major cause of adult disability in the United States (US) [1]. Though many strategies exist for primary and secondary stroke prevention, only one drug has been approved for acute treatment: intravenous (IV) tissue plasminogen activator (tPA). Yet, only a minority of patients in the US and far fewer worldwide receive the medication [2]. Though delay in patient arrival is the main reason cited for this dismal statistic, other factors including physician knowledge, perceptions and fears, hospital delays, and lack of clarity and confusion about inclusion and exclusion criteria may also be implicated. The complex decision-making is further compounded by the lack of a practical "gold standard" diagnostic test for ischemic stroke in the hyperacute setting that places a premium on accurate clinical diagnostic skills. Other dilemmas and pitfalls occur after tPA administration and include monitoring for rare but serious complications. In this review, cases will be presented that illuminate several of these common pitfalls and provide tips on avoiding the "traps."

Case 1. Accurate history

Case description

A 55-year-old man with hypertension and smoking history was noted by his wife at 8 a.m. to be unable to understand her or speak clearly. He was brought in by ambulance and arrived at 8:30 a.m. Initial blood pressure was 175/95 mmHg and computed tomography (CT) of the head was normal. He was unable to provide any meaningful history due to the receptive aphasia. His wife noted, however, that he was in his usual state of health the prior evening when they went for dinner and

retired to bed around 11 p.m. In the morning, when she awoke at 7 a.m., her husband was not in the bedroom. He was later seen in the living room, lying on the sofa, which was unusual for him on a weekday. After she finally had occasion to speak with him at 8 a.m., she immediately noted that his speech was nonsensical. Given that the time of last known normal was perhaps as long as 9 hours earlier (11 p.m.) and without another account that could shorten the time window to within the previous 4.5 hours, the treating physician decided against tPA administration. Later that evening, after admission to the stroke unit, neurologic consultation ascertained through the wife and her review of her husband's cell phone records concluded that the patient spoke with his son by phone around 7:30 a.m. The son was able to verify that his father was speaking normally at that time as they made plans for the following day.

Discussion

Not uncommonly, key historical data are not available directly from the patient due to neurologic deficits such as aphasia or coma. In this instance, the critical information related to time of last known normal or presumed stroke onset time. A frequent error made by physicians is equating onset time as discovery time. While in many instances these are identical (i.e., as in witnessed onset of stroke symptoms), patients in whom symptoms are noted with wakefulness (i.e., wake-up stroke) represent about 25% of all stroke patients [3]. For these patients, studies suggest that the majority likely had symptoms that began shortly before awakening; however, the exact time can only be estimated with modest accuracy, even with advanced imaging [4]. Outside of clinical trials evaluating imaging-based selection of wake-up stroke patients for thrombolysis, a conservative approach must be taken that assumes the

Common Pitfalls in Cerebrovascular Disease: Case-Based Learning, ed. José Biller and José M. Ferro. Published by Cambridge University Press. © Cambridge University Press 2015.

last known normal time to be time of stroke symptom onset. Obtaining advanced neuroimaging that could delay time to tPA treatment is not recommended.

In this case, attempting to gain historical data from family members was not initially attempted. The initial interview in the emergency department (ED) suggested the patient was ineligible based on an erroneous last known normal determination. However, verification of the timeline and potential collateral history using cell phone call inventories and contacting other family, friends, neighbors, and colleagues are useful strategies in these situations. A thorough investigative approach in this case altered the time of onset from 11 p.m. the prior evening to 7:30 a.m. the morning of the stroke. Such information, if available during the hyperacute evaluation, would have changed the course of management. He was, in fact, eligible for IV tPA and could have been treated within the 3-hour window. Compared to placebo, IV tPA if provided within 3 hours of stroke onset affords an absolute 12% improved chance of minimal or no disability at 3 months [5].

Tip

It is critical that a thorough questioning be made of all witnesses, family members, and friends to ascertain the best estimate of last known normal in patients with wake-up stroke and who cannot provide the history themselves. Any evidence that "moves the clock" forward could help re-classify a patient initially ineligible for thrombolysis as eligible.

Case 2. Basilar artery thrombosis

Case description

A 29-year-old woman without known medical history presented to the hospital after her roommate found her unresponsive in their apartment. The woman reportedly was well and last seen to be normal that afternoon at work, where she departed for home at 5:15 p.m. Her roommate found her around 7 p.m. lying on the floor. There were no external signs of trauma. Emergency medical services (EMS) arrived around 7:15 p.m. and noted that she was having spasms of both arms and that her eyes were crossed. They administered lorazepam 1 mg intravenously and brought her to the ED. Her initial blood pressure was elevated at 160/90 mmHg and she was noted to have posturing motions of her limbs that were triggered by even slight tactile stimulation. Initial examination was notable for dysconjugate or

skewed eyes and limited upgaze, fixed pinpoint pupils, and no response to pain except for bilateral extensor posturing. A head CT was negative for intracranial hemorrhage. She was intubated for airway protection, treated with phenytoin loading intravenously, and admitted to the intensive care unit. Upon neurologic consultation the next day, her roommate provided no history of seizure disorder, drug abuse, or recent exposures but noted that the patient had been complaining of some neck pain for about 1 week. She remained comatose and exam was unchanged despite phenytoin loading. MRI of the brain (Figure 7.1a) was performed and showed extensive bilateral midbrain and pontine and scattered left temporal occipital infarcts on diffusion-weighted imaging (DWI). MRA of the head and neck demonstrated no flow in the distal basilar artery and irregular stenosis in the proximal left vertebral artery suggestive of dissection. The patient remained on the ventilator, ultimately required a tracheostomy and gastrostomy, and was discharged to a long-term nursing facility. She regained eye opening but was not interactive with her environment or capable or moving her limbs voluntarily at 3-month follow-up.

Discussion

Basilar artery occlusion is associated with significant morbidity and mortality, especially in the absence of recanalization [6]. Identifying basilar artery thrombosis can be challenging and confusing. The symptoms may vary from very mild presentations such as slurred speech to very severe ones such as coma; in other patients, symptoms may be vaguely characterized or bizarre (i.e., behavioral symptoms such as agitated delirium or hallucinosis). Some patients may present with focal deficits initially and cause clinicians to consider lacunar or hemispheric localization. The so-called herald hemiparesis that was described by C. Miller Fisher refers to such a presentation whereby initial hemiparesis leads subsequently to bilateral symptoms including locked-in state, coma, or death [7]. Greater recognition and urgency in stuttering or gradual onset presentations are critical to early diagnosis and management of this condition.

Not uncommonly, cognitive anchoring can occur in acute neurologic diagnostic formulation when clinicians over-emphasize certain details of the presentation and/or ignore others, having already approached the patient with preconceived biases and expectations [8]. In this instance, the presumed diagnosis in

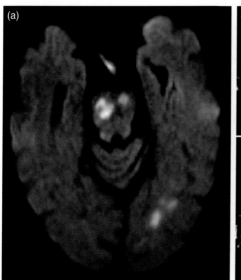 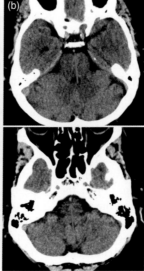

Figure 7.1 (a) Bilateral pontine and left temporo-occipital infarcts on diffusion-weighted imaging consistent with acute infarct in basilar artery and posterior cerebral artery territories. (b) Dense basilar artery on initial CT head (arrows).

a young, previously healthy woman who is unresponsive and posturing is often seizures or toxic exposure. While this patient displayed no seizure activity (i.e., actual convulsions), it should be noted that extensor posturing can be frequently confused with seizures by untrained witnesses and even physicians [9].

Several other clinical clues, however, suggested basilar artery thrombosis. First, fixed pinpoint pupils and limited upgaze are indicative of pontine and midbrain injury, respectively. This should not be confused with pinpoint pupils that are observed with opiate intoxication. A rapid urine drug screen could exclude drug intoxication. Second, dysconjugate and skewed gaze is unusual in supratentorial or diffuse cerebral disorders such as hemispheric stroke, metabolic disturbances, and seizures. In seizures, conjugate gaze abnormalities are notable either in the active or ictal phase (away from the seizure focus) or in the post-ictal phase (toward the seizure focus if a Todd's paralysis is occurring). Lastly, formal neurologic assessment should include detailed brainstem function testing such as papillary, corneal, oculocephalic, oculovestibular, gag, and cough reflex testing in addition to motor response testing with noxious stimulation. These would localize the presentation to the bilateral pons in this patient.

Rapid imaging with CT head is essential to exclude hemorrhage and evaluate for early ischemic signs in the brainstem, cerebellum, thalami, and/or occipital lobes, and also assess for basilar artery thrombosis by dense artery identification. If early ischemic changes are present, these would indicate duration of ischemia of at least 6 hours duration. If CT head is normal, further imaging with MRI brain and MRA head and neck, if emergently available, or CT angiography of the head and neck, are mandatory. In this case, CT head was negative for hemorrhage but further review suggested a dense basilar artery was indeed present on the initial scan (Figure 7.1b).

Had the diagnosis of ischemic stroke been made in this case, the patient would have been eligible for intravenous thrombolysis with tPA. Though poor outcome (modified Rankin scale 4–6) occurred in more than two-thirds of patients, a recent prospective study found that IV tPA reduced the odds of poor outcome by 20% compared to antithrombotic therapy and was equivalent to intra-arterial or endovascular therapy [10]. These data suggest that recognition, early diagnosis, and thrombolytic treatment could reduce the disability and death associated with basilar artery thrombosis.

Tip

Diagnostic suspicion for basilar artery thrombosis should be high in any presentation of coma and tetraparesis given the high morbidity and mortality associated with the condition. Delay in diagnosis or misdiagnosis can have grave consequences. IV tPA, if provided within 3 hours, can improve outcomes and is recommended in all patients with suspected basilar artery thrombosis. Intra-arterial therapy is also reasonable and should be considered on a case-by-case basis.

Case 3. Rapidly improving symptoms

Case description

A 65-year-old woman with hypertension and diabetes presented with right hemiparesis that had been fluctuating since onset 1 hour earlier. Initially, she had stumbled to the floor at her home due to right leg weakness, noted her arm and leg could not move for 10 minutes, and then improved to the point she was able to walk to the other room and call the emergency services. Upon arrival in the ED, she had mild deficits with minimal right facial droop and right arm pronator drift (NIHSS score 2). Her blood pressure was 165/95 mmHg. She underwent prompt CT of the head, which was negative for brain hemorrhage or space-occupying lesion. Upon re-examination following the scan, however, she was noted to have right hemiplegia and significant dysarthria (NIHSS score 12). Intravenous fluids were started and the physician discussed the risks and benefits of tPA with the patient, who agreed with proceeding. Approximately 10 minutes later, the nurse notified the physician that her weakness had improved such that her NIHSS score was now 6 (facial droop 2, dysarthria 1, 2-right arm 2, right leg 1). The physician cancelled the tPA order on the basis that the patient had made a "rapid improvement," which disqualified her from thrombolysis. The patient remained stable in the ED but subsequently worsened on the ward with severe right hemiplegia again 12 hours after the initial onset. Imaging confirmed a left internal capsule infarct and work-up concluded that the mechanism was lacunar or small artery disease. She was discharged to acute inpatient rehabilitation with persistent right hemiplegia.

Discussion

Since its approval by the FDA in 1996, tPA use has been limited and even curtailed by misinterpretations of the many inclusion and exclusion criteria affixed to the drug label. Rapid improvement is one of the most common reasons for withholding thrombolysis in otherwise eligible patients [11]. The rationale for exclusion on this basis in the original trial was clear: to avoid treating patients with transient ischemic attack or non-disabling strokes (near complete or complete recovery) as they were expected to have excellent outcomes without treatment. However, substantial or dramatic improvement, rather than mild or moderate improvement, is required to satisfy this definition of rapid improvement and exclude a patient from thrombolysis. It should also be noted that early improvement often heralds subsequent deterioration [12], which has been speculated to be due to thrombus instability or collateral blood flow compromise. Patients with significant deficits despite moderate improvement, who are likely to be disabled at follow-up such as this patient, should be offered tPA.

The recent Re-examining Acute Eligibility for Thrombolysis (TREAT) taskforce unanimously recommended that patients with moderate–severe deficits who do not improve to non-disabling state should be offered IV tPA unless other contraindications are found [13]. Isolated symptoms such as moderate aphasia, hemianopsia, spatial neglect, and gait ataxia should be considered disabling and may justify thrombolysis. However, non-disabling deficits that should not be treated at this time pending ongoing trial evidence include isolated facial droop, non-dominant arm drift without hand weakness, hemisensory deficits without neglect, and isolated mild dysarthria (Table 7.1).

Table 7.1 Some examples of potential disabling versus likely non-disabling mild stroke presentations (NIHSS score <6)

Likely disabling	Likely non-disabling
Cortically blind (NIHSS score 3)	Isolated facial droop
Monoplegic or severely paretic arm or leg (NIHSS 2–4)	Mild hemimotor deficit (NIHSS score 2)
Complete hemianopsia (NIHSS score 2)	Partial or mild hemianopsia (NIHSS score 1)
Severe aphasia (NIHSS score 2)	Isolated mild aphasia (NIHSS score 1)
Neglect (NIHSS score 1 or 2)	Hemisensory deficit (NIHSS 1 or 2)
Gait or limb ataxia (NIHSS score 2)	Mild hemiataxia (NIHSS score 1)
Dominant cortical hand (NIHSS score 0)	Non-dominant cortical hand without drift (NIHSS score 0)

Furthermore, it was advised that clinicians not delay tPA administration to allow for continued extended observation or monitoring.

In patients who present with fluctuating lacunar stroke, the so-called capsular warning syndrome, wild fluctuations in severity have been known to occur, even within minutes. It is critical that such patients be carefully monitored for deterioration since the majority of such patients complete the stroke and are left with disabling deficits. It is imperative that treating physicians recognize that stroke patients will often fluctuate in the hyperacute setting, anticipate the potential for neurologic deterioration after initial improvement, and measure deficits for their impact on long-term disability when approaching thrombolysis decision-making.

Tip

Exclusion from thrombolysis by rapid improvement implies complete or near-complete recovery. It should not be applied in patients with mild or moderate fluctuations or improvements. Deferring treatment on the basis of mild or moderate improvement to a level that remains disabling is not advised given the likelihood of long-term disability. A suggested approach to determine whether symptoms may be disabling at the time of presentation is to consider whether the patient could perform basic activities of daily living (ADLs) and/or return to work. For example, a right-handed 55-year-old carpenter who has profound right-hand weakness without other deficits should be considered potentially disabled as it will likely impair performance of ADLs and recreational and vocational tasks.

Case 4. Misdiagnosis

Case description

A 70-year-old Chinese man with hypertension was brought in by his son who found the patient on the floor in the kitchen of their apartment at 9 p.m. He was last seen normal at 8:45 p.m. following dinner. He was Cantonese speaking only, appeared confused, and was unable to provide details of history. He was not moving his left arm and leg as briskly as the right side but had no facial droop. There was no gaze deviation, sensory loss, visual field cut, or neglect. His blood pressure initially was 100/70 mmHg. CT head showed no signs of intracranial hemorrhage or skull fracture though a small hematoma was noted beneath his scalp. Given the possible stroke diagnosis and since

he was within the 3-hour window, the neurology-on-call physician decided to treat with IV tPA. Three hours later, the patient developed some minor expansion of the left frontal subcutaneous hematoma requiring compression and also minor tongue and mouth bleeding but his exam remained unchanged with left-sided weakness and ataxia. The following morning, examination revealed he now had bilateral moderate arm and leg weakness, sensory changes to pinprick to the C7 level, and urinary retention. An emergent MRI of the brain and spine demonstrated mid-lower cervical cord edema along with ligamentous injury and paravertebral swelling at the same level secondary to acute trauma (Figure 7.2); no acute stroke was seen on brain imaging. Neurosurgery was consulted, tPA was reversed with cryoprecipitate, and he was taken to the operating room for spinal stabilization. Postoperatively, he continued to have mild to moderate quadriparesis and was ultimately discharged to an acute inpatient rehabilitation facility. Subsequent interviews with family informed the treating team that he regularly consumed large amounts of alcohol after dinner and that he was likely intoxicated leading to a mechanical fall in the kitchen.

Discussion

In this patient, an unwitnessed mechanical fall occurred leading to initial hemi-cord symptoms of arm and leg weakness. Recent intracranial or

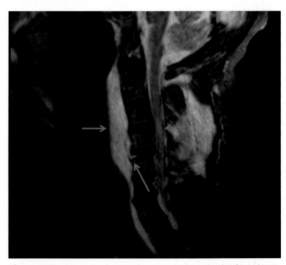

Figure 7.2 MRI cervical spine showing pre-vertebral soft tissue edema, C5–6 level ligamentous tear, and central cord edema (arrows).

intraspinal trauma is considered a contraindication to thrombolysis [14]. However, initial survey was negative for these major findings. Limited history and language barriers in the hyperacute setting further confused this situation as details of the onset of the symptoms were not assessed. Nevertheless, all efforts should be made to acquire pertinent historical details that would inform diagnosis and potentially important contraindications to thrombolysis. In this case, the absence of facial droop, the presence of mild (though at the time clinically ignored) weakness and ataxia on the right side, external trauma to the scalp, and relative hypotension should have alerted the neurologist to the possibility of mechanical fall leading to spinal cord injury.

The importance of reducing time to thrombolysis in acute ischemic stroke treatment is well-established [15] and the success of national quality initiatives to reduce door-to-needle (DTN) time has recently been demonstrated [16]. A potential unintended consequence of rapid thrombolysis is administration of tPA to non-vascular conditions that simulate stroke. While treatment of stroke mimics with IV tPA appears to have a low risk of complication [17], rare and serious complications could result in significant harm to patients without stroke [18].

This case provides a cautionary example of real harm that occurred as a result of initial diagnostic error that led to inappropriate thrombolytic decision-making. Given the emphasis on rapid diagnosis of stroke that relies completely on clinical skills of history and examination and does not provide the luxury of confirmatory tests that would force time delays, neurological examination and careful screening for potential harmful contraindications and stroke mimics is more relevant than ever before. While bedside tools to increase diagnostic certainty of stroke have been posited [19], no one score or finding can supplant clinical intuition, experience, and judgment.

Tip

Diagnostic error in hyperacute stroke evaluation can be extremely dangerous. While rapid neurologic assessment to reduce DTN times is increasingly emphasized, this should not be at the price of forgoing a detailed, focused history and careful physical examination. Attempts to ensure the diagnostic accuracy of stroke and exclude high-risk contraindications remain a priority in thrombolytic decision-making.

Case 5. Informed consent

Case description

A 45-year-old man presented with global aphasia and right hemiplegia. He was in a bank when bystanders witnessed him collapse to the ground. EMS was called immediately and he arrived in the emergency room within 30 minutes of symptom onset. Initial CT scan was negative for hemorrhage but showed a dense left middle cerebral artery sign. Laboratory tests were normal except mild hyperglycemia to 130 mg/dL. Examination noted severe aphasia (mute), left gaze deviation, right visual field deficit, right facial droop, and right hemiplegia (NIHSS score 25). No family was available and no contact information was discovered with the patient's belongings. The treating physician debated whether or not to give tPA without informed consent as the patient lacked decisional capacity and surrogates were not available. Concerned about the liability of administering the drug without informed consent, the physician decided against treatment. The patient developed severe brain edema over the course of 48 hours, requiring left hemicraniectomy for malignant cerebral infarction and edema to save his life. He later required a gastrostomy for nutrition and was discharged to a skilled nursing facility with persistent global aphasia and right hemiplegia.

Discussion

Decision capacity is often impaired in acute stroke patients due to aphasia, neglect, executive dysfunction affecting judgment, decreased level of arousal, and/or pre-existing cognitive impairment [20]. Proxy decision-making is therefore common. While in non-time critical medical scenarios, establishment of durable power of attorney or legal proxy for impaired patients is appropriate, these are rarely achieved, or for that matter, practical in time-critical diseases like stroke. Reasonable attempts, therefore, should be made to contact next of kin (wife, children, parents, siblings) and establish surrogate consent. In such situations when the patient lacks decisional capacity and a legally authorized representative or surrogate is unavailable, proceeding without informed consent is considered legal and ethical. Clear documentation of attempts to reach surrogates in a timely manner should be made in the medical record. Multiple organizations including the American Heart Association/American Stroke Association and American Academy of Neurology have statements regarding this practice [14]. It is advised that two physicians concur and document their decision to proceed without informed consent from patient or proxy given the benefits outweigh the risks and in keeping with reasonable decision-making by a majority of patients.

In a recent survey of older adults, over 75% expressed that they would want thrombolysis for acute ischemic stroke, a similar rate as expressed for cardio-pulmonary resuscitation for cardiac arrest [21]. These data support emergency exemption from informed consent in situations when patients are not capable of providing it and reasonable attempts to contact surrogates fail. Given the strong time dependency of the benefits of tPA in ischemic stroke, reasonable attempts to contact surrogates should not delay thrombolysis in eligible patients by more than 10 minutes.

In patients with decisional capacity or when surrogate consent is possible, informed consent should take place. However, it should be noted that informed consent does not equate with written or signed consent. The latter is discouraged since it may delay or deter thrombolysis needlessly. Rather, standardized and simple culturally adapted language explaining the risks and benefits of tPA and the importance of time should be conveyed verbally. Visual aids may facilitate the discussion and ensure patient or proxy understanding in an emergency setting [22].

Tip

Informed consent should be provided to all patients or legally authorized representatives whenever possible. However, exceptions to informed consent can be made when patients lack decisional capacity and reasonable attempts to contact proxies fail. It is important to document clearly the decision-making process. A statement as follows would suffice: "As an FDA approved therapy, IV tPA was emergently administered using implied consent since the patient does not have decisional capacity and surrogates are unavailable despite multiple attempts."

Case 6. Laboratory delays

Case description

An 83-year-old woman with hypertension presented to the ED at 11:30 p.m. with 2 hours of right arm and leg weakness and sensory loss and slurred speech. Initial examination confirmed right hemiparesis,

hemisensory loss, and dysarthria (NIHSS score 9); her blood pressure was 170/90 mmHg and fingerstick glucose was 111 mg/dL. She was taking only hydro-chlorothiazide for blood pressure. CT of the head was unremarkable except for mild cerebral atrophy and chronic mild-moderate leukoaraiosis. She was eligible for tPA and understood risks and benefits. However, before proceeding, the ED physician asked that laboratory tests for coagulation and complete blood count be drawn and sent to the laboratory. Despite "STAT" orders and rapid blood draw by an experienced nurse, the results were not available when the physician called for them at 12:30 a.m., the end of the 3-hour treatment window. Therefore, he decided against thrombolysis and counseled the patient that "the risks of treatment outweigh the benefits since you could bleed to death." Fifteen minutes later, her laboratory tests revealed normal platelet count and coagulation studies. The patient was admitted to the ward where her deficits persisted. At discharge, she was unable to walk and required acute inpatient rehabilitation.

Discussion

Typical laboratory testing for blood count, chemistry, and coagulation may require 45–60 minutes from initial draw to receipt and processing to final reporting. Current requirements for primary stroke centers mandate that rapid laboratory testing be available all hours of the day and results available within 45 minutes. However, recent guidelines and initiatives such as the Target Stroke Program have made clear recommendations that although laboratory tests are an important component of the initial diagnostic evaluation of suspected stroke patients, the only required laboratory value to inform thrombolytic decision-making in the vast majority of patients is a glucose level. A glucose value above 50 mg/dL is needed to exclude hypoglycemic attacks mimicking focal deficits of stroke.

Several studies have assessed the yield of finding unsuspected thrombocytopenia or coagulopathy in tPA eligible patients and determined its occurrence is extremely low (<0.5%) [23,24]. A screening checklist (Table 7.2) could be adopted to identify patient groups in whom laboratory results are required prior to tPA administration. Indications for obligatory laboratory test confirmation of coagulation status include patients taking traditional (i.e., heparin or warfarin) or novel (i.e., factor Xa or direct thrombin inhibitors) anticoagulants and patients in whom a high index of

Table 7.2 A checklist to determine pre-test probability of coagulopathy of thrombocytopenia and need for laboratory results prior to tPA administration

Question	Laboratory test required
Taking warfarin or novel anticoagulant?	Prothrombin time, partial thromboplastin time, international normalized ratio, thrombin time, factor Xa level
Taking heparin or low-molecular-weight heparinoid?	Partial thromboplastin time, factor Xa level
On hemodialysis or post-angiography?	Partial thromboplastin time
Active malignancy?	Prothrombin time, partial thromboplastin time, platelet count
Liver dysfunction?	Prothrombin time, partial thromboplastin time, platelet count
No medical history?	Prothrombin time, partial thromboplastin time, international normalized ratio, platelet count

suspicion exists for coagulopathy or thrombocytopenia. Point-of-care testing for these patients could offer a considerable time saving in these instances and avoid unnecessary delays while awaiting laboratory test results [25].

Thrombolytic efficacy is time dependent with rapid decline in benefit with increasing time from onset of symptoms. Given the considerable harm introduced by delaying treatment and the negligible risk (<0.5%) of inadvertently treating a patient with unsuspected thrombocytopenia or coagulopathy, it is recommended that physicians not delay tPA administration while awaiting laboratory test results in the vast majority of patients without suspicion of thrombocytopenia or coagulopathy.

Tip

Clinicians should consider the pre-test probability that a stroke patient eligible for tPA harbors a laboratory contraindication such as platelet count <100 000 or elevated international normalized ratio (INR) >1.7. Simple checklists of common conditions associated with these findings aid in decision-making. Clinicians should not delay tPA administration in otherwise eligible patients on the basis that complete laboratory results are not available.

Case 7. Orolingual angioedema

Case description

A 59-year-old man with hypertension presented with right hemiparesis and expressive aphasia. His symptoms started 2 hours earlier. His CT scan excluded hemorrhage and major early infarct signs and examination confirmed moderate deficits (NIHSS score 6 for

moderate expressive aphasia, right facial droop, and right arm weakness). He was treated with IV tPA within 3 hours of symptom onset. One hour after tPA infusion and while still in the emergency department awaiting admission to the intensive care unit, he was noted to have trouble breathing by the nurse. The physician evaluated and noticed labored breathing and swelling around the mouth and tongue. A respiratory code is activated and intubation is attempted without success. Fiberscopic views of the posterior pharynx revealed edema and near complete closure of the vocal cords. An emergent tracheostomy was performed, which was complicated by severe bleeding from the site and required fibrinolytic reversal with cryoprecipitate and platelets.

Discussion

Orolingual angioedema is a rare but potentially fatal complication of tPA treatment. Though its incidence is nearly as common as the more feared intracranial hemorrhage after tPA, angioedema is perhaps underreported and underdiagnosed. Its incidence ranges from 1% to 5% in the literature [26]. Anaphylactoid response to tPA includes vasodilation, urticaria, orolingual edema, and/or hypotension. However, since most cases are mild and transient occurring within hours of tPA infusion, it is likely that many such occurrences are simply missed. The association with premorbid angiotensin-converting enzyme inhibitor (ACEI) use and appearance contralateral to the ischemic hemisphere is well-established in multiple reports. Unless the astute clinician is aware of this unique complication and is specifically evaluating for its occurrence, only severe cases involving airway compromise will be detected, often too late.

All patients should, therefore, be monitored for angioedema post-tPA, especially within the first

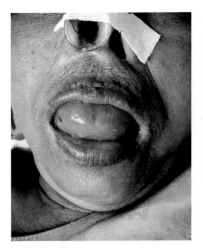 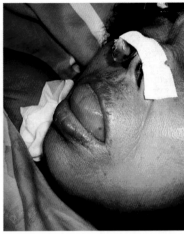

Figure 7.3 Severe example of orolingual angioedema.

several hours. Nurses and physicians should be trained to assess for subtle findings such as contralateral lip or tongue swelling. For mild cases, observation for airway compromise is essential. Histamine antagonists and corticosteroids may be considered. For moderate to severe cases (Figure 7.3), intravenous doses of diphenhydramine or ranitidine and methylprednisone should be administered. Epinephrine may also be required in severe cases. In patients with airway compromise, surgical services may be required including emergency consultation with anesthesiology for careful placement of endotracheal tube or tracheostomy when intubation is not possible. Reversal of tPA with crypoprecipitate and platelets is often needed given bleeding complications upon attempting intubation or tracheostomy.

Tip

Angioedema is not uncommon after tPA administration. The subtle features that typically involve the contralateral oropharynx, lips, and tongue need to be assessed at the bedside in the immediate hours after thrombolysis. In particular, infarcts that involve the frontal and insular cortices have been associated with this occurrence. A strong risk factor is baseline ACEI use and should mark those patients in whom heightened surveillance is mandatory. Moderate to severe presentations of orolingual angioedema require prompt intervention to avoid catastrophic outcomes.

References

1. Go AS, Mozaffarian D, Roger VL, et al. Heart disease and stroke statistics–2013 update: a report from the American Heart Association. *Circulation* 2013;127(1):e6–e245.

2. Schwamm LH, Ali SF, Reeves MJ, et al. Temporal trends in patient characteristics and treatment with intravenous thrombolysis among acute ischemic stroke patients at get with the guidelines-stroke hospitals. *Circ Cardiovasc Qual Outcomes* 2013;6:543–9.

3. Rimmele DL, Thomalla G. Wake-up stroke: clinical characteristics, imaging findings, and treatment option – an update. *Front Neurol* 2014;5:35.

4. Cheng B, Brinkmann M, Forkert ND, et al. Quantitative measurements of relative fluid-attenuated inversion recovery (FLAIR) signal intensities in acute stroke for the prediction of time from symptom onset. *J Cereb Blood Flow Metab* 2013;33(1):76–84.

5. The National Institute of Neurological Disorders and Stroke rt-PA Stroke Study Group. Tissue plasminogen activator for acute ischemic stroke. *N Engl J Med* 1995;333(24):1581–7.

6. Lindsberg PJ, Sairanen T, Strbian D, Kaste M. Current treatment of basilar artery occlusion. *Ann N Y Acad Sci* 2012;1268:35–44.

7. Fisher CM. The herald hemiparesis of basilar artery occlusion. *Arch Neurol* 1988;45(12):1301–3.

8. Brosinski CM. Implementing diagnostic reasoning to differentiate Todd's paralysis from acute ischemic stroke. *Adv Emerg Nurs J* 2014 Jan–Mar; 36(1): 78–86.

9. Ropper AH. Convulsions in basilar artery occlusion. *Neurology* 1988;38(9):1500–1.

10. Schonewille WJ, Wijman CA, Michel P, et al. Treatment and outcomes of acute basilar artery occlusion in the Basilar Artery International Cooperation Study (BASICS): a prospective registry study. *Lancet Neurol* 2009;8(8):724–30.

11. Barber PA, Zhang J, Demchuk AM, Hill MD, Buchan AM. Why are stroke patients excluded from TPA therapy? An analysis of patient eligibility. *Neurology* 2001;56(8):1015–20.

12. Smith EE, Fonarow GC, Reeves MJ, et al. Outcomes in mild or rapidly improving stroke not treated with intravenous recombinant tissue-type plasminogen activator: findings from Get With The Guidelines-Stroke. *Stroke* 2011;42(11):3110–15.

13. Levine SR, Khatri P, Broderick JP, et al. Review, historical context, and clarifications of the NINDS rt-PA stroke trials exclusion criteria: Part 1: rapidly improving stroke symptoms. *Stroke* 2013;44(9):2500–5.

14. Jauch EC, Saver JL, Adams HP, Jr., et al. Guidelines for the early management of patients with acute ischemic stroke: a guideline for healthcare professionals from the American Heart Association/American Stroke Association. *Stroke* 2013;44(3):870–947.

15. Lees KR, Bluhmki E, von Kummer R, et al. Time to treatment with intravenous alteplase and outcome in stroke: an updated pooled analysis of ECASS, ATLANTIS, NINDS, and EPITHET trials. *Lancet* 2010;375(9727):1695–703.

16. Fonarow GC, Zhao X, Smith EE, et al. Door-to-needle times for tissue plasminogen activator administration and clinical outcomes in acute ischemic stroke before and after a quality improvement initiative. *JAMA* 2014;311(16):1632–40.

17. Zinkstok SM, Engelter ST, Gensicke H, et al. Safety of thrombolysis in stroke mimics: results from a multicenter cohort study. *Stroke* 2013;44(4):1080–4.

18. Saver JL, Barsan WG. Swift or sure?: The acceptable rate of neurovascular mimics among IV tPA-treated patients. *Neurology* 2010;74(17):1336–7.

19. Hand PJ, Kwan J, Lindley RI, Dennis MS, Wardlaw JM. Distinguishing between stroke and mimic at the bedside: the brain attack study. *Stroke* 2006;37(3):769–75.

20. White-Bateman SR, Schumacher HC, Sacco RL, Appelbaum PS. Consent for intravenous thrombolysis in acute stroke: review and future directions. *Arch Neurol* 2007;64:785–92.

21. Chiong W, Kim AS, Huang IA, Farahany NA, Josephson SA. Inability to consent does not diminish the desirability of stroke thrombolysis. *Ann Neurol* 2014;76(2):296–304.

22. Gadhia J, Starkman S, Ovbiagele B, Ali L, Liebeskind D, Saver JL. Assessment and improvement of figures to visually convey benefit and risk of stroke thrombolysis. *Stroke* 2010;41:300–6.

23. Rost NS, Masrur S, Pervez MA, Viswanathan A, Schwamm LH. Unsuspected coagulopathy rarely prevents IV thrombolysis in acute ischemic stroke. *Neurology* 2009;73(23):1957–62.

24. Cucchiara BL, Jackson B, Weiner M, Messe SR. Usefulness of checking platelet count before thrombolysis in acute ischemic stroke. *Stroke* 2007;38(5):1639–40.

25. Walter S, Kostopoulos P, Haass A, et al. Point-of-care laboratory halves door-to-therapy-decision time in acute stroke. *Ann Neurol* 2011;69:581–6.

26. Lin SY, Tang SC, Tsai LK, et al. Orolingual angioedema after alteplase therapy of acute ischaemic stroke: incidence and risk of prior angiotensin-converting enzyme inhibitor use. *Eur J Neurol* 2014;21(10):1285–91.

Dilemmas in endovascular stroke therapy

David A. Stidd, Erwin Z. Mangubat, and Demetrius K. Lopes

Introduction

Historical data have shown that large cerebral artery occlusion is a devastating disease associated with a poor clinical outcome [1]. Fortunately, management of acute ischemic stroke (AIS) has had major transformative changes over the last two decades starting with the transition from supportive medical care to intervention with intravenous (IV) thrombolysis. In 1995, a landmark prospective randomized trial demonstrated a 39% favorable outcome defined as a modified Rankin scale (mRS) of 1 or less at 90 days for acute stroke patients treated with IV tissue plasminogen activator (tPA) within 3 hours of symptom onset relative to the 26% favorable outcome observed for the placebo group [2]. The therapeutic window for IV tPA was later extended to 4.5 hours in 2009 by the American Heart Association/American Stroke Association (AHA/ASA) with additional exclusion criteria [3]. However, recanalization rates of large cerebral artery occlusion are as low as 10% using IV tPA alone [4].

Introduced in 1999, the first endovascular therapy for AIS was intra-arterial chemical thrombolysis with the advantage of delivering a lower dose of a thrombolytic agent directly to the clot, and safely extending the therapeutic window up to 6 hours after symptom onset [1]. However, this treatment option has not been widely adopted into clinical practice. Despite the major advances in stroke management, multiple barriers exist for thrombolytic therapy including delayed recognition of AIS, delayed presentation, and multiple contraindications to systemic thrombolytic treatment [5]. Currently, it is estimated that only 2% of patients presenting with AIS are treated with IV tPA [6].

Rapid technological developments over the past 10 years have made mechanical thrombectomy an increasingly important option for the management of AIS. Recent results from the Interventional Management of Stroke III (IMS III) [7] and SYNTHESIS Expansion [8] trials demonstrated non-inferiority of mechanical thrombectomy over IV tPA. These trials have taught us a lot about selection of patients for endovascular treatment. Post-hoc analyses of each of these trials suggest that endovascular treatment for AIS may be indicated for a select patient population. Early generation thrombectomy devices with lower recanalization rates relative to newer devices were used for the majority of both trials. The majority of the endovascular arm in the IMS III trial only received a lower, bridging dose of IV tPA, while the SYNTHESIS endovascular arm received no IV tPA. A post-hoc analysis of IMS III participants with carotid artery terminus occlusion demonstrated higher recanalization rates and better outcomes in the endovascular arm relative to the IV tPA arm [9]. Moreover, a number of recent trials demonstrate promising outcome data for the latest thrombectomy devices [10,11]. High quality multicenter clinical trials comparing combined thrombectomy with stent retrievers and IV tPA to IV tPA alone have been completed, demonstrating the efficacy of endovascular management for a carefully selected group of patients. Mechanical thrombectomy may become the standard of care for a select cohort of patients. Therefore, technical proficiency will be required of practicing neuroendovascular interventionalists.

This chapter reviews some of the challenges and technical considerations of providing neuroendovascular interventions for AIS. First, the institutional organizational requirements for effectively providing mechanical thrombectomy to patients presenting with AIS are reviewed in detail. Without an established infrastructure and detailed planning, expedient endovascular intervention for acute stroke cannot be adequately provided. Next, periprocedural

Common Pitfalls in Cerebrovascular Disease: Case-Based Learning, ed. José Biller and José M. Ferro. Published by Cambridge University Press. © Cambridge University Press 2015.

complications of endovascular stroke intervention and strategies to avoid complications are examined. A case of a basilar artery occlusion is then presented along with a discussion of the unique characteristics of posterior circulation stroke. Finally, a case of pediatric acute ischemic stroke is presented and the challenges specific to this population of patients are reviewed.

Case 1. Coordinated stroke care

Case description

A 71-year-old woman with history of hypertension and atrial fibrillation (AF) noncompliant with oral anticoagulants presented with acute onset of right hemiparesis, right facial droop, left gaze preference, and aphasia. Prior to this event, she had no deficits. The patient was last known to be normal at approximately 6:00 p.m. Her husband found her on the bedroom floor at approximately 6:30 p.m. Emergency medical services (EMS) transported her to a local community hospital. Her initial National Institutes of Health Stroke Scale (NIHSS) score on arrival was 18. A CT scan of the head demonstrated no acute intracranial process. The emergency department (ED) physician initiated a stroke telemedicine consult to a stroke neurologist via a call center at a comprehensive stroke center. After reviewing the clinical presentation, past medical history, and radiographic findings, the patient was administered a total of 0.9 mg/kg of IV tPA starting at 8:50 p.m. (baseline INR 0.9). Transportation arrangements were promptly made by the ED physician for the patient to this comprehensive stroke center. At the community hospital, while waiting for and during transportation, her vital signs were obtained every 15 minutes and blood pressure was tightly controlled, maintaining systolic blood pressure below 180 mmHg and the diastolic blood pressure below 105 mm.

In anticipation of the patient's arrival, the on-call stroke neurologist reviewed the history and presentation with the on-call neuro-interventionalist. The stroke neurologist then informed the transfer center administrator of the incoming admission, who would be directly going to the MRI suite from the ED. The transfer center then sent a page-out to the on-call stroke team, which consisted of the neuro-interventionalist, stroke neurologist, neuro-interventional nurse, neuro-interventional radiology technician, and research coordinator. The transfer center also coordinated with EMS to ensure adequate notification to the stroke team of patient arrival by sending regularly updated pager

texted messages of the approximated estimated time of arrival (ETA). Upon receiving the stroke page, each member of the stroke team sent as a group text message confirmation of the page and their en-route status to the hospital. The neuro-interventionalist informed the anesthesiologist on-call of the incoming stroke patient and ETA, per the emergency transportation service estimates. The neuro-interventionalist also contacted the radiology technician to ready an MRI suite for the arriving patient.

Upon the stroke team's arrival at the hospital, the neuro-interventional radiology technician began to prepare the neuroendovascular suite for possible intervention. Simultaneously, the neuro-interventional nurse contacted the nurse at the outside hospital for patient report, including an MRI screening questionnaire. The neuro-interventionalist and research coordinator discussed the patient's history and presentation with consideration for recruitment into a research protocol. Given the patient's criteria, she was tentatively eligible for the Solitaire™ FR as Primary Treatment for Acute Ischemic Stroke "SWIFT PRIME" trial and the research coordinator contacted the patient's family to obtain informed consent for enrollment with the help of the local community hospital personnel.

Coordinated by the ETA alerts, the stroke neurologist, neuro-interventionalist, neuro-interventional nurse, and research coordinator arrived at the comprehensive stroke center ED to accept the patient when she arrived at 10:00 p.m. An identification band was placed onto the patient after confirming the patient's identity and a baseline exam was obtained. Her right hemiparesis and aphasia were unchanged and her NIHSS score at 10:02 p.m. was 16. The vital signs were continuously monitored and blood pressure tightly controlled. By 10:05 p.m., the patient arrived at the MRI suite and the MRI technician was prepared for the patient's arrival. The patient was quickly transferred to the MRI bed and MRI-compatible monitors were applied in order to monitor vital signs during image acquisition. Acquisition of the predefined set of stroke MRI image sequences was completed by 10:42 p.m., which demonstrated a complete occlusion of the left M1 segment at its origin. There was a minimal area of restricted diffusion involving the posterior limb of the internal capsule, but an estimated volume of 34 mL of ischemic parenchyma was seen surrounding this area with decreased perfusion (Figure 8.1). The patient was formally enrolled into the SWIFT PRIME trial and randomized to the intervention treatment arm.

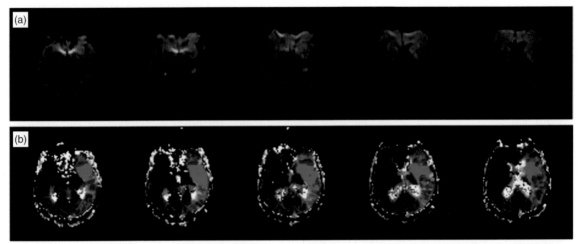

Figure 8.1 MRI scans of the head. (a) Diffusion-weighted MRI scan demonstrated minimal restricted diffusion involving the left posterior limb of the internal capsule. (b) The perfusion-weighted MRI demonstrated a larger area of hypoperfusion deep within the left cerebral hemisphere, indicating a large mismatch volume ratio of ischemic brain parenchyma to infarction.

The anesthesiologist was prepared for the patient's arrival at the neuroendovascular suite at 10:45 p.m. She was quickly transferred from the transport gurney to the procedure table and access to the right common femoral artery was achieved at 10:53 p.m. A 6F sheath was introduced into the femoral artery. Using an exchange length 0.035″ Glidewire (Terumo, Shibuya, Tokyo), the 6F sheath was then exchanged for an 8F Neuron MAX 088 guide catheter (Penumbra, Alameda, CA) and was advanced into the aortic arch. After removing the exchange length wire from the 8F

guide catheter, a Neuron 5F Berenstein select catheter (Penumbra) loaded with a 0.035″ wire was introduced into the 8F guide catheter. The left common carotid artery was selected with fluoroscopic visualization and the 8F guide catheter was advanced into the left internal carotid artery (ICA). The 5F inner select catheter and 0.035″ wire were removed.

An angiogram of the left intracranial ICA distribution demonstrated a complete occlusion of the left mid M1 segment (Figure 8.2a). Using a roadmap technique, a 5Max ACE guide catheter (Penumbra) was

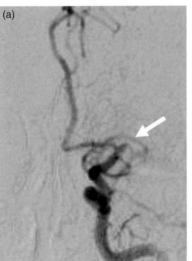

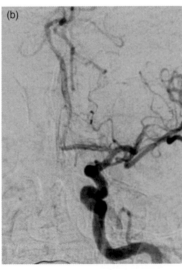

Figure 8.2 Anterior-posterior catheter angiograms of the left ICA before (a) and after (b) mechanical thrombectomy. The left M1 segment occlusion is indicated by the arrow.

advanced into the ICA over a Marksman microcatheter (Covidien, Dublin, Ireland) loaded with a Synchro-14 guidewire (Stryker, Kalamazoo, MI). Under fluoroscopic visualization, the guidewire was advanced through the left M1 thrombus. The microcatheter was then carefully advanced through the M1 thrombus over the guidewire, and the guidewire was removed.

An angiogram obtained by a microinjection through the microcatheter confirmed the microcatheter was distal to the thrombus. A 4 × 20 mm Solitaire Retriever stent (Covidien) was deployed across the M1 thrombus. The microcatheter was removed while the stent retriever was deployed. Continuous aspiration was applied to the 5Max ACE catheter, and the stent retriever was retracted after 2 minutes. An angiogram obtained of the left ICA demonstrated only partial recanalization. The stent retriever was used a second time resulting in complete recanalization of the left M1 segment at 11:10 p.m. (Figure 8.2b). The catheters were removed from the patient and the right femoral arteriotomy was closed with an 8F Angio-Seal closure device (St. Jude Medical, Saint Paul, MN).

The patient was admitted to the neuroscience intensive care unit (NSICU) for stroke management. Immediately after the patient was safely transferred to the NSICU, the neuro-interventionalist, neuro-interventional nurse, neuro-interventional radiology technician, and research coordinator met before leaving the hospital to debrief the case, discussing and documenting any issues encountered during the management of the case. This documentation was then later reviewed at a monthly stroke quality review conference to identify problems and potential solutions for future cases.

After the mechanical thrombectomy, the patient's examination rapidly improved. On the following morning, she was alert and following commands with full strength in all of her extremities. Her NIHSS score improved from 16 to 1. The patient was evaluated for modifiable stroke risk factors, and she was started on simvastatin immediately and, after a 24-hour period after IV tPA administration, was started on a daily aspirin and prophylactic dose of enoxaparin for deep vein thrombosis (DVT) prevention. Cardiology was consulted due to her AF, which was rate controlled with propranolol. By hospital day 7, the patient was transferred to an acute rehabilitation facility with mild dysarthria and a slow gait that required assistance.

Discussion

Providing endovascular intervention for patients presenting with AIS does not start with a groin puncture, but rather begins with careful preparation and coordination among many different healthcare providers and organizations well before a stroke occurs. Efforts to provide improved stroke care delivery began after the approval of IV tPA by the US Food and Drug Administration (FDA) in 1996. Regional disparities in public awareness, acute stroke care teams, and stroke units were identified by the year 2000 and served as the motivation for a substantial reorganization of regional stroke care in the United States. By 2003, The Joint Commission (TJC) in the United States began to formally certify and recognize hospitals as primary stroke centers based on recommendations from the AHA/ASA, the National Stroke Association, and the Brain Attack Coalition (BAC). Primary stroke centers serve as regional focal points providing standardized care to patients that present with acute stroke in a timely manner. Primary stroke centers provide care to most patients with acute stroke, have the ability to provide some acute therapies such as IV tPA, and provide admission to a designated stroke unit. Table 8.1 summarizes the requirements defined by TJC for a primary stroke center designation [12]. Primary stroke centers have been shown to reduce stroke-related deaths by 14%, death or institutionalized care by 18%, and death or dependency by 18% [13].

Just as the need to rapidly administer IV tPA to patients with AIS within a strict therapeutic time period prompted the development of primary stroke centers, the evolution of mechanical thrombectomy technologies helped to provide an impetus to recognize comprehensive stroke center facilities. In 2012, TJC began to certify and recognize comprehensive stroke centers based on guidelines outlined by the BAC. In addition to the requirements for primary stroke center certification, designated comprehensive stroke centers have available resources needed to treat stroke patients who require a higher level of medical, surgical, and interventional care. This population includes large hemispheric ischemic strokes, intraparenchymal hemorrhages, and atraumatic subarachnoid hemorrhages. Requirements for a comprehensive stroke center designation (Table 8.1) include onsite, 24-hour coverage of specialized healthcare providers including vascular neurology, vascular neurosurgery, critical care medicine, and a neuro-interventionalist. The requirements

Table 8.1 Comparison summary of primary versus comprehensive stroke center features

Stroke center features	Primary stroke center	Comprehensive stoke center
Neurology availability	Optional	Required
Neurosurgical availability	Neurosurgical service available within 2 hours	Onsite neurosurgical service required
Cerebrovascular surgery	ns	Required
Stroke team	Required	Required
Neuro-interventional capabilities	ns	Required
Advanced practice nurse	ns	Required
Written care protocols	Required	Required
Emergency department	Required	Required
Intensive care unit		
Stroke unit	Optional	Required
Neurocritical care unit	Optional	Required
Neuroimaging	Required	Required
Rehabilitation therapy	Required	Required
Speech/swallow assessment	ns	Required
Performance measure collection and analysis	Required	Required
Participation in clinical research	ns	Required

ns: not specified.

also specify available infrastructure including neuro-intensive care unit, operating suite, and an interventional suite. Advanced neuroimaging that is available 24 hours a day is required of comprehensive stroke centers including perfusion imaging.

This case presentation exhibits the carefully orchestrated sequence of events that occur at a comprehensive stroke center once an acute stroke patient is identified at another community emergency department. Prior to the presentation of the stroke patient, representatives from the stoke team at the comprehensive stroke center met with and provided education regarding management of stroke patients to community ED personnel, including the ED physician who initially managed the patient from the case presentation. Thus, when the referral call was placed from the ED physician to the stroke neurologist taking call at the comprehensive stroke center, cooperation was already established and the decision to administer IV tPA at the community ED was made more efficiently after the clinical history and CT imaging was reviewed. Prior to the stroke presentation, a working relationship was also established with a local emergency transport service to ensure the patient was carefully monitored during the transfer

and that regular ETAs were forwarded to the transfer center of the comprehensive stroke center, allowing the accepting stroke team to efficiently prepare for the patient's arrival.

An essential concept illustrated by the case presentation is the importance of predefined responsibilities of each stroke team member. These predetermined roles helped streamline patient care, which was facilitated by constant communication of information among the stroke team members, the transfer center, and the transferring facility. For example, the neuro-interventional nurse being the only member to contact the outside facility's ED nurse for report regarding the patient in-transit, who then informed the rest of the stroke team, epitomizes elimination of unwanted redundancy. These established responsibilities of each member are essential to provide efficient and expedient patient care.

The post-procedure debriefing following the interventional case is another important point illustrated by the case presentation. This step is crucial to identify and document difficulties that occurred during the management of the patient. These issues were then reviewed at a monthly quality control conference to remedy problems and implement solutions to avoid repeating the same difficulties with future patients. Lastly, the research coordinator continued to track outcomes based on ongoing data analysis to aid in implementing improvements.

Tip

Rapid identification and treatment of acute stroke is associated with improved clinical outcomes. Coordinated care is imperative.

Case 2. Periprocedural complications

Case description

A 41-year-old woman with morbid obesity, congestive heart failure (CHF), status post automatic implantable cardioverter defibrillator (AICD) placement, hypertension, type 2 diabetes mellitus, pulmonary hypertension, and sarcoidosis presented to a community ED with acute onset of difficulty speaking and right hemiplegia that started at 11:45 p.m. At the community hospital, her initial NIHSS score was 23. A CT scan of the head did not demonstrate an acute intracranial process. The ED physician initiated a stroke telemedicine consult at a comprehensive stroke center. After the patient's presentation was reviewed with the stroke neurologist on-call, IV tPA was administered and arrangements for transfer were made.

On arrival at the comprehensive stroke center at 3:40 a.m., almost 4 hours since the patient was last known to be normal, her NIHSS score remained 23.

She was lethargic, requiring painful stimuli to remain awake. She had a global aphasia, left gaze deviation, right facial droop, and right hemiplegia. She did not follow commands, but had purposeful movements of her left arm and leg. Given the presence of the AICD, the patient was transferred to the CT scanner suite where a non-contrast CT scan showed a hypodensity within the deep left hemisphere. CT perfusion imaging of the head demonstrated decreased cerebral blood volume (CBV) and cerebral blood flow (CBF) within the left basal ganglia, left insula, and left temporal lobe consistent with cerebral infarction. The mean transit time (MTT) of the entire left middle cerebral artery (MCA) distribution was significantly increased, consistent with a large penumbra of ischemia within the remaining left MCA territory. A computed tomography angiography (CTA) scan of the head revealed an occlusion of the left ICA terminus with robust opacification of the left anterior cerebral artery (ACA) distribution from a patent anterior communicating artery (Figure 8.3) and some opacification of the distal left MCA distribution via retrograde leptomeningeal collateral circulation. The patient was then immediately transferred to the endovascular suite.

At 4:08 a.m., the patient arrived at the endovascular suite and was positioned supine on the procedure table. The patient's airway could not be adequately protected while lying supine and general endotracheal tube anesthesia was started, ensuring that the systolic blood pressure remained around 140–160 mmHg. The patient was prepped and draped. A 6F sheath was inserted into the right common femoral artery. An exchange length 0.035″ Glidewire (Terumo) was introduced into the

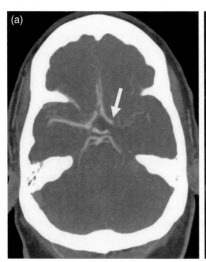
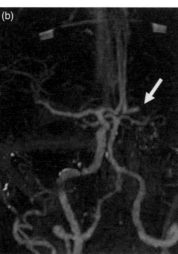

Figure 8.3 CT angiography (a) and 3D reconstruction (b) of left ICA terminus occlusion. The left ACA fills through a patent anterior communicating artery. There is retrograde filling of the left A1 segment to the left ICA terminus occlusion (arrow).

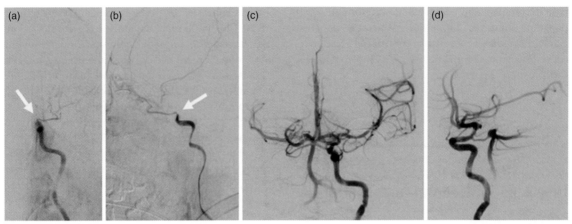

Figure 8.4 Anterior-posterior (a) and lateral (b) projections of a left ICA catheter angiogram demonstrating occlusion of the left ICA distal to the ophthalmic segment (arrows). Complete recanalization of the left ICA is demonstrated anterior-posterior (c) and lateral (d) in left ICA angiogram after mechanical thrombectomy.

sheath. The sheath was exchanged for an 8F Neuron 088 guide catheter (Penumbra) and, under direct visualization, the guide catheter was advanced to the aortic arch. A Neuron 5F Berenstein select catheter over a 0.035″ Glidewire was used to help guide the guide catheter into the left ICA under fluoroscopic visualization. The 5F Berenstein select catheter and guidewire were removed.

An angiogram of a left ICA injection demonstrated complete occlusion of the supraclinoid segment of the left ICA (Figures 8.4a and 8.4b). A 5Max ACE catheter over a 0.014″ Synchro microwire (Stryker) was carefully advanced through the left ICA to engage the proximal portion of the thrombus. The guidewire was removed and continuous aspiration was applied to the catheter as the catheter was carefully advanced to the ICA terminus.

The catheter was then withdrawn back into the cavernous ICA and an angiogram demonstrated complete recanalization of the left ICA, but a thrombus fragment remained in the left MCA. After a failed attempt to aspirate the MCA thrombus using aspiration through the catheter, a 0.025″ Velocity microcatheter (Penumbra) was loaded with a 0.014″ Synchro microwire (Stryker) and introduced into the 5Max catheter. The microcatheter was then advanced through the M1 segment passed the thrombus and a 6 × 20 mm Solitaire FR stent retriever (Covidien) was deployed across the clot. The microcatheter was removed. With aspiration applied to the 5Max catheter, the stent retriever was withdrawn after 2 minutes. The resulting angiogram of the left ICA at 4:50 a.m. demonstrated

complete recanalization of the left anterior circulation (Figures 8.4c and 8.4d). The catheters were removed from the patient and the right femoral arteriotomy was closed with an Angio-Seal closure device (St. Jude Medical). The patient remained intubated at the end of the procedure and was admitted to the NSICU.

The patient's examination was unchanged from her initial presentation when she arrived at the NSICU. She was intubated, had a left gaze deviation and her pupils were bilaterally equal and reactive. She still had right hemiplegia and purposeful movements of the left arm and leg. A new hyperdensity deep within the left hemisphere concerning for hemorrhagic conversion of infarcted brain parenchyma was noted on routine post-procedure CT imaging (Figure 8.5). A dual-energy CT scan of the head was then obtained, characterizing the hyperdensity as contrast media used during the intra-arterial (IA) recanalization rather than acute hemorrhage (Figure 8.6). The patient was medically optimized, and permissive hypertension was allowed, keeping the systolic blood pressure below 180 mmHg.

By 1:45 a.m. on the following morning, the patient's neurologic examination acutely changed. The right pupil was found to be dilated and non-reactive, and she exhibited extensor posturing. An emergent CT scan showed that the left cerebral hyperdensity was stable in size. There was increased cerebral edema of the left hemisphere with a resulting midline shift indicative of a malignant MCA infarction. Following the CT scan, 116 g of IV mannitol was administered and IV 3% NaCl with goal sodium of 155–165 mmol/L saline was

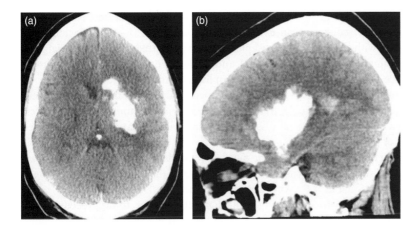

Figure 8.5 Axial (a) and sagittal (b) CT images of the head demonstrating a hyperdensity deep within the left hemisphere after a mechanical thrombectomy.

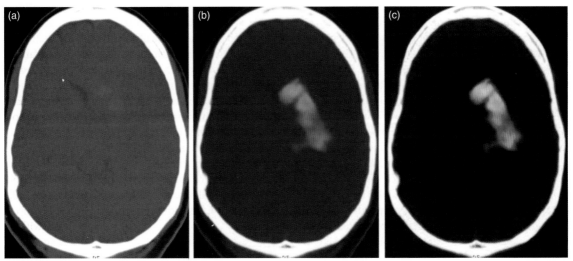

Figure 8.6 Dual-energy CT imaging. Based on the different attenuation characteristics of acute hemorrhage and iodine at two different X-ray spectra, a virtual non-contrast image (a), mixed (b), and iodine overlay map (c) was reconstructed demonstrating that the hyperdensity within the right cerebral hemisphere was iodine contrast media rather than hemorrhage.

started. The neurosurgical service recommended an emergent left hemicraniectomy. After carefully reviewing the risks and benefits of the surgical procedure and the long-term prognosis of the patient, the patient's next of kin, her mother, elected to decline both surgical intervention and further medical management in favor of comfort care measures. A do-not-resuscitate order was initiated. Later in the day, the AICD was deactivated, ventilation support was stopped, and the patient expired.

Discussion

Improvements of technology and greater experience have made periprocedural complications associated with endovascular intervention of AIS equivalent to medical management of AIS, including the administration of IV tPA [6]. The IMS III trial, for instance, showed no significant difference for mortality, symptomatic intracerebral hemorrhage (ICH), or other non-intracerebral bleeding complications between the endovascular therapy treatment arm and the IV tPA treatment arm [6]. Periprocedural complications of IA stroke therapy can be broadly classified into five categories: vascular access complications, complications of medication and contrast media, systemic complications, complications associated with anesthesia, and device-related complications [14].

Hemorrhagic complications, which significantly increase morbidity and mortality, are the most frequent complications and are usually associated with the use of thrombolytic agents or reperfusion injury [14]. The IMS III trial reported a 6.2% incidence of symptomatic ICH within 30 hours of endovascular therapy for stroke [6]. Clinical trials of mechanical thrombectomy for treatment of AIS have established a safe treatment window of 5–8 hours from the onset of initial stroke symptoms. ICH most likely occurs as the blood–brain barrier (BBB) breaks down resulting in reperfusion injury, but may represent a technical error such as a vessel perforation caused by a catheter, microwire, or device. Careful patient selection for endovascular intervention is important in order to identify patients at higher risk of hemorrhagic complications. Extent of infarction demonstrated on initial neuroimaging [15] and time interval from symptom onset to recanalization are predictors of hemorrhagic transformation. Advanced neuroimaging techniques such as CT perfusion, MRI, and MRI perfusion imaging capable of defining the extent of core infarction relative to the volume of ischemic penumbra may improve patient selection for endovascular intervention by establishing safe, objective pathophysiologic parameters for intervention, instead of relying on clinical history that may at times be unreliable.

Early recognition of ICH is crucial. Many contemporary endovascular suites have the capability to obtain flat panel detector CT imaging with acquisition quality comparable to multidetector CT imaging if ICH is clinically suspected prior to conclusion of an endovascular procedure. During angiography, the mass effect of an ICH may also become evident as distortions of the intracranial vascular anatomy or visualized extravasation of contrast media. As illustrated by the case presentation, leakage of iodine contrast media into brain parenchyma resulting from increased permeability of the BBB documented on routine post-procedure CT imaging may be mistaken for periprocedural ICH.

Continuing anticoagulation therapy is dependent on early differentiation of contrast leakage versus ICH. Distinguishing contrast material leakage from ICH is difficult because of the similar Hounsfield densities of iodine and acute hemorrhage. Serial imaging is necessary to demonstrate gradual resolution of iodine contrast from an increase of stable volume of ICH. A dual-energy CT scan can differentiate iodine from hemorrhage with a single scan [16]. In our practice, management of intracranial hemorrhage includes early

surgical decompression when indicated, placement of an external ventricular drain (EVD) for evidence of hydrocephalus or suspected elevated intracranial pressure (ICP), and, although not evidence-based, consideration for prophylactic antiepileptic therapy.

Other periprocedural complications of endovascular treatment for AIS are less common. Iatrogenic arterial dissection is a rare complication with a reported incidence of 0.4% [17]. Angioplasty with possible stenting may be required for flow-limiting dissections; otherwise, small arterial dissections may be managed with antiplatelet therapy. Distal emboli can occur during a mechanical thrombectomy procedure as a thrombus or thrombus fragment migrates into smaller branches during manipulation. The use of aspiration either through large-bore soft catheters [18] or balloon guide catheters [19] has decreased the incidence of distal emboli. The incidence of air emboli is less than 0.1% and can be avoided with meticulous technique during the endovascular procedure [20]. Published recommendations for the management of symptomatic air embolism are limited. Elevated mean arterial pressure greater than 100 mmHg, ventilation with 100% oxygen, IA verapamil infusion, and prophylactic antiepileptic therapy should be considered for symptomatic air embolism. Arterial vasospasm can occur after manipulation of catheters, wires, and devices within the intracranial vasculature and can be managed with IA vasodilator infusion or angioplasty.

Tip

Symptomatic ICH is the most common periprocedural complication associated with endovascular intervention for acute stroke. Early differentiation of iodine leaking through a disrupted BBB from true hemorrhage dictates management strategy and can be accomplished quickly with dual-energy CT imaging. Other periprocedural complications are rare. Neuro-interventionalists should be aware of these rare complications and familiar with treatment strategies.

Case 3. Basilar artery occlusion

Case description

A 58-year-old man with atrial fibrillation, coronary heart disease status post a four-vessel bypass 7 years prior, a minimally invasive maze procedure, and placement of an implantable cardioverter defibrillator 6 years prior, abruptly developed severe nausea and emesis at approximately 5:00 p.m. on the day prior to presentation. He had been noncompliant on his oral anticoagulation with rivaroxaban secondary to the patient's confusion with his own prescriptions and has been off of any oral anticoagulation for a long period of time. He did not initially seek medical attention after onset of his symptoms. At approximately 1:00 a.m. after a restless night, his symptoms progressed to a right hemiplegia, prompting him to contact the EMS who transported the patient to a community hospital. There, a CT scan of the head demonstrated a hyperdense basilar artery (BA) suggestive of a possible embolic occlusion. A stroke telemedicine consult was initiated at a comprehensive stroke center and the patient's initial NIHSS score was determined to be 12 due to right hemiplegia and dysarthria. He was not a candidate for IV tPA since onset of symptoms was well beyond the 4½ hour window of time for systemic therapy, and he was transported to a comprehensive stroke center for possible endovascular intervention.

On arrival at the comprehensive stroke center at 6:30 a.m., the patient became increasingly somnolent and his NIHSS score increased to 13. A CT angiogram of the head demonstrated complete occlusion of the intradural segment of the right vertebral artery (VA) and proximal BA. The distal third of the BA was supplied by a patent right posterior communicating artery (Figure 8.7a). The entire course of the left vertebral artery was not visualized, presumably representing a congenitally absent left VA. The patient had a generalized tonic-clonic seizure during the acquisition

of the CT angiogram and received a 1 gram IV bolus of levetiracetam and was promptly brought to the endovascular suite.

In the endovascular suite, the patient was quickly positioned, prepped, and draped. Access to the right common femoral artery was obtained with a 6F sheath using local anesthesia and mild sedation. An Envoy DA guide catheter (Codman Neuro, Raynham, MA) with a 0.035″ Glidewire (Terumo) was introduced into the sheath and the right vertebral artery was selected under fluoroscopic guidance. An angiogram showed delayed filling of the proximal right VA indicative of a distal occlusion of the distal VA (Figure 8.7b). Through the guide catheter, a Trevo Pro 18 microcatheter (Stryker) was advanced through the thrombus within the right VA extending into the BA over a Synchro-14 microwire (Stryker). A 4 × 20 mm Trevo XP ProVue Retriever stent (Stryker) was deployed across the thrombus. After 5 minutes, aspiration was applied to the guide catheter and the stent was withdrawn through the guide. An angiogram demonstrated complete opacification of the posterior circulation (Figure 8.7c). The guide catheter was withdrawn and the groin puncture site was closed with a 6F Angio-Seal device (St. Jude Medical) after the sheath was removed. The patient was transferred to the NSICU afterward.

The patient was medically optimized and spent a total of 5 days in the NSICU. Full recanalization of the right vertebral artery and basilar artery was demonstrated on a post-procedure CT angiogram

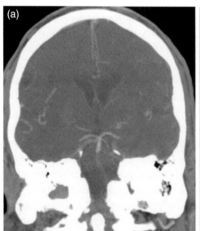
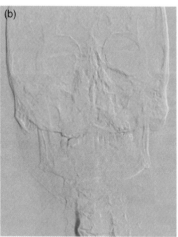
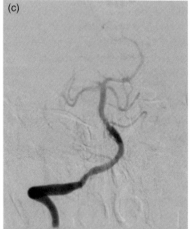

Figure 8.7 (a) Coronal CT angiogram demonstrating vertebral-basilar occlusion with retrograde filling of the distal BA. (b) Anterior-posterior catheter angiogram of a right VA injection demonstrating occlusion. (c) Anterior-posterior catheter angiogram of a right VA injection after mechanical thrombectomy.

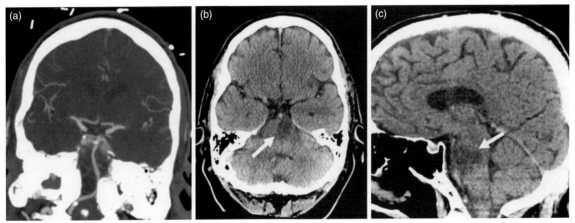

Figure 8.8 Coronal CT angiogram (a) demonstrating recanalization of the right VA and proximal BA. CT scan axial (b) and sagittal (c) views showing a left pontine stroke (arrows) after mechanical thrombectomy of the BA occlusion.

(Figure 8.8a). However, a non-contrast CT scan did show a left pontine hypodensity indicative of a brainstem infarction (Figures 8.8b and 8.8c). The patient was restarted on his anticoagulation in the form of rivaroxaban 10 days after his stroke. Over his hospitalization course, he gained some strength in his right leg, but his dysarthria remained unchanged. He was deemed to be an excellent candidate for physical rehabilitation and was ultimately discharged to an inpatient rehabilitation center. His discharge medications included levetiracetam, aspirin, prophylactic dose of enoxaparin, and rivaroxaban. At the time of discharge, his NIHSS score was 11.

At a 3-month outpatient follow-up visit, he was requiring some assistance at home from his sister. His left hemiparesis had improved and he was able to independently ambulate with a cane. He continued to receive physical therapy and occupational therapy twice a week. Although he declined speech therapy, his dysarthria had improved since discharge.

Discussion

Posterior circulation ischemic strokes account for nearly 20% of all strokes. A number of characteristics distinguish AIS involving the posterior circulation from anterior circulation stroke. The brainstem is a critical neurologic structure that receives arterial supply mostly from the BA, the main vessel of the posterior circulation. Acute BA occlusion (BAO) is a catastrophic event with a grave prognosis if left untreated. Acute BAO treated with supportive therapy along with antiplatelets, antithrombotics, or a combination of the

two has an associated 40% mortality and 65% severe disability for survivors [21].

The BA can potentially receive additional collateral circulation through patent posterior communicating arteries aside from leptomeningeal collateral circulation analogous to ischemic stroke involving the anterior circulation. This potential collateral circulation from the circle of Willis, along with other factors including the level of occlusion and the extent of the thrombus, makes the clinical presentation of BAO more variable. Also, greater than 60% of patients with BAO have prodromal symptoms including vertigo, nausea, headache, hemiparesis, and diplopia weeks prior to onset of stroke [22]. These prodromata prior to BAO may confound the timing for effective intervention.

Most large clinical trials for mechanical thrombectomy as a treatment for cerebrovascular occlusion to date have included mainly anterior circulation stroke and established a safe treatment window of 5–8 hours from the onset of any stroke symptoms. A recent large prospective observation registry of BAO demonstrated that the time period for optimal, safe intervention for BAO should begin with the onset of severe neurologic deficit clinically consistent with BAO, rather than the start of any minor stroke symptoms as would be considered for anterior circulation stroke onset [23].

The case vignette illustrates a typical presentation of BAO with non-focal symptoms including severe nausea and emesis, which presented 12 hours prior to admission to a comprehensive stroke center. As per the indications of the stent retriever used in the case, the patient would not have been a candidate for mechanical thrombectomy as the patient's stroke symptoms were over 8 hours. Ultimately, the patient tolerated the procedure well and being made a favorable recovery, returning to his home and being able to ambulate independently with a cane. This case supports endovascular intervention for this disease process that bears a potentially devastating prognosis.

Tip

Acute BAO is a devastating disease with a dismal prognosis. Intervention for BAO may be warranted beyond the 5–8 hour time period established for acute anterior circulation stroke.

Case 4. Pediatric acute ischemic stroke

Case description

A 2-year-old boy with history of hypoplastic left heart syndrome requiring multiple cardiothoracic reconstructive surgeries and heterozygosity for the prothrombin G20210A mutation managed with warfarin presented with acute left hemiplegia. At baseline, the patient was without neurologic deficits. At 2:30 p.m. on the day of presentation, his mother initially noticed that his gait progressively worsened from walking normally, to having a limp on the left, to becoming non-ambulatory. She attributed this to her son being defiant, and the child was set down for a nap. Fifteen minutes later, he awoke with a persistent left hemiplegia. The patient's mother brought him to the ED for evaluation.

On presentation to the ED, the patient was alert and appropriately irritable. He had a left facial droop and left hemiplegia. He did not withdraw to noxious stimuli applied to the left arm or leg. His INR was found to be 1.57, which was subtherapeutic to his goal of 1.8–2.5. A CT scan of the head demonstrated an area of hypodensity in the right hemisphere concerning for an AIS. Consults were made to the stroke neurology service and neuro-interventionalist. The patient was electively intubated. An MRI/MRA of the head demonstrated an occlusion of the proximal right M1 segment with restricted diffusion within the right lentiform nucleus and posterior limb of the internal capsule (Figure 8.9). After the MRI, the patient was transferred to the endovascular suite.

Under general endotracheal tube anesthesia, a 10 cm 4F sheath was inserted into the right common femoral artery using a micropuncture technique. A 65-cm 4F angled Glidecath (Terumo) was introduced into the sheath and advanced to the aortic arch over a 0.035″ Glidewire (Terumo) under direct visualization. The right common carotid artery was selected without difficulty despite the previous aortic arch reconstruction. The right ICA was selected using a roadmap technique and the guidewire was withdrawn. An angiogram obtained of the right ICA confirmed the occlusion of the proximal M1 segment (Figure 8.10a). A Trevo Pro 14 microcatheter (Stryker) was loaded with a 0.014″ Synchro microwire (Stryker) and introduced into the 4F guide catheter. The microwire was carefully advanced through the M1 thrombus followed by the microcatheter. The microwire was withdrawn and successful positioning of the microcatheter completely through the thrombus was confirmed by an angiogram obtained from a microinjection through

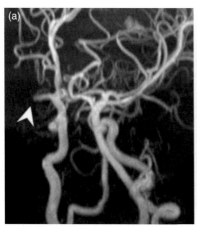
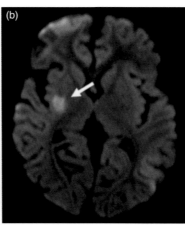

Figure 8.9 (a) MRA demonstrating an occlusion of the right M1 segment (arrowhead). (b) Diffusion-weighted MRI scan showing restricted diffusion within the right lentiform nucleus and posterior limb of the internal capsule (arrow).

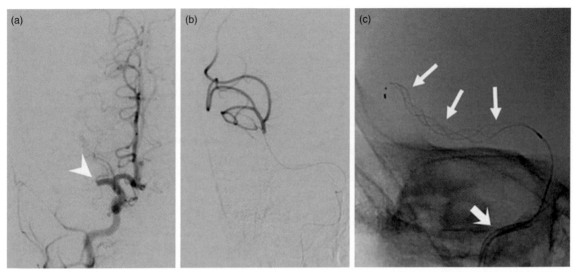

Figure 8.10 (a) Anterior-posterior catheter angiogram of a right ICA injection demonstrating a right M1 segment occlusion (arrowhead). (b) Microinjection angiogram through a microcatheter passed though the right M1 thrombus, confirming that the distal end of the catheter is distal to the thrombus. (c) Anterior-posterior fluoroscopic image demonstrating a stent retriever (arrows) deployed within the right M1 segment. The 4F guide catheter is visible within the intracranial ICA (thick arrow).

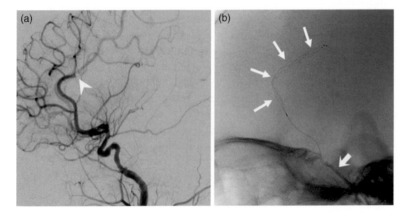

Figure 8.11 (a) Lateral catheter angiogram of a right ICA injection showing an ACA occlusion (arrowhead). (b) Lateral fluoroscopic image depicting a stent retriever (arrows) within the right ACA. The 4F guide catheter is seen within the intracranial ICA (thick arrow).

the microcatheter (Figure 8.10b). The 3 × 20 mm Trevo XP ProVue Retriever stent (Stryker) was then deployed through the thrombus (Figure 8.10c). After allowing the stent retriever to incorporate into the clot, the stent and microcatheter were retracted as a unit back into the 4F guide catheter. A subsequent angiogram of the right ICA demonstrated that the M1 segment remained occluded and a fragment of clot had migrated into the right ACA (Figure 8.11a).

After the initial failed thrombectomy attempt using the 3 × 2 mm stent retriever, a Trevo Pro 18 microcatheter (Stryker) loaded with a 0.014″ microwire was introduced into the 4F guide catheter. Again, the microwire was carefully advanced through the M1 thrombus and the microcatheter was then advanced past the thrombus over the wire. A 4 × 20 mm Trevo XP ProVue Retriever stent (Stryker) was then deployed across the M1 thrombus. While the stent retriever incorporated into the clot over 5 minutes, the microcatheter was withdrawn, increasing the space between the stent retriever pusher wire and the inner wall of the 4F guide catheter. While gentle aspiration was applied to the 4F guide catheter, the stent retriever was then withdrawn through the 4F guide catheter. The resulting angiogram of the right ICA demonstrated a partial recanalization of the right M1 segment. Ultimately,

(a) 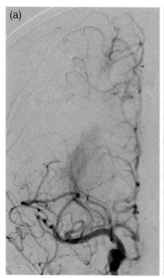 (b)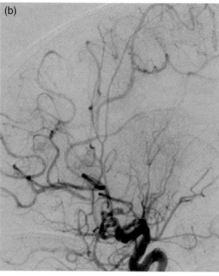

Figure 8.12 Anterior-posterior (a) and lateral (b) catheter angiogram projections of a right ICA injection after mechanical thrombectomy demonstrating recanalization of the right MCA and right ACA.

a third pass using a larger 4 × 20 stent retriever and aspiration through the 4F guide catheter successfully recanalized the right M1 segment (Figure 8.12a).

The same mechanical thrombectomy technique was then used to retrieve the thrombus fragment that migrated into the right ACA (Figure 8.11a). A microcatheter was loaded with a 0.014″ microwire and introduced into the 4F guide catheter that still remained in the right ICA. The microwire was carefully advanced past the thrombus followed by the microcatheter. The microcatheter was confirmed with an angiogram obtained by an injection through the microcatheter. A 4 × 20 mm stent retriever was then introduced into the microcatheter and deployed across the thrombus. The microcatheter was then carefully removed, leaving only the 4F guide catheter and the stent retriever in position (Figure 8.11b). After incorporating into the clot over 5 minutes, the stent retriever was carefully withdrawn while gentle aspiration was applied to the guide catheter. The subsequent right ICA angiogram revealed a complete recanalization of the right ACA distribution (Figure 8.12b). The guide catheter was then removed from the patient and direct pressure was applied to the groin for 15 minutes. The total puncture to recanalization time for the procedure was 55 minutes and time from symptom onset to full recanalization was 7 hours.

At the conclusion of the procedure, the patient was extubated and admitted to the pediatric intensive care unit. He was alert and crying, but consolable. He moved all extremities purposefully, but his left arm and leg were weaker than the right arm and leg. An MRI obtained on the following day revealed an increased area of restricted diffusion deep to the right insular cortex. To manage his thrombophilia, a heparin IV drip was started as a bridge as his warfarin was restarted with goal INR of 2.0–2.5. The left hemiparesis improved over his hospitalization course. He was discharged home by hospital day 7. At a 30-day outpatient follow-up visit, the patient was walking normally with only a mild motor deficit of his left hand and a slight facial droop. His mRS at that time was 1.

Discussion

Pediatric AIS is rare with only an estimated incidence of 2.5–13 cases per 100 000 per year [24]. The mortality rate for pediatric AIS is only estimated to be 3–6%, but pediatric AIS is associated with a 70% morbidity, resulting in lifelong neurologic deficits [25]. This makes pediatric AIS an important medical health issue that has received little attention. The higher morbidity associated with pediatric AIS relative to the estimated 50% morbidity associated with surviving patients of adult AIS [26] may be a consequence of delayed diagnosis. On average, there is an approximately 25-hour delay from clinical onset to radiologic confirmation of pediatric AIS [27]. Low clinical suspicion and community awareness delay prompt diagnosis. Accurate diagnosis is confounded by other more common pediatric pathologies that share similar symptoms to AIS, such as post-ictal paresis, demyelinating pathologies, and migraine headaches [28]. The recognition of the stroke in the presented case was initially mistaken for a temper tantrum.

Currently, management recommendations for pediatric AIS are extrapolated from available adult literature. To date, pediatric patients have been excluded from major clinical stroke trials. Formal management recommendations for pediatric AIS are limited to supportive care and anticoagulation using aspirin or heparin [29,30]. Thrombolysis with IV tPA at present is only recommended in the setting of clinical research protocols [31]. However, optimal dosing of tPA in the pediatric population is difficult to establish. The maturation of the hemostatic system occurs throughout childhood, resulting in a poorly understood dose-related pediatric response to tPA as a function of age [32]. There are currently no recommendations for the roles of IA tPA or mechanical thrombectomy in the management for pediatric AIS as evidence is limited to published case reports.

Given that pediatric AIS can be more difficult to recognize and treatment delayed, mechanical thrombectomy may serve an important primary treatment strategy for pediatric AIS. There are a growing number of case reports that demonstrate the successful application of mechanical thrombectomy in the pediatric population, suggesting that this procedure can be safely performed. Vascular anatomy may limit the size of guide catheter that can be used to for the procedure, particularly in the very young patients. As in the case vignette, a 4F guide catheter was the largest catheter that could be safely inserted into the common femoral artery of this 2-year-old patient. Aspiration through the guide catheter is paramount to prevent small embolization into the distribution distal to the thrombus or to prevent thrombus migration during its retrieval. If a 4F guide catheter is used, it is recommended that the microcatheter used to deliver the stent retriever should first be withdrawn providing enough space within the guide catheter to allow adequate aspiration. Stent retrievers are available in a number of different dimensions and the size should be tailored to the specific anatomy of the patient.

Tip

Pediatric AIS is a rare event associated with a high morbidity, likely due to diagnostic delay. Treatment recommendations are limited and are extrapolated from adult clinical trials. Mechanical thrombectomy can be safely performed on pediatric patents.

Case 5. Difficult access

Case description

A 79-year-old man with a complex past medical history of coronary artery disease (CAD) status post angioplasty, peripheral artery disease (PAD) status post bilateral femoral-popliteal bypass, chronic kidney disease, diabetes mellitus type 2, hypertension, and renal cell carcinoma status post left nephrectomy was initially transferred from an outside institution with acute coronary syndrome and was found to have 95% left main occlusion on catheterization. The patient underwent a three-vessel coronary artery bypass graft (CABG) and placement of an intra-aortic balloon pump (IABP) uneventfully. However, on postoperative day 1 at approximately 11:20 a.m., the patient was found to be aphasic with a dense right hemiplegia. The on-call stroke neurology team was quickly notified and was at bedside by 11:39 a.m. His exam was consistent with a left MCA syndrome likely cardioembolic in nature given his recent procedures. NIHSS score was found to be 26. CT scan of the head was obtained, which was negative for any acute intracranial process. Unfortunately, a CT angiography of the head could not be acquired due to his elevated creatinine level (2.46 mg/dL). The stroke service deemed administration of tPA to be unsafe due to the recent surgery.

The case was then discussed with the neuro endovascular team, who agreed that the next best step in management was to take the patient quickly to the angiography suite for diagnostic cerebral angiogram with plan for mechanical thrombectomy. Due to the patient's recent IABP placement as well as extensive lower extremity revascularization surgeries, femoral arterial access would be difficult. A right radial approach was decided as the best alternative.

An Allen test was first performed, ensuring adequate collateral blood supply to the hand. The patient was positioned, prepped, and draped. A 12-cm 6F sheath was cut to 3 cm and was used to achieve access to the right radial artery using local anesthetic and mild sedation (Figure 8.13). The patient was then infused with 5000 IU of heparin, 10 mg of verapamil, and 200 µg of nitroglycerin through the introducer sheath to prevent vasospasm. A 5F Internal Mammary Tight (IMT) guide catheter (Medtronic, Minneapolis, MN) over a 0.035″ Glidewire was used to selectively catheterize the left common carotid artery. An angiogram demonstrated a complete left M2 occlusion

(Figure 8.14). A 0.027″ Marksman microcatheter (Covidien) and a 0.014″ Synchro standard microwire (Stryker) was then used to selectively catheterize the left M2 branch using a roadmap technique. With fluoroscopic guidance, the microwire was passed through the thrombus, which was followed by the microcatheter. An angiogram through the microcatheter was done to ensure complete passage through the thrombus (Figure 8.15). A Trevo XP ProVue Retriever stent (Stryker) was deployed across the thrombus. After 5 minutes, the stent was withdrawn through the guide catheter with continuous manual aspiration of the guide catheter. Another angiogram through the guide catheter demonstrated successful revascularization of the M2 branch (Figure 8.16). The guide catheter was then removed and moderate compression was applied to the right radial pulse to obtain hemostasis. This procedure was complete at 2:15 p.m., which was less than 3 hours from stroke onset.

Immediately after the procedure, the patient was now lifting his right upper extremity against gravity, moving the toes of his right lower extremity to command, and attempting to verbalize. By 4 p.m.,

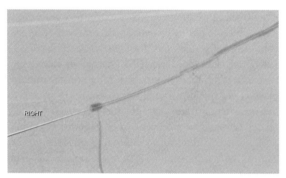

Figure 8.13 Right radial angiogram through a 3 cm 6F sheath.

his NIHSS score was 7, and by post-stroke day 2, his NIHSS score was 1. Immediately post thrombectomy, the patient was started on 81 mg of aspirin. On further work-up, he was found to have a patent foramen ovale (PFO) with a flat thrombus in the anteroapical wall. The patient was then started on a heparin bridge to warfarin and taken off aspirin. On post-stroke day 15, the patient was transferred to an acute rehabilitation facility.

Discussion

Due to the wide-caliber of the femoral artery to facilitate use of large-diameter catheters and other endovascular devices, the transfemoral approach is the most common access route for endovascular procedures. Moreover, this approach allows access to all arteries originating from the aortic arch. However, anatomic factors, such as aortoiliac occlusive disease and tortuosity of the aortic or brachiocephalic vessels may hinder angiography and may increase risk of intervention [33], prompting the need for alternative access. In the presented case vignette, access was limited by a recently placed IABP and complicated by prior lower extremity revascularization procedures. Alternative approaches for endovascular procedures have been described in the past, including transradial [34,35], transbrachial [36–38], transaortic [33], and transcarotid [39].

The transradial approach has been suggested as a more attractive alternative for arterial access. The superficial anatomic location of the radial artery facilitates hemostasis by local compression, minimizing potential hematoma formation. Radial artery occlusion is a well-tolerated complication in the presence of an intact palmar arcade and a competent ulnar artery, which is assessed with an Allen test [40,41]. In a study

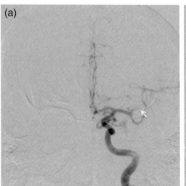
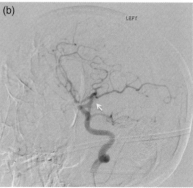

Figure 8.14 Anterior-posterior (a) and left anterior oblique (b) projections of a left ICA angiogram demonstrating occlusion of a left M2 branch (arrow).

of 1360 patients, no radial artery occlusions occurred after immediate sheath removal [42].

The transradial approach has been extensively described as a safe and effective means of access in the peripheral vascular and cardiovascular literature [43–48]. Numerous authors have reported using the transradial approach for coronary angiography and stenting with favorable results and minimal complications [44,46]. In a randomized comparison of transradial, transfemoral, and transbrachial approaches for coronary stenting, there was no statistically significant difference in complication rates or length of stay [49]. A randomized comparison of 900 patients undergoing percutaneous transluminal coronary angioplasty demonstrated that a significantly lower complication rate is associated with radial artery access (0%) compared

with that of brachial artery access (2.3%) or femoral artery access (2%) [50].

In the neuro-interventional literature, this the transradial approach has been used for cerebral angiography [51–53], cervical carotid and extracranial vertebral angioplasty and stenting [54–56], and intracranial interventions involving the posterior circulation [34,35]. Yoo et al. [55] reported successful use of a transradial approach for cervical carotid stenting in a patient with total occlusion of the distal abdominal aorta, with no long-term complications. Bendock et al. [34] reported successful application of this approach in four patients whose brachiocephalic ectasias limited access to pathologies involving the posterior circulation. Endovascular interventions in these patients included coiling of a basilar apex aneurysm remnant and angioplasty and/or stenting of the vertebral and basilar arteries. Eskioglu et al. [35] reported successful utilization of the transradial approach to successfully treat a number of intracranial pathologies in nine patients, which included five posterior circulation aneurysms, a mid-basilar artery stenosis, a ruptured dural arteriovenous fistula, and a posterior frontal arteriovenous malformation via a large posterior communicating artery.

Despite the feasibility of the transradial approach, it does bear limitations. Firstly, radial artery vasospasm may cause significant patient discomfort and prevent successful completion of the procedure [57,58]. Kiemeneij et al. [50] reported higher failure rates when performing percutaneous transluminal coronary angioplasties via the transradial approach as compared to the transfemoral and transbrachial approaches, likely related to radial artery spasm and narrow vessel caliber. To limit this complication, numerous authors administer a "radial cocktail," which may include heparin, verapamil, and nitroglycerin [34,51]. Secondly, certain

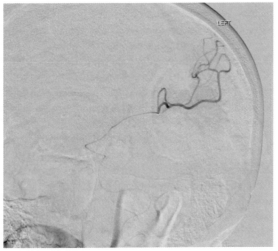

Figure 8.15 Microcatheter injection into M2 branch, ensuring complete passage through the thrombus.

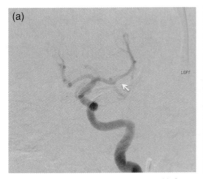
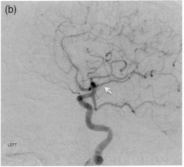

Figure 8.16 Anterior-posterior (a) and left anterior oblique (b) projections of a left ICA angiogram demonstrating successful revascularization of the left M2 (arrows) with a single pass of the Trevo XP ProVue Retriever stent.

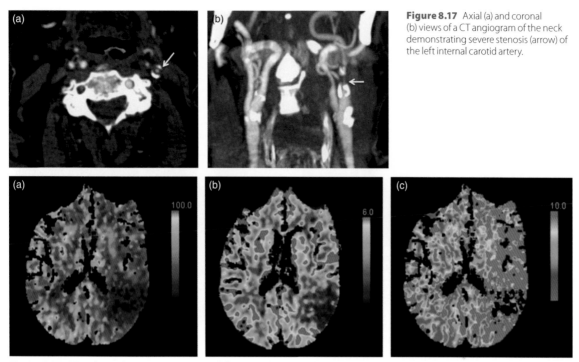

Figure 8.17 Axial (a) and coronal (b) views of a CT angiogram of the neck demonstrating severe stenosis (arrow) of the left internal carotid artery.

Figure 8.18 CT perfusion demonstrating an acute left temporal-parietal infarct. Cerebral blood flow map (a); cerebral blood volume map (b); mean transit time map (c).

anatomic variations of the radial artery that can be found in up to 7.8% of patients [59], such as a radioulnar loop or hypoplasia of the radial artery, may hinder access. Thirdly, the transradial approach is also limited by the greater difficulty in accessing other arch vessels, particularly the contralateral vertebral artery. Lastly, the small caliber of the radial artery may occasionally limit the application of a number of endovascular devices.

Tip

Despite the transfemoral route being the route of choice for most neuro endovascular procedures, challenges may arise, necessitating other means of access. A comprehensive stroke center should have the protocols and clinical expertise to choose the radial approach when necessary. It can be a safe and effective alternative.

Case 6. Radiation-induced carotid disease

Case description

A 73-year-old man with a past medical history including hypertension, alcohol abuse, and oropharyngeal cancer status post neck radiation presented to an ED with acute onset of aphasia and right-sided hemiplegia that began at approximately 2 p.m. that day. By the time he arrived at the ED at 6:30 p.m., he had dysarthria, right facial droop, and right upper and lower extremity weakness. He was given an NIHSS score 14. A non-contrast CT scan of the head was negative for any acute intracranial process. An MRI could not be acquired because the patient had a pacemaker. The ED team proceeded to administer tPA at approximately 6:45 p.m. (baseline INR 1.13). At approximately 8 p.m., the ED reported that the patient's exam had improved with only slight dysarthria and his right extremities were stronger. The patient was then transferred to a comprehensive stroke center for further evaluation.

The patient arrived at the comprehensive center at approximately 10 p.m. The patient was extremely agitated with worsened aphasia and more profound right-sided weakness than initially reported; his NIHSS score on arrival was 16. A CT angiogram of the neck demonstrated a 90% stenosis of the ICA at the level of the cervical carotid bifurcation (Figure 8.17). The cerebral blood volume component of the CT perfusion was consistent with a small left temporal-parietal

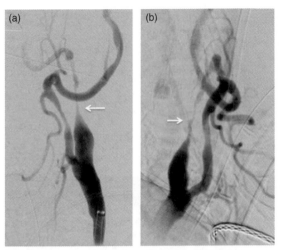

Figure 8.19 Left anterior oblique (a) and lateral (b) projections of a cervical carotid angiogram demonstrating severe stenosis (arrow) of the left internal carotid artery.

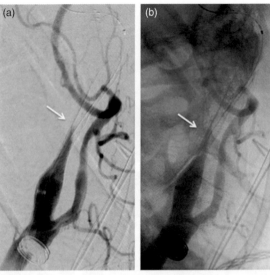

Figure 8.20 Lateral projection (a) and native view (b) of a cervical carotid angiogram at the time of stent placement and subsequent acute thrombosis (arrow). Lack of flow is evident in the distal two-thirds of the stent and beyond. The distal protection device can be seen without evidence of blood flow.

infarct (Figure 8.18). A 24-hour post tPA administration CT scan of the head confirmed an acute infarct without any acute hemorrhagic component. The patient was started on 325 mg of aspirin 24 hours after tPA administration.

The neuroendovascular team was consulted for the patient's severe carotid stenosis. Given the patient's history of prior radiation to the mouth and neck, the endovascular team agreed that carotid artery stenting would be a more reasonable strategy than carotid endarterectomy. The procedure was performed on post-stroke day 3 following administration of 600 mg of clopidogrel and 650 mg of aspirin on the day prior.

Due to the patient's agitated state, the procedure was performed under general anesthesia. Access to the right femoral artery was achieved with a 6F sheath. A 5F catheter was used to perform a diagnostic angiogram, confirming a 90% left carotid stenosis (Figure 8.19). The 6F sheath and 5F diagnostic catheter were exchanged for an 8F Neuron Max 088 guide catheter (Penumbra) that was positioned in the left common carotid artery. At this point 5000 IU of IV heparin were administered, and at 5 minutes after administration, the activated clotting time was 305 s. A 5.5-mm Angioguard distal protection device (Cordis, Miami, Florida, USA) was deployed in the left ICA approximately 2 cm distal to the stenosis and a Precise carotid stent (Cordis) was deployed across the stenosis. Post-stent angioplasty was performed using a 5-mm Viatrac balloon catheter (Abbott Vascular, Abbott Park, Illinois, USA).

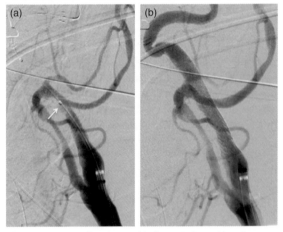

Figure 8.21 Lateral projection (a) of a cervical carotid angiogram at the time of aspiration with the Penumbra 4Max catheter. The aspiration catheter (arrow) can be seen within the stent and blood flow can be seen distal to the site of occlusion in Figure 8.20. Lateral projection (b) after successful revascularization following aspiration of the acute thrombus. Minimal residual stenosis is observed within the stent and good blood flow is observed distal to the stent and site of the distal protection device.

The cervical carotid angiogram after balloon angioplasty demonstrated complete occlusion of the left ICA within the stent and distal to it (Figure 8.20). An intra-arterial injection of 10 mg of verapamil and 10 mg abciximab was unsuccessful in obtaining recanalization. Since it was unclear if there was occlusion within the stent or due to debris within the distal protection device, the distal protection device was not just simply recaptured. A 4Max aspiration catheter (Penumbra) was introduced over the existing Angioguard wire and across the in-stent thrombus to the level of the distal protection device (Figure 8.21). Thrombus was aspirated at the distal protection device and within the stent. Macroscopic inspection of the aspirated content from the stent suggested an acute thrombus rather than embolized plaque. A follow-up angiogram demonstrated complete recanalization with restoration of blood flow. There was residual stenosis of approximately 25–30% (Figure 8.20b) and no evidence of intracranial vessel occlusion. Following the procedure, the aspirin and clopidogrel levels were confirmed to be therapeutic.

The patient did not suffer any new neurological injury immediately after the procedure. The patient's postoperative course was complicated by a groin hematoma at the puncture site, requiring injection of thrombin into a pseudoaneurysm, and aspiration pneumonia, requiring a course of antibiotics. The patient was transferred to an acute rehabilitation facility on post-stroke day 20 on aspirin and clopidogrel. His NIHSS score was 10 at the time of discharge.

Discussion

Carotid artery stenting (CAS) has become widely employed for the treatment of carotid artery stenosis, particularly in those who bear high surgical risk [60]. Intraprocedural in-stent or distal protection device occlusion are recognized potential complications, occurring in 0.5–2% of cases [61] and up to 30% of cases [62–64], respectively.

These complications may be considered on a continuum of acute thrombotic events that may occur during carotid stenting as they are attributed to similar etiologies and similar rescue strategies have been described. Factors that may be involved in these complications may include inadequate pretreatment with antiplatelet drugs, under-herparinization intra-procedurally, underlying hypercoagulable states, local factors (e.g., vessel dissection, plaque protrusion), or technical factors (e.g., poor apposition of stent along vessel wall, inadequate angioplasty) [63,65,66]. Furthermore, trauma to the luminal plaque by stent deployment and angioplasty may expose thombogenic factors, thereby promoting local thrombosis within the

stent and remotely at the distal protection device [67]. The most likely cause of distal protection device occlusion is the debris burden in the filter, leading to blood flow stagnation and eventual occlusion of the artery.

Literature remains sparse in treatment of such potentially devastating complications. Tong et al. [61] reported that administration of abciximab (glycoprotein IIb/IIIa antagonist) has been an effective intervention in the setting of acute in-stent thrombosis. Steiner-Boker et al. [68] described successfully revascularizing acute in-stent thrombosis via a "combined thrombolysis and dethrombolysis" approach by locally administering intra-arterial tPA, abciximab, and heparin. Balloon angioplasty is a potential intervention, but risks showering distal emboli to an already hemodynamically compromised cerebral parenchyma and may theoretically risk disrupting the stent's construct and stability. Open surgical thrombectomy and removal of the occluded stent may be an effective option [69,70]; however, this approach is generally a salvage procedure and may be particularly risky in those patients already deemed poor surgical candidates. In cases of distal protection device occlusion, simple device retrieval may lead to thromboembolic complications attributed to release of embolic material within the device during manipulation [64].

Utilization of an aspiration catheter could be a viable option in both in-stent and distal protection device occlusion. In cases of protection device occlusion, the use of an aspiration catheter to suction debris prior to filter retrieval may be a safer strategy to empty the filter prior to recapturing the device, theoretically reducing potential embolic complications. Although aspiration catheters, such as the Penumbra 4Max catheter that was used in the above case vignette, are devices often utilized in mechanical thrombolysis during acute stroke settings, they may be used as a rescue strategy for in-stent thrombosis.

Regardless of the strategy, in cases of either in-stent thrombosis or distal protection device occlusion, efficient re-establishment of arterial flow in a timely manner is paramount. Delay in recanalization of the vessel or incorrect technique could lead to ischemia and neurologic injury.

Tips

Acute in-stent and distal protection device thrombosis are potential complications that may occur during carotid artery stenting. Effective treatment strategies for these complications are necessary to prevent potentially devastating neurologic consequences.

References

1. Furlan A, Higashida R, Wechsler L, Gent M, Rowley H, Kase C, et al. Intra-arterial prourokinase for acute ischemic stroke. The PROACT II study: a randomized controlled trial. Prolyse in Acute Cerebral Thromboembolism. *JAMA* 1999;282(21):2003–11.

2. Tissue plasminogen activator for acute ischemic stroke. The National Institute of Neurological Disorders and Stroke rt-PA Stroke Study Group. *N Engl J Med* 1995;333(24):1581–7.

3. Del Zoppo GJ, Saver JL, Jauch EC, Adams HP, Jr. Expansion of the time window for treatment of acute ischemic stroke with intravenous tissue plasminogen activator: a science advisory from the American Heart Association/American Stroke Association. *Stroke* 2009;40(8):2945–8.

4. Akins PT, Amar AP, Pakbaz RS, Fields JD. Complications of endovascular treatment for acute stroke in the SWIFT trial with solitaire and Merci devices. *AJNR Am J Neuroradiol* 2014;35(3):524–8.

5. Mokin M, Snyder KV, Siddiqui AH, Hopkins LN, Levy EI. Endovascular management and treatment of acute ischemic stroke. *Neurosurg Clin N Am* 2014;25(3):583–92.

6. Hassan AE, Chaudhry SA, Grigoryan M, Tekle WG, Qureshi AI. National trends in utilization and outcomes of endovascular treatment of acute ischemic stroke patients in the mechanical thrombectomy era. *Stroke* 2012;43(11):3012–17.

7. Broderick JP, Palesch YY, Demchuk AM, Yeatts SD, Khatri P, Hill MD, et al. Endovascular therapy after intravenous t-PA versus t-PA alone for stroke. *N Engl J Med* 2013;368(10):893–903.

8. Ciccone A, Valvassori L, Nichelatti M, Sgoifo A, Ponzio M, Sterzi R, et al. Endovascular treatment for acute ischemic stroke. *N Engl J Med* 2013;368(10):904–13.

9. Demchuk AM, Goyal M, Yeatts SD, Carrozzella J, Foster LD, Qazi E, et al. Recanalization and clinical outcome of occlusion sites at baseline CT angiography in the Interventional Management of Stroke III Trial. *Radiology* 2014;273(1):202–10.

10. Pereira VM, Gralla J, Davalos A, Bonafe A, Castano C, Chapot R, et al. Prospective, multicenter, single-arm study of mechanical thrombectomy using Solitaire Flow Restoration in acute ischemic stroke. *Stroke* 2013;44(10):2802–7.

11. Saver JL, Jahan R, Levy EI, Jovin TG, Baxter B, Nogueira RG, et al. Solitaire flow restoration device versus the Merci Retriever in patients with acute ischaemic stroke (SWIFT): a randomised, parallel-group, non-inferiority trial. *Lancet* 2012;380(9849):1241–9.

12. Janjua N, Katzan I, Badruddin A, Nguyen TN, Abou-Chebl A, Zaidat OO. Endovascular comprehensive stroke center designation parameters. *Neurology* 2012;79(13 Suppl 1):S239–42.

13. Gorelick PB. Primary and comprehensive stroke centers: history, value and certification criteria. *J Stroke* 2013;15(2):78–89.

14. Darkhabani Z, Nguyen T, Lazzaro MA, Zaidat OO, Lynch JR, Fitzsimmons BF, et al. Complications of endovascular therapy for acute ischemic stroke and proposed management approach. *Neurology* 2012;79(13 Suppl 1):S192–8.

15. Larrue V, von Kummer R, Muller A, Bluhmki E. Risk factors for severe hemorrhagic transformation in ischemic stroke patients treated with recombinant tissue plasminogen activator: a secondary analysis of the European-Australasian Acute Stroke Study (ECASS II). *Stroke* 2001;32(2):438–41.

16. Tijssen MP, Hofman PA, Stadler AA, van Zwam W, de Graaf R, van Oostenbrugge RJ, et al. The role of dual energy CT in differentiating between brain haemorrhage and contrast medium after mechanical revascularisation in acute ischaemic stroke. *Eur Radiol* 2014;24(4):834–40.

17. Cloft HJ, Jensen ME, Kallmes DF, Dion JE. Arterial dissections complicating cerebral angiography and cerebrovascular interventions. *AJNR Am J Neuroradiol* 2000;21(3):541–5.

18. Turk AS, Spiotta A, Frei D, Mocco J, Baxter B, Fiorella D, et al. Initial clinical experience with the ADAPT technique: a direct aspiration first pass technique for stroke thrombectomy. *J Neurointerv Surg* 2014;6(3):231–7.

19. Nguyen TN, Malisch T, Castonguay AC, Gupta R, Sun CH, Martin CO, et al. Balloon guide catheter improves revascularization and clinical outcomes with the Solitaire device: analysis of the North American Solitaire Acute Stroke Registry. *Stroke* 2014;45(1):141–5.

20. Gupta R, Vora N, Thomas A, Crammond D, Roth R, Jovin T, et al. Symptomatic cerebral air embolism during neuro-angiographic procedures: incidence and problem avoidance. *Neurocrit Care* 2007;7(3):241–6.

21. Schonewille WJ, Algra A, Serena J, Molina CA, Kappelle LJ. Outcome in patients with basilar artery occlusion treated conventionally. *J Neurol Neurosurg Psychiatry* 2005;76(9):1238–41.

22. Ferbert A, Bruckmann H, Drummen R. Clinical features of proven basilar artery occlusion. *Stroke* 1990;21(8):1135–42.

23. Schonewille WJ, Wijman CA, Michel P, Rueckert CM, Weimar C, Mattle HP, et al. Treatment and outcomes of acute basilar artery occlusion in the Basilar Artery International Cooperation Study (BASICS): a prospective registry study. *Lancet Neurol* 2009;8(8):724–30.

24. Arnold M, Steinlin M, Baumann A, Nedeltchev K, Remonda L, Moser SJ, et al. Thrombolysis in childhood stroke: report of 2 cases and review of the literature. *Stroke* 2009;40(3):801–7.

25. Ellis MJ, Amlie-Lefond C, Orbach DB. Endovascular therapy in children with acute ischemic stroke: review and recommendations. *Neurology* 2012;79(13 Suppl 1):S158–64.

26. Di Carlo A. Human and economic burden of stroke. *Age Ageing* 2009;38(1):4–5.

27. Srinivasan J, Miller SP, Phan TG, Mackay MT. Delayed recognition of initial stroke in children: need for increased awareness. *Pediatrics* 2009;124(2):e227–34.

28. Hu YC, Chugh C, Jeevan D, Gillick JL, Marks S, Stiefel MF. Modern endovascular treatments of occlusive pediatric acute ischemic strokes: case series and review of the literature. *Childs Nerv Syst* 2014;30(5):937–43.

29. Monagle P, Chalmers E, Chan A, DeVeber G, Kirkham F, Massicotte P, et al. Antithrombotic therapy in neonates and children: American College of Chest Physicians Evidence-Based Clinical Practice Guidelines (8th Edition). *Chest.* 2008;133(6 Suppl):887S–968S.

30. Roach ES, Golomb MR, Adams R, Biller J, Daniels S, Deveber G, et al. Management of stroke in infants and children: a scientific statement from a Special Writing Group of the American Heart Association Stroke Council and the Council on Cardiovascular Disease in the Young. *Stroke* 2008;39(9):2644–91.

31. Dubedout S, Cognard C, Cances C, Albucher JF, Cheuret E. Successful clinical treatment of child stroke using mechanical embolectomy. *Pediatr Neurol* 2013;49(5):379–82.

32. Kuhle S, Male C, Mitchell L. Developmental hemostasis: pro- and anticoagulant systems during childhood. *Semin Thromb Hemost* 2003;29(4):329–38.

33. Glower DD, Clements FM, Debruijn NP, Stafford-Smith M, Davis RD, Landolfo KP, Smith PK. Comparison of direct aortic and femoral cannulation for port-access cardiac operations. *Ann Thorac Surg* 1999;68:1529–31.

34 Bendock BR, Przybylo JH, Parkinson R, Hu Y, Awad IA, Batjer HH. Neuroendovascular interventions for intracranial posterior circulation disease via the transradial approach: technical case report. *Neurosurgery* 2005;56(3):E626.

35. Eskioglu E, Burry MV, Mericle RA. Transradial approach for neuroendovascular surgery of intracranial vascular lesions. *J Neurosurg* 2004;101:767–9.

36. Gritter KJ, Laidlaw WW, Peterson NT. Complications of outpatient transbrachial intraarterial digital subtraction angiography: work in progress. *Radiology* 1987;162:125–7.

37. Yip KM, Yurianto H, Lin J. False aneurysm with median nerve palsy after iatrogenic brachial artery puncture. *Postgrad Med J* 1997;73:43–4.

38. Zaldat OO, Szeder V, Alexander MJ. Transbrachial stent-assisted coil embolization of right posterior inferior cerebellar artery aneurysm: technical case report. *J Neuroimaging* 2007;17(4):344–7.

39. Berkmen T, Troffkin N, Wakhloo AK. Direct percutaneous puncture of a cervical internal carotid artery aneurysm for coil placement after previous incomplete stent-assisted endovascular treatment. *AJNR Am J Neuroradiol* 2003;24:1230–3.

40. Mandel M, Dauchet P. Radial artery cannulation in 1,000 patients: precautions and complications. *J Hand Surg* 1977;6:482–5.

41. Slogoff S, Keats AS, Arlund C. On the safety of radial artery cannulation. *Anesthesiology* 1983;59:42–7.

42. Saito S, Miyake S, Hosokawa G, Tanaka S, Kawamitsu K, Kaneda H, Ikei H, Shiono T. Transradial coronary intervention in Japanese patients. *Catheter Cardiovasc Interv* 1999;46:37–42.

43. Kiemeneij F, Laarman GJ, de Melker E. Transradial artery coronary angioplasty. *Am Heart J* 1995;129:1–7.

44. Lotan C, Hasin Y, Mosseri M, Rozenman Y, Admon D, Nassar H, Gotsman MS. Transradial approach for coronary angiography and angioplasty. *Am J Cardiol* 1995;76:164–7.

45. Mann JT III, Cubeddu G, Bowen J, Schneider JE, Arrowood M, Newman WN, Zellinger MJ, Rose GC. Stenting in acute coronary syndromes: a comparison of radial versus femoral access sites. *J Am Coll Cardiol* 1998;32:572–6.

46. Otaki M. Percutaneous transradial approach for coronary angiography. *Cardiology* 1992;81:330–3.

47. Scheinert D, Brèaunlich S, Nonnast-Daniel B, Schroeder M, Schmidt A, Biamino G, Daniel WG, Ludwig J. Transradial approach for renal artery stenting. *Catheter Cardiovasc Interv* 2001;54:442–7.

48. Shuck J, Khan A, Cavros N, Galanakis S, Patel V. Transradial renal angioplasty: initial experience. *Catheter Cardiovasc Interv* 2001;54:346–9.

49. Benit E, Missault L, Eeman T, Carlier M, Muyldermans L, Materne P, Lafontaine P, De Keyser J, Decoster O, Pourbaix S, Castadot M, Boland J. Brachial, radial, or femoral approach for elective Palmaz-Schatz stent implantation: a randomized comparison. *Cathet Cardiovasc Diagn* 1997;41:124–30.

50. Kiemeneij F, Laarman GJ, Odekerken D, et al. A randomized comparison of percutaneous transluminal coronary angioplasty by the radial, brachial and femoral approaches: the access study. *J Am Coll Cardiol* 1997;29:1269–75.

51. Levy EI, Boulos AS, Fessler RD, Bendok BR, Ringer AJ, Kim SH, Qureshi AI, Guterman LR, Hopkins LN. Transradial cerebral angiography: an alternative route. *Neurosurgery* 2002;51:335–40.

52. Iwasaki S, Yokoyama K, Takayama K, et al. The transradial approach for selective carotid and vertebral angiography. *Acta Radiol* 2002;43:549–55.

53. Nohara AM, Kallmes DF. Transradial cerebral angiography: technique and outcomes. *AJNR Am J Neuroradiol* 2003;24:1247–50.

54. Fessler RD, Wakhloo AK, Lanzino G, Guterman LR, Hopkins LN. Transradial approach for vertebral artery stenting: technical case report. *Neurosurgery* 2000;46:1524–7.

55. Yoo BS, Lee SH, Kim JY, Lee HH, Ko JY, Lee BK, Hwang SO, Choe KH, Yoon J. A case of transradial carotid stenting in a patient with total occlusion of distal abdominal aorta. *Catheter Cardiovasc Interv* 2002;56:243–5.

56. Levy EI, Kim SH, Bendok BR, et al. Transradial stenting of the cervical internal carotid artery: technical case report. *Neurosurgery* 2003;53:448–52.

57. Goldberg SL, Renslo R, Sinow R, French WJ. Learning curve in the use of the radial artery as vascular access in the performance of percutaneous transluminal coronary angioplasty. *Cathet Cardiovasc Diagn* 1998;44:147–52.

58. Hildick-Smith DJ, Lowe MD, Walsh JT, Ludman PF, Stephens NG, Schofield PM, Stone DL, Shapiro LM, Petch MC. Coronary angiography from the radial artery: experience, complications and limitations. *Int J Cardiol* 1998;64:231–9.

59. Yokoyama N, Takeshita S, Ochiai M, Koyama Y, Hoshino S, Isshiki T, Sato T. Anatomic variations of the radial artery in patients undergoing transradial coronary intervention. *Catheter Cardiovasc Interv* 2000;49:357–62.

60. Yadav JS, Wholey MH, Kuntz RE, et al. Protected carotid artery stenting versus endarterectomy in high-risk patients. *N Engl J Med* 2004;351(15):1493–501.

61. Tong FC, Cloft HJ, Joseph GJ, et al. Abciximab rescue in acute carotid stent thrombosis. *AJNR Am J Neuroradiol* 2000;21(9):1750–2.

62. Angelini A, Reimers B, Della Barbera M, et al. Cerebral protection during carotid artery stenting: collection and histopathologic analysis of embolized debris. *Stroke* 2002;33(2):456–61.

63. Bonaldi G, Aiazzi L, Baruzzi F, et al. Angioplasty and stenting of the cervical carotid bifurcation under filter protection: a prospective study in a series of 53 patients. *J Neuroradiol* 2005;32(2):109–17.

64. Kwon OK, Kim SH, Jacobsen EA, et al. Clinical implications of internal carotid artery flow impairment caused by filter occlusion during carotid artery stenting. *AJNR Am J Neuroradiol* 2012;33(3):494–9.

65. Castellan L, Causin F, Danieli D, et al. Carotid stenting with filter protection. Correlation of ACT values with angiographic and histopathologic findings. *J Neuroradiol* 2003;30(2):103–8.

66. Iancu A, Grosz C, Lazar A. Acute carotid stent thrombosis: review of the literature and long-term follow-up. *Cardiovasc Revasc Med* 2010;11(2):110–13.

67. Jeong MH, Owen WG, Staab ME, et al. Porcine model of stent thrombosis: platelets are the primary component of acute stent closure. *Cathet Cardiovasc Diagn* 1996;38(1):38–43.

68. Steiner-Boker S, Cejna M, Nasel C, et al. Successful revascularization of acute carotid stent thrombosis by facilitated thrombolysis. *AJNR Am J Neuroradiol* 2004;25(8):1411–13.

69. Markatis F, Petrosyan A, Abdulamit T, et al. Acute carotid stent thrombosis: a case of surgical revascularization and review of treatment options. *Vascular* 2012;20(4):217–20.

70. Owens EL, Kumins NH, Bergan JJ, et al. Surgical management of acute complications and critical restenosis following carotid artery stenting. *Ann Vasc Surg.* 2002;16(2):168–75.

Choosing the right patients for carotid artery procedural interventions

Michael J. Schneck, Paul D. Ackerman, and Christopher M. Loftus

This chapter discusses the diagnosis and management of symptomatic and asymptomatic carotid atherosclerotic artery disease. Six cases illustrating the importance of proper case definition, diagnostic evaluation, and appropriate intervention are discussed. Variations in clinical factors critical in determining which patients should undergo carotid artery intervention are reviewed. The cases highlight potential pitfalls involved in the diagnosis of carotid artery disease and some of the complexities of clinical decision-making.

Case 1. Symptomatic carotid artery disease

Case description

A 79-year-old woman presented to her primary physician with complaints of visual blurring that started early that morning. The blurring involved her right eye only. She had no other neurologic complaints. She described the visual blurring as a gray area that involved the lower half of her right eye. The blurring occurred abruptly and resolved over 30 minutes. The blurring was painless and not associated with any headache, neck pain, or focal neurologic symptoms. She had no systemic complaints.

The medical history included well-controlled arterial hypertension and hyperlipidemia with a remote history of cigarette smoking. The family history was only remarkable for coronary artery disease (CAD).

On examination, the patient had a soft, rumbling sound on the left cervical region, and she also had a soft systolic heart murmur. Mental status examination was normal. Cranial nerve examination was normal, but the optic discs were poorly visualized secondary to cataracts. There was facial symmetry with normal bilateral

extremity strength and sensation. Coordination and gait were unremarkable. Muscle stretch reflexes were also normal with bilateral flexor plantar responses.

The primary physician ordered a carotid artery ultrasound that showed 50–74% right carotid artery stenosis and 50–74% left carotid artery stenosis. The patient was subsequently referred for surgical evaluation for consideration of left carotid endarterectomy (CEA). The surgeon declined to perform a procedure as he deemed the carotid artery stenosis to be asymptomatic and, in turn, referred the patient to a local neurologist who obtained a magnetic resonance imaging (MRI) of the brain. This showed infarctions including a left occipital lobe infarct (Figure 9.1). Cardiac evaluation, including a transthoracic echocardiogram (TTE) and prolonged cardiac monitoring, was unrevealing. The patient was then referred to the stroke clinic for evaluation of stroke of "undetermined etiology." Additional examination showed an inconsistent right visual field defect, subsequently confirmed by formal visual field testing. CT angiogram (CTA) confirmed "moderate to high-grade" left extracranial carotid artery stenosis at the bifurcation, and bilateral "take-off" of the posterior cerebral arteries (PCA) from the intracranial carotid arteries. Therefore, the patient underwent a left CEA for symptomatic carotid artery atherosclerotic disease.

Discussion

This case highlights the critical importance of a detailed history and physical examination in the evaluation of patients with extracranial atherosclerotic carotid arterial disease. In evaluating a patient with an ischemic stroke or transient ischemic attack (TIA), there are a number of important variables. The degree of carotid artery luminal narrowing and the appropriate

Common Pitfalls in Cerebrovascular Disease: Case-Based Learning, ed. José Biller and José M. Ferro. Published by Cambridge University Press. © Cambridge University Press 2015.

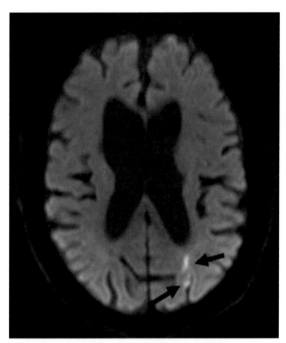

Figure 9.1 Axial MRI brain with evidence of multiple left hemispheric infarcts (arrows) on diffusion-weighted imaging (DWI).

clinical correlation between the patient's symptoms and their purported pathology are the most critical factors because the benefit of a carotid artery revascularization procedure is determined by the degree of stenosis, and the symptomatic/asymptomatic status of the patient. For patients with high-grade symptomatic carotid artery stenosis (defined as 70–99% luminal stenosis), the number needed to treat (NNT) is eight procedures to prevent one stroke at 2 years. For symptomatic patients with 50–69% carotid artery stenosis, the NNT is 20. For symptomatic patients with <50% carotid artery stenosis, the NNT is 67. The benefit is much less for asymptomatic patients with >60% carotid artery stenosis – with an NNT ratio of 87 at 2 years [1,2]. Thus, identification of symptomatic status and degree of arterial stenosis has profound implications when determining who should undergo a carotid artery intervention.

Defining symptomatic disease thus determines the relationship between the stenotic vessel and the need for intervention. A patient with a left retinal artery TIA, but right carotid artery stenosis, has asymptomatic carotid artery disease. Furthermore, a patient with moderate-grade carotid artery stenosis who has symptoms of a hemispheric TIA may benefit more from a carotid procedure than a patient with moderate-grade

carotid artery stenosis and a retinal TIA. Frequently, patients who present for evaluation may not immediately realize they have experienced a minor ischemic stroke or TIA. Patients referred for evaluation of asymptomatic carotid artery stenosis may, on careful examination, have unrealized sensory deficits that are directly attributable to a small subcortical infarct in the vascular territory of a previously assumed asymptomatic stenotic carotid artery.

The illustrative case above also highlights the importance of complete extracranial and intracranial cervicocerebral arterial imaging in all patients being evaluated for ischemic stroke or TIA. In patients with extracranial carotid artery stenosis, there is little benefit for carotid artery intervention if the distal extracranial or intracranial internal carotid artery (ICA) has a tandem stenosis or occlusion that is more severe than the stenosis of the proximal ICA bifurcation. Knowledge of anatomic variants is also important. For example, the prevalence of a "fetal PCA" ranges from 15% to 32% in healthy subjects, and from 5% to 36% in patients with cerebral infarction [3,4]. In this case, our patient might otherwise have been excluded from a beneficial carotid artery revascularization procedure because of lack of awareness of an important variant of cerebral vascular anatomy.

Tip

The clinical case presentation suggested a retinal TIA. However, brain imaging and imaging of the entire cervicocerebral vasculature is important as one needs to consider the possibility of an occipital lobe TIA or infarct due to vertebrobasilar disease or, alternatively, because of a PCA territory lesion in the context of a posterior cerebral artery (PCA) origin off the carotid artery: a "fetal PCA."

Case 2. Symptomatic carotid artery disease and a middle cerebral artery (MCA) stroke with concomitant atrial fibrillation: exclusion factors and timing of carotid interventions

Case description

A 63-year-old left-handed woman experienced the sudden onset of a headache. Shortly thereafter, her secretary found her confused in her office with difficulty walking. She was taken to the nearby emergency department where her blood pressure was 170/90 mmHg and her pulse was 80, but irregular. Telemetry confirmed she was in atrial fibrillation (AF).

The general examination suggested bilateral cervical bruits versus a transmitted cardiac murmur. On neurologic examination, she was awake and appeared alert, but was confused and was perseverating. She had no gaze difficulties. There was right arm and leg weakness with preserved antigravity strength. Sensory examination showed decreased pin-prick and temperature sensation on the right side. The National Institutes of Health Stroke Scale (NIHSS) score was 7.

Because she had last been seen "normal" within 2 hours prior to admission, she was given intravenous tissue plasminogen activator (tPA). Within the next 2–3 hours, she had resolution of her symptoms except for some mild speech impairment. Diagnostic evaluation showed a left insular infarct. Magnetic resonance angiogram (MRA) of the head was normal. MRA of the cervical vessels showed high-grade left bifurcation extracranial carotid artery stenosis. This was confirmed by carotid duplex ultrasonography. A TTE showed normal left ventricular ejection fraction (LVEF) and normal valve function with left atrial enlargement (LAE), and mild diastolic dysfunction. No atrial or ventricular thrombi were seen.

Neurology, cardiology, and surgery consults were requested to determine whether the patient should undergo CEA or should, instead, be started on anticoagulation for AF. Because of AF, the decision was made to first anticoagulate the patient. The patient then underwent inpatient rehabilitation and an outpatient cardiac stress test that was unremarkable. Six weeks later, the patient had a CTA to confirm there was no interval change in the degree of left ICA stenosis (Figure 9.2). The patient had a left CEA, the following day, without complications.

Discussion

Benefits of CEA

The benefit of CEA for stroke risk reduction was established in symptomatic carotid artery disease by two major randomized clinical trials, NASCET (North American Symptomatic Carotid Endarterectomy Trial) and ECST (European Carotid Surgery Trial) [2,5–8]. Subsequently, the Asymptomatic Carotid Artery Study (ACAS) and the Asymptomatic Carotid

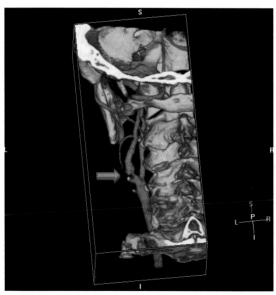

Figure 9.2 CTA (reconstructed 3D image) showing high-grade left ICA stenosis just distal to the carotid artery bifurcation (arrow).

Surgery Trial (ACST) showed similar, but lesser benefits of CEA in asymptomatic carotid artery disease [2,5,9,10].

The ipsilateral stroke and any perioperative stroke or death aggregate 5-year risk rate in the ACAS study for patients with >60% stenosis was 4.8% for surgery plus medical therapy, and 10.6% for medical therapy alone (absolute risk reduction (ARR) 5.8%; $P = 0.04$) [9]. Perioperative surgical risk was 2.3%. For ACST, the perioperative 30-day stroke or death rate was 3%, and the 5-year stroke risk (excluding perioperative events and non-stroke mortality) was 4.1% in the surgical arm versus 10.0% in the control arm ($P < 0.0001$) [10].

For patients in the NASCET study with 50–69% carotid artery stenosis, the ipsilateral stroke and death 5-year aggregate risk rate was 15.7% for surgery plus medical therapy, and 22.2% for medical therapy alone (ARR 6.5%; $P = 0.045$) [8]. For patients in the NASCET study with <50% carotid artery stenosis, the ipsilateral stroke and death 5-year aggregate risk rate was 14.9% for surgery plus medical therapy, and 18.7% for medical therapy alone – a finding that was not statistically significant ($P = 0.16$) [8]. The all stroke and death aggregate 2-year risk rate in the NASCET study for patients with >69% stenosis was 14.6% for surgery plus medical therapy and 35.6% for medical therapy alone (ARR 21%) [6]. Perioperative surgical risk was 6%. For symptomatic carotid artery stenosis, but not

Table 9.1 Summary of NASCET stroke rates at 18 months by percent carotid artery stenosis

% Carotid stenosis	% Stroke control	% Stroke surgical	Absolute % difference
90–99	33	6	27
80–89	28	8	20
70–79	19	7	12
Overall	25	7	18

Adapted from NASCET, 1991 [6].

for asymptomatic carotid artery stenosis, there was a gradient effect: symptomatic patients with a greater degree of carotid artery stenosis accrued more benefit from a carotid intervention (Table 9.1). Similar risk reduction rates were reported in the ECST study with a 3-year major stroke and death aggregate risk of 14.9% in the surgical arm, and 26.5% rate in the medical arm, with a similar gradient in benefit based on severity of carotid artery stenosis [8].

The current accepted outcome rates for symptomatic or asymptomatic carotid artery stenosis are based on 1990s data from the North American and European surgical trials. The accepted 30-day risk of perioperative stroke or death is 6% in the context of symptomatic carotid artery disease, and 3% in the context of asymptomatic carotid artery disease [5]. The ACAS study reported a perioperative risk of about 1% related to catheter cervicocerebral angiography, and 2% related to the actual surgical procedure. Arguably, therefore, the postsurgical complication rate, in the absence of preoperative angiography, should probably be held to a standard rate of 2% or less.

Timing of a procedure

Timing of carotid artery revascularization after stroke or TIA is not well defined. There are no strong prospective data, and this continues to be an issue of major clinical concern. In addition, the data are derived from the randomized clinical trials that enrolled patients with TIA or minor disabling stroke with only a few medical comorbidities [11–14]. Thus, decisions about when to intervene are currently based on subjective impressions of various clinical factors.

Retrospective data from observational studies and post-hoc analysis of randomized trials suggest that the reduction of stroke and death following a symptomatic carotid artery event was greatest when the patient was evaluated and treated within 2 weeks of symptom onset [12–14]. In a pooled analysis of the randomized symptomatic carotid endarterectomy clinical trials,

the NNT to prevent a subsequent stroke in 5 years was 5 for patients randomized within 2 weeks, versus 125 for patients randomized after 12 weeks [12,13]. There is a slightly greater risk of infarct extension or cerebral hemorrhage with early surgery that presumably can be mitigated with tight control of blood pressure, and other risk factors (i.e., glucose and lipid control) [11]. Among the associated clinical factors governing early versus late surgery are size of infarction on head CT, clinical deficits including level of consciousness, and extent of residual tissue at risk in the ipsilateral carotid artery territory following stroke. Since carotid artery flow is greatest to the MCA under ordinary anatomic conditions, MCA cortical strokes may subsequently have a greater risk of hemorrhagic conversion following an ipsilateral carotid artery procedure, as compared with strokes in other vascular territories supplied by the carotid artery.

In general, patients with TIA or minor clinical stroke, with only small areas of infarction on CT or MRI, are good candidates for early carotid artery intervention within a few days of presentation. For patients who have larger strokes, greater degrees of clinical deficits, or significant medical comorbidities that require stabilization, a more nuanced approach may be appropriate with delays of 4–6 weeks to address medical comorbidities, and define the degree of post-rehabilitation recovery prior to carotid artery intervention.

Tip

While patients with AF were excluded from the original CEA trials, this is not an absolute contraindication to surgery (see also Case 6 about patient selection factors). Ideally, all patients being considered for carotid artery surgery should undergo a formal cardiac evaluation, as there is a high incidence of concomitant CAD in patients with atherosclerotic carotid artery disease.

Case 3. Asymptomatic carotid artery disease

Case description

A 79-year-old right-handed woman presented to her primary physician with complaints of "dizziness." She described the symptoms as a "woozy" feeling and noted that the dizziness had occurred several times over the past three consecutive days. The dizziness seemed worse with changes in position from sitting to standing but it was not consistently associated with positional changes. She had no prior history of dizziness. She had experienced bilateral visual blurring with the last episode and this was the symptom that prompted her to go to her primary physician. She had no symptoms of chest pain, shortness of breath, or palpitations and her symptoms were not worse with exertion. She had no focal neurologic symptoms.

Medical history included well-controlled arterial hypertension and hyperlipidemia. She was on lisinopril, atorvastatin, and aspirin. She had no prior cardiac history. Her mother died of complications of Alzheimer's disease, and her father's cause of death was unknown. She had one sister with a history of heart problems and a brother with a history of CEA for unknown reasons. Surgical history was remarkable for a knee replacement 2 years earlier, and bilateral cataract surgery.

On examination, she had bilateral, soft cervical bruits, the one on the left more prominent. She had an unremarkable cardiac examination. Distal pulses were present in both feet though diminished on the right side compared with the left side. She had a normal mental status examination. Cranial nerve examination was unremarkable. She had normal facial and extremity strength and sensation. Coordination and gait were normal. Muscle stretch reflexes were normoreactive and symmetric. Plantar responses were flexor bilaterally.

The primary physician ordered a head CT that showed scattered areas of subcortical ischemic changes. A carotid artery duplex ultrasound report showed high-grade bilateral carotid artery stenosis (Figure 9.3). The patient was then referred to a stroke specialist for possible ischemic strokes in the context of high-grade asymptomatic carotid artery disease. The neurologist obtained an MRI of the brain that also showed bilateral subcortical ischemic white matter changes without evidence of acute ischemic disease on diffusion-weighted imaging (DWI) sequences. MRA also confirmed high-grade extracranial ICA stenoses at the bifurcations. Complete metabolic panel, lipid profile, and glycated hemoglobin (hemoglobin A_{1c}) were unremarkable.

The stroke neurologist met with the patient to review the imaging findings and the options for carotid artery intervention. The patient elected to undergo a CEA. The surgeon recommended that she undergo a left CEA, with consideration of right CEA at a later date.

Discussion

The benefit of intervention in asymptomatic patients is no greater than for symptomatic patients with <50% carotid artery stenosis for whom carotid interventions typically are not recommended [2,5]. Still, in selected low surgical risk asymptomatic patients with high-grade carotid artery stenosis (arbitrarily >80% to some clinicians, but 60% to one of us, CML, predicated on the ACAS/ACST data) many physicians do offer patients the option of a procedure based on the ACAS clinical trial data (see also discussion in Case 2).

The risk of stroke in people with asymptomatic carotid bruits is relatively low, with an estimated risk of stroke of 1.5% annually [1,2,5,15]. Approximately 4% of the population has an asymptomatic cervical bruit, but a bruit is not a strong predictor of ipsilateral high-grade carotid artery stenosis [15]. Routine screening for asymptomatic carotid artery disease is not recommended because of lack of cost-effectiveness, the small benefit of carotid artery intervention in asymptomatic individuals, and the risk of false-positive or false-negative tests [15–18]. While identification of a cervical bruit may prompt physicians to obtain carotid ultrasound studies, the detection of a bruit does not correlate well with hemodynamically consequential carotid artery stenosis. Even though auscultation of the cervical arteries for bruits is a standard part of the physical examination of adults, detection of a cervical bruit correlates more closely with systemic atherosclerosis than with carotid artery stenosis. For detection of ipsilateral >70% stenosis, the sensitivity of a cervical bruit was only 63% and the specificity was 61% [5,15]. Cervical bruits, however, are a marker of significant CAD; half of persons with a cervical bruit have significant CAD.

Ultrasonography may be appropriate as a screening tool in high-risk populations, but quality and accuracy of vascular laboratories varies widely, and testing

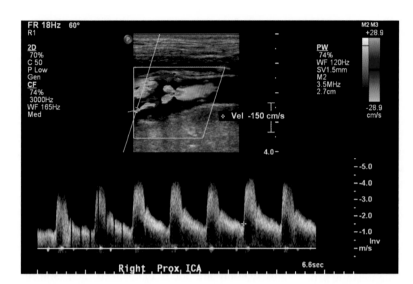

FR 18Hz 60°
R1
2D
 70%
C 50
P Low
Gen
CF
 74%
 3000Hz
WF 165Hz
Med

Vel -150 cm/s

4.0

M2 M3
+28.9

PW
 74%
WF 120Hz
SV1.5mm
M2
3.5MHz
2.7cm

-28.9
cm/s

-5.0
-4.0
-3.0
-2.0
-1.0
Inv
m/s

Right Prox ICA

6.6sec

Figure 9.3 Example of carotid duplex image showing right high-grade carotid artery stenosis.

should only be performed at certified vascular ultra-sound laboratories. Screening might be considered in people aged 65 or older with multiple vascular risk factors or known CAD. However, the benefits of carotid artery disease screening are controversial, and the United States Preventive Services Task Force (USPSTF) report suggested that carotid duplex ultrasonography had significant limits in sensitivity and reliability [18]. The USPSTF report noted that confirmation by angiography for positive tests would expose patients to a 1% risk of stroke and a 30-day perioperative stroke risk of 1.6–3.7% for asymptomatic patients with variations in risk between 1.4% and 6.7% for the combined rate of perioperative stroke and death. In an estimate of "the magnitude of net benefit," the USPSTF report suggested that 23 strokes would be prevented over 5 years following screening of 100 000 persons. The number needed to screen was 4348 persons to prevent one stroke after 5 years, and 8696 persons screened to prevent one disabling stroke. These rates, however, also presuppose that carotid duplex ultrasonography is accurate enough to identify appropriate persons at risk.

Tip

If there is high-grade bilateral asymptomatic carotid artery stenosis, and there is equal evidence for silent cerebral ischemia on MRI, with no difference in collateral blood flow on either side, the left carotid artery should be preferentially considered for CEA first. If, however, the burden of silent cerebral ischemia is

greater on the right side, then one might consider first doing a right CEA preferentially. All patients with a cervical bruit should, however, undergo cardiac stress testing for possible underlying coronary heart disease.

Case 4. Imaging in extracranial carotid artery disease

Case description

A 60-year-old right-handed man presented for consideration of CEA or carotid artery angioplasty and stenting (CAS) after he had a carotid ultrasound that, by report, at an outside vascular laboratory showed 70–95% stenosis of the extracranial right ICA and 50–69% stenosis of the extracranial left ICA with plaque ulceration. There was also high-grade stenosis of the left external carotid artery just distal to the bifurcation. The ultrasound had been done, following a routine physical examination by the patient's cardiologist, when a cervical bruit was identified on the left side. The patient had no clinical history of strokes or TIAs and no focal neurologic or ophthalmologic symptoms.

Medical history was remarkable for arterial hypertension, hyperlipidemia, and prior history of myocardial infarction 10 years earlier treated with coronary angioplasty and deployment of one coronary artery stent. He was on simvastatin for lipid-lowering therapy, metoprolol, clopidogrel, and aspirin. He was also on pantoprazole for gastrointestinal reflux disease. He had a strong family history of cardiac disease and stroke. He did not smoke cigarettes and drank one glass of red wine daily with meals.

Physical examination showed a blood pressure of 134/84 mmHg and pulse rate of 64 beats per minute and regular. He had a normal cardiac examination with a soft left cervical bruit. Distal extremity pulses were normal. Mental status and cranial nerve examinations were unremarkable. Extremity strength, tone, and coordination, bulk, and gait were normal. Sensory examination was completely normal. There were normal muscle stretch reflexes, and both plantar responses were flexor.

A TTE showed normal LVEF with mild left ventricular diastolic dysfunction and left ventricular hypertrophy. A cardiac stress test 2 years earlier was normal.

MRI of the brain showed a few scattered T2 and FLAIR hyperintensities in the subcortical hemispheric regions bilaterally. MRA of the intracranial circulation showed no intracranial stenosis. MRA of the extracranial circulation showed high-grade left ICA stenosis (Figure 9.4). CT angiogram (CTA) showed moderate- to high-grade bilateral extracranial carotid artery stenosis with significant bifurcation plaque with calcification. At that point, the option for a left CEA was discussed.

Prior to CEA, however, a conventional catheter cervicocerebral angiogram was obtained. This revealed only moderate-grade stenosis bilaterally with an estimated 60% right ICA stenosis, by NASCET criteria, and 45% left ICA stenosis. A repeat ultrasound was then obtained that confirmed the findings of moderate-grade carotid artery stenosis bilaterally (with lower velocities than seen on the outside carotid artery duplex ultrasound). The patient had a follow-up carotid duplex one year later, with no significant progression in carotid artery disease.

Discussion

Imaging of the extracranial carotid arterial bifurcation is necessary to determine patient eligibility for possible carotid artery revascularization. One of the most common "pitfalls," however, is reliance solely on a single imaging modality for determination of eligibility for carotid artery revascularization. Many surgeons have resorted to offering patients CEA simply on the basis of one diagnostic carotid ultrasound study. Another common approach for patients with stroke or TIA has been MRI and MRA imaging of the brain, but

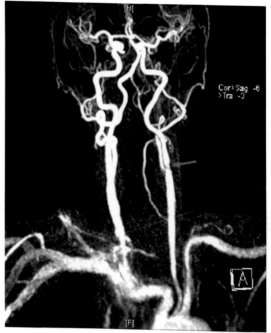

Figure 9.4 MRA demonstrating extracranial left internal carotid artery stenosis (arrow).

only carotid duplex ultrasound imaging of the cervical arterial vessels. Both of these approaches for asymptomatic or symptomatic carotid artery disease are woefully inadequate. All patients with stroke or TIA should have brain imaging (preferably MRI of the brain unless there are contraindications), and all screened asymptomatic patients who are then being referred for possible carotid artery revascularization should also have preoperative structural brain imaging to screen for silent cerebral ischemia.

The "gold-standard" by which all other modalities are measured is catheter-guided cervicocerebral contrast angiography [5]. While this modality provides the most accurate imaging measure of stenosis, it is an invasive procedure with associated potential nephrotoxicity and allergic reactions due to contrast dye, as well as potential injury to blood vessels. Cost and the requirements for adequately trained teams also limit the availability of this modality.

The most problematic complication is catheter-related stroke embolism. While the ACAS study reported a catheter-associated complication rate of approximately 1.2%, the rate is probably now much lower at experienced centers.

The most accepted methodology for measuring the degree of carotid artery stenosis is based on NASCET criteria where the length of the residual lumen at the point of maximal carotid artery stenosis is divided by the length of the extracranial carotid artery lumen distal to the stenosis beyond any point of post-stenotic dilatation. Angiography is typically employed when there are conflicting results among the various non-invasive studies, when significant calculation obscures the accuracy of the non-invasive study results, when there are questions about anatomic variations (such as very tortuous carotid artery segments), or in the context of planned CAS. Otherwise, non-invasive imaging has, for the most part, supplanted, invasive catheter angiography in the screening or determination of patient eligibility for a surgical procedure.

Carotid artery duplex ultrasonography is the preferred screening modality for patients with asymptomatic carotid artery disease [15–18]. The threshold of a peak systolic velocity (PSV) >129 centimeters/second (cm/s) has been associated with a sensitivity of 98% and a specificity of 88% for >49% angiographic stenosis [17]. The ultrasonography PSV >199 cm/s has been associated with a sensitivity of 90% and a specificity of 94% for greater than 69% stenosis. However, there were wide measurement criteria variations among laboratories, and the authors implied differences in patients, study design, equipment, techniques, or training [17].

MRA and CTA complement ultrasound in imaging the carotid bifurcation but give additional information about the entire carotid and vertebrobasilar circulation. As such, these modalities are the preferred approach for initial evaluation of patients with possible stroke or TIA symptoms. CTA is limited by costs, problems with post-processing imaging quality, risks of nephrotoxicity from contrast dye, and radiation. MRA is similarly limited by costs, risks of contrast-induced nephrotoxicity, and patient-related factors such as claustrophobia, obesity, presence of MR non-compatible medical devices, and patients not medically able to lie still for MR imaging. Thus, MRA and CTA are not suitable screening tools for asymptomatic carotid artery disease. Nevertheless, in lieu of catheter angiography, MRA or CTA should be obtained to complement carotid ultrasonography in all patients being considered for carotid artery intervention.

CTA may have 100% sensitivity and 63% specificity compared to catheter angiography and may have higher specificity using more advanced scanners or post-processing techniques [5,19]. It has been our clinical experience that in the presence of calcification at the cervical carotid bifurcation, which is very common in this patient group, CTA often overestimates the degree of stenosis. For >69% carotid artery stenosis, one report suggested 100% sensitivity and 100% specificity for CTA, compared with catheter angiography. In that report, MRA had 100% sensitivity and 97% specificity for >69% carotid artery stenosis, compared with catheter angiography [19]. Overall, when done under optimal conditions, MRA has been reported to have a sensitivity of 97–100%, and a specificity of 82–96%, for >50% carotid artery stenosis [5,19]. These data presume that all studies are of high quality. MRA is most useful at ruling out significant carotid artery stenosis, and one benefit of MRA is that it is less subject to artifact problems related to calcifications, as compared with CTA or ultrasonography. However, the pitfalls of MRA are overestimation of the degree of arterial stenosis, and limitations in identifying total versus subcortical carotid artery occlusions.

Tip

As discussed in Case 1, imaging of the brain should be performed on all patients. Additionally, carotid artery revascularization should never be performed based on a single diagnostic imaging study. Furthermore, patients with extracranial carotid artery atherosclerosis, especially with significant bifurcation calcifications, may need formal catheter angiography to determine the true degree of carotid artery stenosis and plaque morphology.

Case 5. Combination CAD and carotid artery disease: the indications for possible combined procedures and the relative indications of CEA versus CAS

Case description

A 60-year-old man presented to the office following a carotid duplex ultrasound report showing evidence of 1–49% stenosis of the extracranial left ICA and 50–69% stenosis of the right ICA. The ultrasound was done as part of a perioperative evaluation for CAD by his cardiologist, who saw the patient because of dyspnea on exertion, and evaluated him for possible coronary artery bypass grafting (CABG). He had no speech, language, cognitive, or visual complaints, and no symptoms of focal weakness or numbness. He had no prior history of TIA or stroke, but had intermittent lightheadedness that he attributed to his cardiac medications.

He had well-controlled arterial hypertension, diabetes mellitus, hyperlipidemia, peripheral vascular disease, and coronary angioplasties with stents deployed 5 and 15 years earlier. He was on statin, clopidogrel, and aspirin in the context of his prior history of coronary artery stents. He was a prior cigarette smoker, and drank beer occasionally.

Physical examination was remarkable for a blood pressure of 155/90 mmHg and a pulse rate of 58 beats per minute. He had a normal S1 and S2 with a positive S4 but no murmurs were heard. There was a very soft right cervical bruit. Distal pulses in the extremities were normal. Neurologic examination was unremarkable.

TTE showed 50% LVEF with evidence of left ventricular hypertrophy, mild anterior wall motion abnormalities with no aneurysmal dilatation, and normal valve function.

Cardiac angiography showed 100% stenosis of the proximal left anterior descending artery, 60% stenosis of the mid right coronary artery, and 70% stenosis of the proximal left circumflex artery. There was evidence of mild anterolateral hypokinesis and mild diaphragmatic hypokinesis. As part of a preoperative evaluation, a selective angiogram of the right carotid artery was also performed. This showed a focal 95%

right ICA stenosis just distal to the carotid bifurcation (Figure 9.5). The lesion was deemed to be complex, eccentric, and mildly calcified.

The cardiologist consulted a stroke neurologist as to whether the patient should undergo a carotid artery procedure prior to any contemplated CABG. Based on the asymptomatic character of the carotid artery lesion, albeit high-grade, one option discussed with the patient was to undergo CABG with treatment of the carotid artery stenosis thereafter. The cardiac surgeon was disinclined to do CABG until after treatment of the carotid artery stenosis, however. The option of CEA followed immediately by CABG was also discussed, but the patient eventually first underwent left CAS based on the preferences of the cardiac surgeon. The patient was then maintained on clopidogrel and aspirin for 6 weeks. The clopidogrel was then discontinued and, one week later, the patient underwent uneventful three-vessel CABG.

Discussion

Carotid artery angioplasty and stenting (CAS) versus carotid artery endarterectomy (CEA)

Recent randomized trials have explored the suitability of CAS as an alternative to CEA. Carotid artery angioplasty and stenting was first purported to be of particular

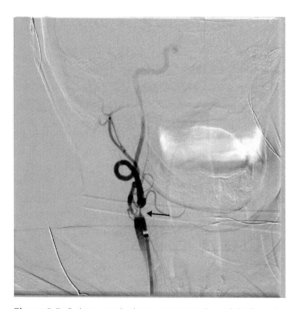
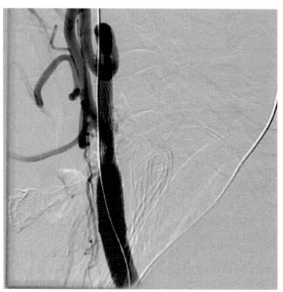

Figure 9.5 Catheter cerebral artery angiography with high-grade (arrow) proximal right extracranial ICA stenosis pre (a) and post (b) angioplasty and stent placement.

benefit in patients at particularly high risk for a surgical procedure. The SAPPHIRE trial was a randomized study that enrolled 156 patients to CAS and 151 to CEA (total N = 307) [20]. Additionally, there was a registry of 407 non-randomized patients deemed at high risk for CEA who had CAS, and 7 patients who had CEA. Patients could have asymptomatic carotid artery disease with >80% carotid artery stenosis by ultrasound or symptomatic carotid disease with >50% carotid artery stenosis; the majority of enrolled patients were asymptomatic. High risk was defined by the presence of at least one of the following features: age >80 years, presence of congestive heart failure (CHF), severe chronic obstructive pulmonary disease (COPD), previous CEA with restenosis, previous radiation therapy, previous radical neck surgery, or carotid artery lesions distal or proximal to the usual cervical location. The primary endpoint (PEP) was death, any stroke, or myocardial infarction (MI) at 30 days post procedure and a major prespecified endpoint was 30-day death, stroke, or MI plus death and ipsilateral stroke between 31 days and 12 months post procedure. The PEP result was that 30-day event rates were 5.8% for CAS compared to 12.6% for CEA (P = 0.047). These results were driven, however, primarily by the 30-day MI rate. At one year, the death rate alone for CAS was 7%, and for CEA was 12.9%.

The SAPPHIRE trial was underpowered and was also limited in that 25% of cases were re-do CEA for which the surgical risk is known to be much higher. Furthermore, there were more patients in the registry arm of the trial than in the randomized arm, and patients in the registry did worse as compared to the randomized patients. A logical conclusion of this trial should have been that patients with high-risk carotid artery stenosis might be better off with medical therapy alone. Subsequently, several European studies (SPACE, EVA-3S, and ICSS) failed to confirm a benefit for CAS [21– 23]. While these trials were criticized for problems of operator selection and training, and failure to procedurally deploy any embolic protection devices, the benefit of CAS remained to be proven.

The subsequent Carotid Revascularization Endarterectomy versus Stenting Trial (CREST) was a large randomized trial of lower-risk carotid artery patients. In this study only 47% of the enrolled subjects had asymptomatic carotid artery disease [24]. The CREST primary endpoint found that the rate of stroke, MI, or any death in the 30-day periprocedural period

(30 days), or any ipsilateral stroke within 4 years after randomization, was 7.2% for CAS and 6.8% for CEA (P = 0.51). The overall outcome of stroke and death favored CEA (4.7% vs. 6.4%; P = 0.03). The periprocedural stroke rate also favored CEA above CAS (2.3% vs. 4.1%; P = 0.01). The major stroke rates, however, were comparable between the two arms (0.9% for CAS vs. 0.6% for CEA; P = 0.52). There was also a trend toward symptomatic patients faring better following CEA as opposed to CAS (6.0% CAS vs. 3.2% CEA; HR 1.89; P = 0.02). Myocardial infarction rates were lower in the CAS arm. Post-intervention, cranial nerve palsies were also less frequent in the CAS arm. The periprocedural MI rate for CAS was 1.1% vs. 2.3% for CEA (P = 0.03). While there may have been trends related to better outcome in the CEA arm for symptomatic patients or female sex (as compared to CAS), the only significant subgroup interaction appeared to be age. In the CREST study, patients in the 40–70 year age group had better outcomes following CAS, driven mainly by the MI rate, whereas patients in the 70–80 year age group had better outcomes following CEA, driven mainly by the stroke event rate.

There have been numerous discussions about how to parse the data further in favor of either CAS or CEA, but the probable major lesson from the CREST study is that patients cared for by skilled proceduralists, using a team-based approach, had a very acceptable rate of periprocedural complications, regardless of the type of procedure. The bigger concern at this time is whether these results are generalizable to the broader non-study populations.

CABG and carotid interventions

The prevalence of cerebrovascular disease in patients with CAD is considerable. In the REACH registry of 26 389 patients with CAD, with an average 4-year follow-up, 460 patients (16.9%) had a history of stroke or TIA [25]. Carotid revascularization, however, is not necessary in all patients being considered for CABG. Moreover, literature is not definitive regarding whether to intervene as well as the role of staged versus combined procedures. Carotid artery angioplasty with stenting (CAS) is an option in this population but the safety and efficacy of CAS compared to CEA is a much-debated topic.

The reported prevalence of carotid artery stenosis in patients (>50%) in patients in need of CABG is described in Table 9.2 [26]. Risk factors for severe carotid stenosis (>80%) include: age >75 years; female

Table 9.2 Prevalence of carotid artery disease in patients being considered for CABG [25]

Degree of carotid artery stenosis	Prevalence (%)
>50%	12–17
>79%	8.5
Unilateral occlusion	0.6
Bilateral occlusion	0.04

Adapted from Ansari et al., 2011 [26].

sex; smoking; peripheral vascular disease; prior history of stroke or TIA; and left main CAD. The risk of stroke, however, is less clear. Carotid artery stenosis in patients undergoing CABG is associated with overall increased stroke risk, but the risk is low for stroke related to ipsilateral carotid artery. Mechanisms of stroke in the post-CABG period include: atheromatous emboli from the aortic arch or heart valves; intraoperative hypoperfusion/hypotension; AF; and fat or air embolism [26–30]. There is no association with side of carotid stenosis and perioperative stroke, with perhaps 40% of perioperative stroke possibly attributable to carotid artery disease with half of these strokes occurring in patients with <50% carotid artery disease. Naylor reported that the stroke risk was <2% in patients with <50% carotid artery stenosis, 3% in patients with 50–99% carotid artery stenosis, 5% in patients with bilateral 50–99% carotid artery stenosis, and 7–11% in patients who a carotid artery occlusion [27]. This did not imply, however, that perioperative strokes were directly related to carotid artery disease. The 2011 ACC/AHA screening guidelines for carotid artery stenosis prior to CABG included age >65 years, history of TIA or stroke, left main CAD, and history of cigarette use. Based on these guidelines 85% of patients >65 years-old would be screened [18].

Overall, there is a low prevalence of significant carotid artery disease on ultrasound in patients proceeding to CABG, and there is limited value for routine preoperative screening carotid duplex ultrasound. Ansari et al. reported there was no significant difference in perioperative strokes compared with non-screened patients (3% vs. 1.2% respectively, P= NS) [26]. Conversely, risk estimates are that 25–60% of patients with moderate- to high-grade carotid artery disease being evaluated for CEA, with no history of cardiac symptoms, have clinically significant CAD detected by cardiac stress testing. In one study of coronary angiography (n=200), 40% of patients being evaluated for CEA had severe CAD (>70% stenosis in at least one coronary artery [27]). Thus, the American Heart Association (AHA) guidelines recommend cardiac stress testing when the diagnostic evaluation of stroke patients reveals carotid artery or other large-vessel atherosclerosis, including some sort of dynamic stress testing [28]. Nawaz et al. reported that, of 198 patients who underwent CEA with no history of preoperative coronary heart disease (CHD), there were no fatalities, and only one case (0.5%) of reversible cardiac ischemia but among 204 patients with preoperative CHD, there were two deaths (1%) and 11 cases of postoperative cardiac ischemia (5.4%) [29]. In this series, the mortality for 60 patients who had a combined procedure was even higher at 6.6%.

Interventional options include treating the more clinically active (either coronary or cerebrovascular) vascular system first in a staged sequence, treating the vascular system with the pathologically more severe vessel stenosis first whether done surgically or percutaneously, or revascularization of the coronary and the carotid arteries at the same time in a combined procedure. These options translate into the following possible sequences: (1) staged procedures with first treatment of whichever vascular bed is most symptomatic; (2) staged procedures with either CEA or CAS done prior to CABG; (3) staged procedures with CABG or coronary artery stenting of the most severe artery being done first followed by a carotid procedure; or (4) combined surgical procedures with the CEA being done under regional anesthesia followed by CABG or, alternatively, general anesthesia for both surgical procedures [27,29,30,31].

There is no generally accepted approach, however, and, in the absence of definitive data, all options are equally valid. Overall stroke morbidity and mortality with combined procedures has variously ranged from approximately 3% to 6%. The rate in combined CEA/CABG procedures favorably compared with the data from the SAPPHIRE study of CAS versus CEA for high-risk patients (who did not undergo CABG) where the 30-day rate of death, stroke, and MI in the CAS arm was 4.8% [20]. Still, CAS preceding CABG is an appealing protocol, and the SHARP study reported a 98% success rate with this protocol in an Italian population with a mean carotid artery stenosis of 80 ± 9% who had staged CAS followed by CABG [32]. It is noteworthy that approximately 55% had bilateral carotid disease and 15% had symptomatic carotid artery stenosis, although patients with stroke in the prior 6 weeks were excluded from the study.

In summary, all patients with moderate- or high-grade carotid artery stenosis should probably undergo cardiac evaluations, including cardiac stress testing. The guidelines also suggest patients undergoing CABG might benefit from screening for carotid artery disease. The sequence of procedural interventions for patients with carotid stenosis and coronary disease remains to be determined. Staged carotid artery procedures prior to CABG are reasonable for patients with stable severe CAD and symptomatic carotid artery disease or asymptomatic high-grade carotid artery disease. Finally, combined procedures should possibly be reserved for patients with both symptomatic CAD and carotid artery stenosis whereas patients with moderate-grade carotid artery disease probably can safely undergo CABG without carotid intervention [26,28,29].

Tip

Regardless of whether a patient undergoes a CEA or CAS, the most important procedural consideration is the skill and experience of the person performing the procedure. As noted previously, the ideal rate of major periprocedural complications should be under 2%. In the best of circumstances, centers would provide verification of complication rates by independent qualified observers but this may not always be possible at all institutions. Referring physicians should only seek out those interventionalists and centers where there is available evidence for high success rates.

Case 6. Clinical variables of importance in selection of patients for carotid artery interventions

Case description

A 71-year-old right-handed woman with a history of medication-controlled glaucoma experienced loss of vision in the right eye described as a gray curtain descending over the eye abruptly and gradually lifting within 10–15 minutes. Her ophthalmologist saw her the next day, reported a normal ophthalmologic examination, and referred the patient to a vascular surgeon after a carotid artery duplex ultrasound study demonstrated a moderate degree of carotid artery stenosis bilaterally.

Medical history was remarkable for arterial hypertension. She was on a beta-blocker and aspirin 81 mg

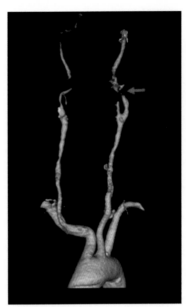

Figure 9.6 CTA showing >90% extracranial ICA stenosis (arrow) of the post-bulbar left ICA.

daily. Surgical history was only remarkable for a total hysterectomy at age 50. Family history included CAD and cerebrovascular disease in her parents and grandparents.

On review of systems, she had no active cardiac, pulmonary, gastrointestinal, or genitourinary symptoms. However, one week prior to presentation, the patient had a 10-minute episode of numbness and tingling on the right side of her face and body that she attributed to "sleeping funny."

The general examination was normal with a regular cardiac rate and rhythm. There were no cervical bruits. Mental status and cranial nerve examinations were unremarkable. The patient had normal strength, tone, bulk, coordination, and sensation. She had normal muscle stretch reflexes and bilateral plantar responses were flexor.

Based on the clinical history, the patient was admitted to hospital for evaluation of TIA related to carotid artery disease. The patient was started on a statin, and continued on aspirin at an increased dose of 325 mg daily. Brain MRI showed a few bilateral T2 and FLAIR hyperintensities. Magnetic resonance angiography confirmed moderate-grade bilateral carotid artery stenosis without calcification, and a CTA confirmed the MRA findings (Figure 9.6). A vascular neurosurgeon was consulted for possible CEA. The stroke neurologist recommended a left CEA for possible left hemispheric sensory TIAs, and that the right carotid artery be followed by serial carotid artery duplex studies for her right retinal artery TIA. There were no complications from the left CEA. Serial carotid artery duplex studies done at 6, 12, and 24 months showed no disease progression with patency of the left CEA site. She has remained symptom-free 2 years post-CEA.

Discussion

There are only a few clinical variables that absolutely preclude carotid artery revascularization. These include complete subacute or chronic carotid artery occlusion, for which the risk of CEA far outweighs any benefit, terminal illness, and certain vascular anatomic considerations of the carotid artery which might intrinsically preclude either CEA or CAS. Otherwise, most clinical factors are, at best, relative contraindications to a procedure. Among high-risk factors for CEA, certain exclusionary factors, such as AF, were only specified in the clinical trials to avoid confounding from alternative stroke mechanisms in the analyses of post-randomization carotid-related stroke or death. There are other clinical factors, such as a high carotid artery bifurcation or radiation-induced carotid artery stenosis, that might make CEA more technically challenging, but for which CAS may still be an option (as discussed in Case 5) [5].

Various analyses suggest there are a number of clinical variables that might modify perioperative morbidity and mortality risk or the benefit of a carotid artery procedure [2,5,13,20,33–35]. These include age, sex, diabetes mellitus, plaque morphology, and contralateral carotid artery occlusion. In post-hoc analyses of the NASCET and ECST trials, age greater than 75 years and male sex were predictors of greater benefit.

Women had a higher risk of perioperative stroke and death as compared with men (odds ratio 1.31, $P < 0.001$) [2,5,33]. A plausible explanation is that women have smaller carotid arteries compared to men. However, women not only had higher perioperative risks, but also fewer events on medical therapy alone. These findings have been consistent for both asymptomatic carotid artery stenosis and moderate symptomatic carotid artery stenosis where there was no clear benefit for CEA in women. For patients with high-grade symptomatic carotid artery stenosis, men and women had similar robust benefits from CEA.

The observation that older patients have a greater benefit from CEA is consistent across the European and North American trials. Furthermore, there is suggestive evidence that patients aged 71–80 had greater benefit from CEA as compared with CAS. One caveat is that we have limited data about patients aged 80 and older, who were excluded from the NASCET and CREST studies. The perioperative stroke and death rate may be reasonable for older patients and, in one series of 2500 octogenarian patients, the perioperative risk was 3.45% [34]. However, the overall non-cerebrovascular disease-related morbidity and mortality rates among octogenarians and nonagenarians must be considered before offering carotid artery interventions. As the crossover point, where the benefit of surgery outweighed the procedural risk, was approximately 3 months for symptomatic carotid artery disease, carotid surgery in this subgroup may be reasonable [1,2]. For asymptomatic carotid artery disease, the crossover point was closer to 3 years, such that intervention in older patients with asymptomatic carotid artery disease should not be routinely recommended.

The type of symptomatic presentation also governs the risk-benefit analysis. In NASCET, those presenting with transient monocular visual symptoms were half as likely to have a stroke as those presenting with hemispheric TIAs. Carotid endarterectomy was of significant benefit only for those subjects with transient monocular visual symptoms who had additional risk factors: age 75–80 years, concomitant symptomatic peripheral vascular disease, or high-grade carotid artery stenosis [2,5,7].

Diabetes mellitus also conveys a higher risk of stroke and death; numerous observational studies and post-hoc analyses of randomized clinical trials suggest diabetes mellitus is associated with a greater risk of perioperative MI or cerebral hemorrhage [5]. Diabetic patients, however, do benefit from CEA, as compared to medical therapy alone, and there is no reason for diabetes mellitus to be an exclusionary risk factor for carotid interventions.

Patients with plaque ulceration may be at higher risk for stroke as shown in analyses of both NASCET and ACAS data. The presence of ulcerated plaque in NASCET was associated with a 2–3 times greater risk of stroke among patients with high-grade carotid artery stenosis randomized to the medical arm [5]. There are no data, however, to support CEA in patients with ulcerated plaque with <50% arterial stenosis. Patients with contralateral ICA occlusion are also thought to be at high risk for stroke in the perioperative period (14% vs. 5%) [35]. The risk, however, of ipsilateral stroke in patients with contralateral arterial occlusion was markedly reduced in the subsequent 2 years in the surgical group as compared to the medical group (22% vs. 69%).

Thus, clinical variables may be considered in the decision-making process regarding the relative risk or benefit of CEA or CAS but should not, a priori, be used to exclude patients from carotid interventions.

Tip

The complexity of patient selection is based on a clear understanding of the risk profile. In this case, a woman with a hemispheric TIA and moderate-grade carotid artery stenosis should undergo a carotid procedure but the occurrence of a retinal TIA in a woman does not absolutely mandate a carotid artery procedure. Careful individualized risk/benefit analysis and patient preference regarding procedural intervention is essential.

References

1. Gorelick PB. Carotid endarterectomy: where do we draw the line? *Stroke* 1999;30:1745–50.

2. Chaturvedi S, Bruno A, Feasby T, et al Carotid endarterectomy – an evidence-based review. Report of the Therapeutics and Technology Assessment Subcommittee of the American Academy of Neurology. *Neurology* 2005;65:794–801.

3. Johnson MJ, Thorisson HM, DiLuna ML. Vascular anatomy: the head, neck, and skull base. *Neurosurg Clin N Am* 2009;20(3):239–58.

4. Shaban A, Albright KC, Boehme AK, et al. Circle of Willis variants: fetal PCA. *Stroke Research and Treatment* 2013. http://dx.doi.org/10.1155/2013/105937.

5. Brott TG, Halperin JI, Abbara S, et al. 2011 ASA/ACCF/AHA/AANN/AANS/ACR/ASNR/CNS/SAIP/SCAI/SIR/SNIS/SVM/SVS Guideline on the Management of Patients With Extracranial Carotid and Vertebral Artery Disease. A Report of the American College of Cardiology Foundation/American Heart Association Task Force on Practice Guidelines, and the American Stroke Association, American Association of Neuroscience Nurses, American Association of Neurological Surgeons, American College of Radiology, American Society of Neuroradiology, Congress of Neurological Surgeons, Society of Atherosclerosis Imaging and Prevention, Society for Cardiovascular Angiography and Interventions, Society of Interventional Radiology, Society of NeuroInterventional Surgery, Society for Vascular Medicine, and Society for Vascular Surgery Developed in Collaboration With the American Academy of Neurology and Society of Cardiovascular Computed Tomography. *Circulation* 2011;124:e54–e130.

6. NASCET Collaborators. Beneficial effect of carotid endarterectomy in symptomatic patients with high grade stenosis. *N Engl J Med* 1991;325:445–53.

7. NASCET Collaborative Group. The final results of the NASCET trial. *N Engl J Med* 1998;339:1415–25.

8. ECST Collaborative Group. Randomised trial of endarterectomy for recently symptomatic carotid stenosis: final results of the MRC European Carotid Surgery Trial (ECST). *Lancet* 1998;351:1379–87.

9. ACAS Study Group. Carotid endarterectomy for patients with asymptomatic internal carotid artery stenosis. *JAMA* 1995;273:1421–8.

10. Halliday A, Mansfield A, Marro J, et al. Prevention of disabling and fatal strokes by successful carotid endarterectomy in patients without recent neurological symptoms: randomised controlled trial. *Lancet* 2004;363:1491–502.

11. Fritz MB. Timing of carotid endarterectomy after stroke. *Stroke* 1997;28:2563–7.

12. Fairhead JF, Mehta Z, Rothwell PM. Population-based study of delays in carotid imaging and surgery and the risk of recurrent stroke. *Neurology* 2005;65:371–5.

13. Rothwell PM, Eliasziw M, Gutnikov SA, et al. Endarterectomy for symptomatic carotid stenosis in relation to clinical subgroups and timing of surgery. *Lancet* 2004; 363(9413):915–24.

14. Schneck MJ, Biller J. How long are delays to carotid imaging and carotid endarterectomy. *Nat Clin Neurol Pract* 2006; 2930 126–7.

15. Sandercock PAG, Kavvadia E. The carotid bruit. *Pract Neurol* 2002;2:221–4.

16. Hill AB. Should patients be screened for asymptomatic carotid artery stenosis? *Can J Surg* 1998;41:208–13.

17. Jahromi AS, Cina CS, Liu Y, Clase CM. Sensitivity and specificity of color duplex ultrasound measurement in the estimation of internal carotid artery stenosis: a systematic review and meta-analysis. *J Vasc Surg* 2005;41(6):962–72.

18. U.S. Preventive Services Task Force. Screening for carotid artery stenosis: U.S. Preventive Services Task Force recommendation statement. *Ann Intern Med* 2007;147:854–9.

19. Randoux B, Marro B, Koskas F, et al. Carotid artery stenosis. Prospective comparison of CT, three-dimensional gadolinium-enhanced MR, and conventional angiography. *Radiology* 2001;220(1):179–85.

20. Yadav JS. Wholey MH, Kuntz RE, et al. Stenting and Angioplasty with Protection in Patients at High Risk for Endarterectomy Investigators. Protected carotid-artery stenting versus endarterectomy in high-risk patients. *N Engl J Med* 2004;351(15):1493–501.

21. Mas JL, Chatellier G, Beyssen B, et al. EVA-3S Investigators. Endarterectomy versus stenting in patients with symptomatic severe carotid stenosis. *N Engl J Med* 2006; 355:1660–71.

22. SPACE Collaborative Group. 30 day results from the SPACE trial of stent-protected angioplasty versus carotid endarterectomy in symptomatic patients: a randomised non-inferiority trial. *Lancet* 2006;368(9543):1239–47.

23. International Carotid Stenting Study Investigators (ICSS). Carotid artery stenting compared with endarterectomy in patients with symptomatic carotid stenosis (International Carotid Stenting Study): an interim analysis of a randomised controlled trial. *Lancet* 2010; 375(9719): 985–91.

24. Brott TG, Hobson RW 2nd, Howard G, et al. Stenting versus endarterectomy for carotid artery stenosis. *N Engl J Med* 2010;363(1):11–23.

25. Ducrocq G, Amarenco P, Labreuche J, et al. A history of stroke/transient ischemic attack indicates high risks of cardiovascular event and hemorrhagic stroke in patients with coronary artery disease. *Circulation* 2013;127(6):730–8.

26. Ansari S, Tan JY, Larcos GS, et al. Low prevalence of significant carotid artery disease on ultrasound in patients proceeding to coronary artery bypass surgery. *Intern Med J* 2011;41(9):658–61.

27. Naylor AR, Mehta Z, Rothwell PM, et al. Carotid artery disease and stroke during coronary artery bypass: a critical review of the literature. *Eur J Vasc Endovasc Surg* 2002;23:283–94.

28. Adams RJ, Chimowitz MI, Alpert JS, et al. Coronary risk evaluation in patients with transient ischemic attack and ischemic stroke: a scientific statement for healthcare professionals from the Stroke Council and the Council on Clinical Cardiology of the American Heart Association/American Stroke Association. *Stroke* 2003; 34:2310–22.

29. Nawaz I, Lord RS, Kelly RP. Myocardial ischaemia, infarction and cardiac-related death following carotid endarterectomy: risk assessment by thallium myocardial perfusion scan compared with clinical examination. *Cardiovasc Surg* 1996;4(5):596–601.

30. Byrne J, Darling RC 3rd, Roddy SP, et al. Combined carotid endarterectomy and coronary artery bypass grafting in patients with asymptomatic high-grade stenoses: an analysis of 758 procedures. *J Vasc Surg* 2006;44:67–72.

31. Venkatachalam S, Gray BH, Mukherjee D, et al. Contemporary management of concomitant carotid and coronary artery disease. *Heart* 2011;97:175–80.

32. Versaci F, Reimers B, Del Giudice C. Simultaneous hybrid revascularization by carotid stenting and coronary artery bypass grafting: the SHARP study. *JACC Cardiovasc Interv.* 2009; 2:393–401.

33. Alamowitch S, Eliasziw M, Barnett HJ. The risk and benefit of carotid endarterectomy in women with symptomatic internal carotid artery disease *Stroke* 2005;36:27–31.

34. Grego F, Lepidi S, Antonello M, et al. Is carotid endarterectomy in octogenarians more dangerous than in younger patients? *J Cardiovasc Surg (Torino)* 2005;46(50):477–83.

35. Gasecki AP, Eliasziw M, Ferguson GG, et al. Long-term prognosis and effect of endarterectomy in patients with symptomatic severe carotid stenosis and contralateral carotid stenosis or occlusion: results from NASCET. North American Symptomatic Carotid Endarterectomy Trial (NASCET) Group. *J Neurosurg* 1995;83(5):778–82.

Chapter 10

Stroke and patent foramen ovale: the conundrum of closure

James R. Brorson

Introduction

Finding a patent foramen ovale (PFO) in the work-up of a stroke patient presents a conundrum to the neurologist. It is clear that with a PFO, cryptogenic stroke can sometimes be caused by paradoxical embolism; beyond that, all consensus ends. The import accorded to the finding of PFO on echocardiography ranges from the main finding mentioned by some trainees in their case presentations, to a fact dismissed as irrelevant by an expert stroke neurologist at a recent national meeting, given the lack of evidence-based treatment implications. Can a middle ground be found?

Some facts about PFO warrant review. An atrial septal opening is a feature of the normal anatomy of the fetal heart, allowing return of oxygenated placental blood to the systemic circulation. Incomplete closure of the PFO after birth occurs in fully a quarter of the population [1]. PFO is found more commonly in young persons with cryptogenic stroke than in controls [2], and certain rare cases of imaging documentation of thrombus penetration through the foramen ovale provide incontrovertible proof that PFO has the potential to allow for paradoxical embolism. However, the finding of PFO alone, in the best evidence from series of cryptogenic stroke in the young, does not imply an increased risk of recurrent stroke [3]. Various associated clinical or cardiac anatomical features, particularly an associated atrial septal aneurysm, have been cited as suggesting a causative role for PFO in the stroke, and possibly an increased risk of recurrence of stroke in follow-up [3,4].

Treatment options for young patients with cryptogenic stroke and PFO might include usual secondary prevention measures with antiplatelets, anticoagulation, or anatomical closure of the PFO with a percutaneously inserted device or even by open surgery. For years the availability of devices to close a PFO have fueled a debate between procedural cardiologists, ready to fix a perceived anatomical flaw, and conservative clinicians noting a lack of any evidence regarding the efficacy of such procedures in preventing secondary strokes. These debates were based on minimal data, however, consisting largely of case series showing the relative success and safety of endovascular PFO closure.

We now have results of randomized controlled trials of PFO closure devices to consider. The CLOSURE I trial described results of randomizing patients with PFO and cryptogenic stroke or transient ischemic attack (TIA) to closure with the Starflex device or to medical therapy [5]. Device placement was accompanied by a modest risk of procedure- or device-related serious adverse events of 3.2%. After 2 years, the hazard ratio for the combined event endpoint was 0.78 in the intention-to-treat analysis comparing the device group to controls, a nonsignificant difference. Of note, 23 patients developed atrial fibrillation in the device group, as compared to 3 patients in the medical group, and 3 of the 12 strokes in the device group occurred in patients with atrial fibrillation. Thus, device-induced atrial fibrillation may have contributed to the lack of benefit in stroke prevention.

The RESPECT trial looked at stroke patients, excluding TIA or lacunar stroke patients, and randomized to closure of PFO with the Amplatzer PFO closure device versus best medical therapy. As in the CLOSURE I study, there was a modest risk of procedure- or device-related serious adverse events, of 4.2%, but there was no detection of increased numbers of patients developing atrial fibrillation with this device. This trial found a relative risk of stroke of 0.49

in the intention-to-treat analysis of comparing the device group to medically treated patients [6]. Again, this was a nonsignificant difference.

The simplistic interpretation of these trials is that the devices are ineffective in preventing stroke associated with PFO. However, in addition to noting that point estimates of device closure effects favored the device in both trials, it is important to realize that a number of the patients randomized to medical therapy ended up receiving device closure during the study, and that some of the recurrent strokes in patients randomized to device placement occurred before device was in place, so that a look at the data from an as-treated perspective produces a different result than the intention-to-treat analysis. In the RESPECT study [6], in an analysis of results in patients as actually treated, PFO closure reduced the risk of recurrent stroke by 73% as compared to the medically treated group, a highly significant difference, both from a statistical perspective and in terms of clinical impact. Furthermore, subgroup analyses showed that the stroke risk reduction by device placement was greatest in patient subgroups with larger right-to-left shunt size and in those with atrial septal aneurysms. This evidence, in total, despite the formal failure to reach pre-defined statistical targets, provides strong support to the thesis that device closure of PFO does effectively prevent recurrent stroke if it can be done safely (with low procedural risks and low risk of inducing atrial fibrillation), and if it is selectively applied to patients in whom the anatomy of the atrial septum creates a significant ongoing risk of paradoxical embolism (i.e., larger shunt, atrial septal aneurysm).

The strict disciple of evidence-based medicine would say, following recent AHA guidelines for secondary stroke protection [7], that "for patients with a cryptogenic ischemic stroke or TIA and PFO without evidence for DVT, available data do not support a benefit for PFO closure" and therefore closure should not be undertaken outside of trials. However, in the clinical world where incomplete evidence is confronted by patients' fears of stroke recurrence and expectations of treatment, as illustrated in the cases below, device closure of PFO continues to be a strong consideration for patients in whom compelling evidence points to a role for PFO in stroke etiology, and in whom risks of recurrent paradoxical embolism loom large.

Case 1. Cryptogenic stroke in a young woman with PFO and atrial septal aneurysm

Case description

A 26-year-old woman in good health, while donating blood plasma, experienced a feeling of warmth, light-headedness, and left arm stiffness, followed by brief loss of consciousness and shaking. After returning home she collapsed in her bathroom, with left hemiparesis. When she presented to the local emergency room, brain MRI showed acute right cerebral hemispheric infarction (Figure 10.1), and MRA showed a filling defect in the distal right M1 segment of the middle cerebral artery (MCA) (Figure 10.2). Further history revealed that she smoked cigarettes and marijuana, and used an oral contraceptive. Personal and

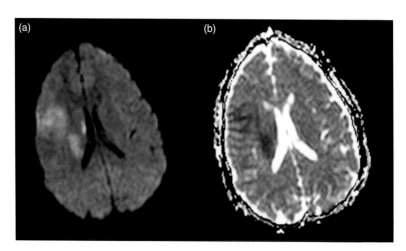

(a)   (b)

Figure 10.1 Acute brain magnetic resonance imaging diffusion-weighted (a) and apparent diffusion coefficient map (b) images showing evidence of acute ischemic lesions in right frontal cortex and para-ventricular white matter areas.

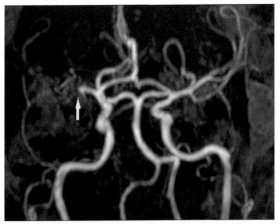

Figure 10.2 Acute head time-of-flight magnetic resonance angiography images suggesting occlusion of mid right MCA M1 segment (arrow).

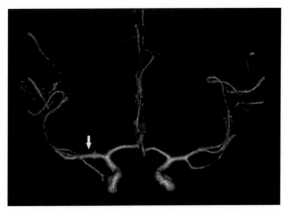

Figure 10.3 CT angiography one week following acute right MCA stroke showed normal findings, consistent with recanalization of the previously occluded right MCA (arrow).

family histories were negative for venous thrombosis. Urinary toxicology screen was positive for marijuana and amphetamines. A transthoracic echocardiogram showed normal valve structures and chamber function, with possible inter-atrial shunt and atrial septal aneurysm. Lower extremity Doppler examination was negative for thrombi.

After 5 days she was transferred to our medical center's cardiology service expressly for consideration of PFO closure. Transesophageal echocardiogram (TEE), with intravenous infusion of agitated saline, confirmed an inter-atrial shunt and visualized a PFO. Hypercoagulable work-up was entirely negative. Repeat imaging with brain CT (not shown) and CT angiogram revealed evolving right hemispheric infarction, without hemorrhagic transformation, and restoration of normal flow in the right MCA (Figure 10.3).

She was treated initially with aspirin and supportive care. Seven weeks later, percutaneous closure was accomplished using a 25 mm Amplatzer cribriform PFO closure device (Figure 10.4). She tolerated the procedure without complication. One day later, transthoracic echocardiography with bubble study showed the device in place at the interatrial septum and "a minimal interatrial shunt." She was discharged, and was lost to subsequent follow-up at our center.

Discussion

Documented proximal MCA occlusion, threatening a devastating stroke, followed by recanalization, as in this case, provides a recognizable pattern highly suggestive

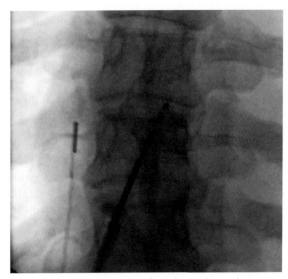

Figure 10.4 Fluoroscopic image from closure-device placement, showing intracardiac echocardiogram transducer and device delivery catheter, attached to hub of closure device, immediately preceding deployment.

of embolic stroke. In a young person with few vascular risk factors, paradoxical embolism rises high on the a priori list of possible etiologies to consider. The findings of a PFO, with atrial septal aneurysm, by Bayesian statistical reasoning, raises this from possible to probable cause, although alternative embolic sources can never be fully ruled out.

It stands to reason that paradoxical embolism must start with venous thromboembolism. The presence of known risks for venous thrombosis, such as smoking and oral contraceptives in this case, are common in patients with paradoxical embolism, even when Doppler examination fails to confirm deep venous thrombosis. A lack of identified venous thrombosis is common even in cases of pulmonary embolism, so that negative findings on lower extremity venous Doppler examination cannot be considered as ruling out paradoxical embolism from a venous source. Some centers advocate additional work-up to include pelvic CT or MRI scanning to search further for venous thrombi, which, when positive, may strengthen the diagnosis of presumed paradoxical embolism. The treatment of such patients must address the risks of recurrent venous thrombosis and pulmonary embolism as well as risks of recurrent stroke.

Best medical therapy for prevention of recurrent stroke in cryptogenic stroke associated with PFO is not well-established. One might rationalize that the supposed etiology of the stroke, due to paradoxical embolism from a venous source, would dictate that anticoagulation must be recommended, as the more effective therapy for prevention of venous thromboembolism. If deep venous thrombosis can be directly identified, then clearly anticoagulation is indicated, at least for 3 months [8]. However, lacking identified venous thrombosis, the balance between risks and benefits of anticoagulation versus antiplatelet therapy may be different. The embolic source might be a superficial vein, or the atrial septum itself. Furthermore, recurrent stroke following cryptogenic stroke in a young person with PFO has been shown to be a relatively low-risk event, substantially less frequent than the early recurrence rate of venous thromboembolism after initial deep venous thrombosis. For long-term prevention of an uncommon event the risk/benefit balance between full anticoagulation and antiplatelet therapy is not the same as that for the short-term prevention of recurrent venous thromboembolism. Thus, many practitioners have chosen to use antiplatelet therapy rather than anticoagulation for secondary prevention in their patients with cryptogenic stroke and PFO.

The finding of atrial septal aneurysm (ASA) with PFO on echocardiography may suggest a higher risk condition than PFO alone. Mas et al. [3] found that PFO with ASA was a marker of increased risk of recurrent stroke in young patients with cryptogenic stroke, associated with a rate of stroke recurrence of 15.2% over 4 years, much more than PFO alone, associated with a 4-year rate of stroke recurrence of 2.3%, not significantly greater than (and numerically less than) the incidence of recurrence in those without either PFO or ASA.

The advisability of recommending PFO device closure for cryptogenic stroke associated with PFO involves all of the issues above, as well as the risks and effectiveness of the devices in preventing recurrent embolization. While randomized controlled trials, as reviewed above, have not successfully demonstrated effectiveness of device closure for stroke prevention in their primary endpoints, in patients with PFO and ASA, in the RESPECT trial [6], there was a strong signal suggesting efficacy of closure over medical treatment. Off-label use of a closure device can be offered on these grounds, with careful explanation to the patient of the lack of conclusive evidence for efficacy and the lack, at the present time, of device approval for stroke prevention.

A confounding factor in decision-making for patients with stroke and PFO is often the influence of the expectations of patients and referring physicians. If told that medical therapy might be a more appropriate course of action for secondary prevention in his/her case, the patient will sometimes respond with the implication that the physician is depriving him or her of the life-saving procedure "to fix the hole in my heart." While these influences must be tempered with careful patient education about what is known and not known about stroke and PFO, and about the effectiveness of device closure, shared doctor–patient decision-making inevitably brings these expectations into play.

The timing of closure following stroke, if it is to be attempted, should be carefully considered. Prior to the dual antiplatelet therapy that is temporarily required after device placement, hemorrhagic conversion of the stroke must be ruled out. A period of recovery of brain tissue from acute effects of ischemia, and restoration of normal autoregulatory function, should be allowed before challenging the patient with an intracardiac procedure. For infarctions of moderate size or larger, a period of at least 4–6 weeks between stroke occurrence and device placement is appropriate.

Tip

When a patient with PFO has been referred directly to the cardiologist, inevitably the final decision regarding PFO device closure occurs between the patient and the physician offering the procedure. The neurologist serving in a consulting role has the responsibility to provide verification of the nature of the cerebral event as ischemic, to ensure that a complete etiological work-up has been completed and has been interpreted correctly, and to fully inform the patient regarding the implications of the finding of PFO and the uncertainties regarding the best approach to secondary prevention.

Case 2. Transient focal neurological symptoms

Case description

A 31-year-old man awoke from a nap during a long ride back from a holiday with family and experienced right hand, arm, and face tingling and numbness, difficulty reaching with the right hand, and garbled word order in expressive speech. Stopping at a gas station, he felt lightheaded and had trouble reading a billboard. These symptoms abated within 10 minutes, but a bifrontal headache occurred. He was admitted to a local hospital and extensive work-up was done, including brain MRI scanning, cervical spine MRI, head and neck MRA, transcranial Doppler (TCD) study, and MRI of pelvis, and antiphospholipid antibody screening, all entirely normal. However, a TEE was positive for left-to-right flow across the interatrial septum, suggestive of PFO (Figure 10.5, not this patient).

Three weeks later he had another event that was similar, but less severe, with trouble talking on the phone, difficulty finding words, and right arm tingling, lasting minutes, without headache. He was referred to our medical center for evaluation for possible PFO closure. Review of medical history revealed only occasional mild headaches associated with a sick feeling in the stomach, and two episodes of syncope, once while fasting, another time at the sight of blood.

On examination he was a thin fit young man, appearing somewhat anxious. His vital signs were normal, with blood pressure 117/78 mmHg, and his entire neurological examination was normal.

He was advised that these events with apparent aphasia and right sensory disturbance were possible TIAs, with alternative possibilities including migrainous events. Based on the clinical features, with uncertainty regarding the diagnosis of cerebral ischemia, and lack of high-risk PFO anatomical features, closure of PFO was not recommended. Instead, continued antiplatelet therapy, and evaluation for hyperlipidemia and need for statin therapy were advised.

Over subsequent 6 years he had recurrent symptoms that he learned to recognize as anxiety-associated, with symptoms of panic attacks. These were successfully treated by his primary physician with low dose alprazolam as needed.

Discussion

Diagnosis of transient events, without lasting signs and without MRI scan correlates, is inherently less certain than diagnosis of stroke with lasting objective signs. Transient symptoms are difficult to assign to specific

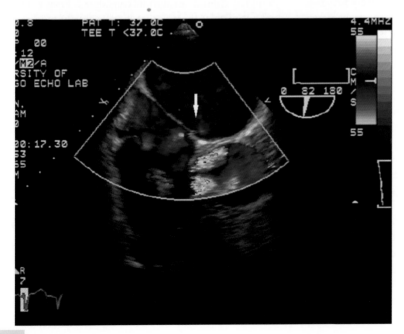

Figure 10.5 Example of transesophageal echocardiogram (not from this patient), with Doppler signal indicating flow across interatrial septum from right atrium to left atrium (arrow).

etiology. Diagnosis is based entirely upon historical characteristics of the symptoms and associated patient factors. Scoring systems using clinical features to provide a numerical score predictive of risk of recurrent stroke, such as the ABCD^2 score, have been validated. The risk stratification they produce is probably based more on classifying transient neurological events in terms of the likelihood of their true thromboembolic nature, rather than finding different risk implications for different kinds of true ischemic events. It is notable that the ABCD^2 score [9] does not award any points for purely sensory symptoms. The features of this case, with primarily sensory symptoms, short duration, and no accompanying vascular risk factors, would produce a low ABCD^2 score, casting doubt on the ischemic nature of the event. Furthermore, recurrent events with stereotypical symptoms are not consistent with a cardiac source of emboli, as flow in the heart is turbulent and emboli from the heart will travel disparate paths. While two successive symptomatic emboli might with some probability go to the same MCA territory, more than two events with similar symptoms should point to a non-embolic cause or intracranial or possibly cervical source of emboli. Finally, the associated headache raises the possibility of migraine as cause. Reports of palpitations or panic might point to anxiety-driven symptoms.

Given these challenges in accurate diagnosis of etiology of transient events, it is notable that TIA was included as an entry criterion for the CLOSURE I study, likely contributing some patients with non-embolic causes for symptoms to the study pool, and decreasing the study's power to detect the effectiveness of device closure for preventing recurrent stroke.

The presence of a PFO in a patient with an event of uncertain nature is not unexpected by chance alone as an incidental finding. An urge to reach premature diagnostic closure, assigning blame for the event to the PFO, must be resisted. The lack of high-risk anatomical features of the PFO in this case, without right-to-left shunt at rest, or associated ASA, are further reasons to discourage an interventional procedure. In other patients, the reason for discovery of a PFO might be the work-up done for a stroke not likely to be cardioembolic in nature, such as a lacunar infarction in a middle-aged patient with hypertension or diabetes, or a stroke in the territory of an artery with documented atherosclerotic plaque. Such patients should not be subjected to PFO device closure.

Tip

In patients with substantial doubts regarding the diagnosis of a cerebral embolic ischemic event, unproven therapies with substantial risk such as endovascular PFO closure or prolonged anticoagulation should be regarded with skepticism. In such cases, the neurologist's role needs to be one of providing clarity of thinking about the etiology of the event, redirecting the focus away from the incidental finding of a PFO and towards the more pertinent risk factors.

Case 3. Cryptogenic stroke with PFO and thrombophilia

Case description

A 30-year-old right-handed woman, with history of hypertension, smoking, preeclampsia, asthma, and spontaneous abortion, and known to carry the factor V Leiden mutation (heterozygous), developed sudden chest pain and dyspnea. At her local hospital, chest CT angiogram was equivocal for pulmonary embolism, and she was not anticoagulated. Three months later, she again experienced sudden severe chest pain, followed 5 minutes later by right-sided numbness involving face, arm, leg, and trunk. The right hand was clumsy and the speech was slurred, with word-finding difficulties. Most symptoms and signs improved within 2 hours, and brain CT and MRI scans were reportedly negative. Repeated chest CT scan showed no sign of pulmonary embolism. Carotid duplex scanning showed no stenosis or disease. Transthoracic echocardiogram showed entirely normal findings. One week later a repeat echocardiogram was performed, this time with infusion of intravenous bubble contrast, and was reportedly entirely normal, without any detection of PFO or right-to-left shunting. She was diagnosed with TIA and released without further treatment. She stopped smoking.

Her physician referred her for a neurovascular opinion. Aspirin was recommended immediately, as well as consideration of long-term anticoagulation for venous thromboembolism prophylaxis, based on clinical suspicion. To further search for paradoxical embolism, TCD study with intravenous bubble infusion was performed. This revealed prominent passage of bubbles into the bilateral MCAs at rest, and markedly increased shunting with Valsalva maneuver (Figure 10.6). Based on this finding, a recommendation

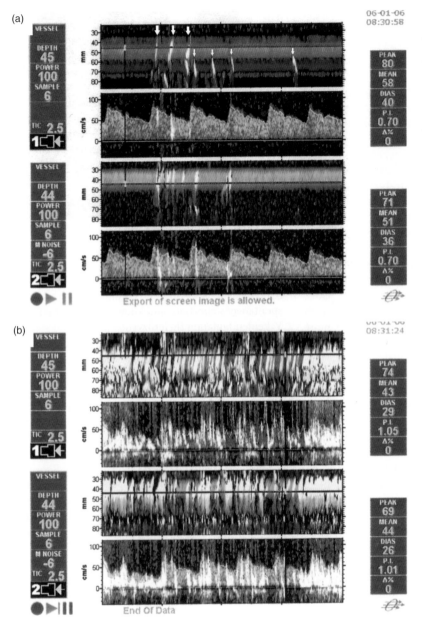

Figure 10.6 Frame shots from TCD recordings during venous infusion of agitated saline bubbles, from a patient with similar findings to those of this case. (a) At rest, frequent individual high-intensity transient signals at depths consistent with MCA or ACA localization are seen (arrows). (b) With a 5-second Valsalva maneuver, the device screen is filled with multiple overlapping high-intensity transient signals.

was made for secondary stroke prevention with either long-term anticoagulation for venous thromboembolism prophylaxis, or device closure of the PFO. The question of whether anticoagulation might also be indicated for prevention of venous thromboembolism was referred to her internist.

A TEE at our center revealed a PFO with right-to-left shunting. PFO closure was performed 2 months after the neurological event with a 30 mm cribriform atrial septal occluder device, without complication (Figure 10.7). Intracardiac echocardiogram post-device deployment showed elimination of atrial shunting. She was treated with aspirin and clopidogrel for 3 months, followed by brief treatment with warfarin, which she did not tolerate, changing to aspirin. Follow-up at 2 years revealed no recurrence of thromboembolism, though she had episodes suggesting migraine with visual aura.

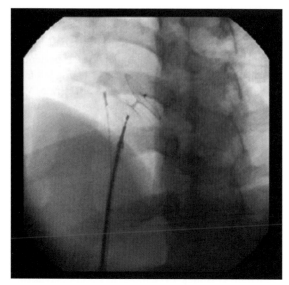

Figure 10.7 Fluoroscopic image from closure-device placement, showing intracardiac echocardiogram transducer and device delivery catheter, near the hub of closure device, immediately following deployment.

Discussion

Sometimes the case for paradoxical embolism as the cause for a stroke is greatly strengthened by near-simultaneous evidence for pulmonary embolism. When pulmonary embolism is confirmed, and no other cause for stroke is identified, parsimonious reasoning would infer that the stroke resulted from the same venous embolic shower. Such cases clearly call for treatment with anticoagulation. In this case, although the clinical symptoms and the patient's risk factors would seem to raise high suspicion for pulmonary embolism, the treating physicians were unconvinced of the diagnosis.

Hereditary thrombophilias increase the risk of venous thromboembolism some two- to eightfold, and are frequently found in young patients with cryptogenic stroke and PFO. The identification of a well-defined hypercoagulable state strengthens the suspicion of a mechanism of paradoxical embolism causing the stroke, and is often taken as an indication for prolonged or lifelong anticoagulation after a stroke. An enhanced propensity for formation of venous thrombi would be expected to increase the future risk associated with right-to-left shunting via the PFO, and at least one study, in a retrospective unblinded analysis, found a significantly higher rate of recurrent cerebral ischemic events in patients with thrombophilia than

in those without, with elimination of the difference in rates after PFO closure [10]. On the other hand, in a substudy (PICSS-APASS study) of the large WARRS trial of warfarin versus aspirin in older stroke patients, presence of the antiphospholipid antibody syndrome with PFO did not reach statistical significance in its effect on risk of recurrent stroke, TIA, or death over 2 years (23.9% vs. 13.9%) [11]. A conundrum is sometimes faced: does an enhanced risk for repeated venous thromboembolism eliminate the need for considering PFO closure, because lifelong anticoagulation will be needed in any case, or does it increase the impetus for PFO closure, to prevent further paradoxical embolization? In a young person with these conditions, facing a lifelong risk of recurrent paradoxical embolism, the latter viewpoint carries weight, given the lack of any fail-safe means to prevent recurrent venous thromboembolism.

It is not uncommon for a young patient to present with cryptogenic stroke and heightened suspicion for paradoxical embolism, yet with echocardiography, including bubble studies for right-to-left shunting, entirely negative. In such cases, TCD studies, with infusion of agitated saline–air mixture, can often detect evidence for paradoxical embolism even when no sign was found on TEE. There may be several reasons for the superior sensitivity of TCD bubble studies, including the ability to detect even a single bubble entering the middle cerebral artery circulation as a high-intensity transient signal (HITS), the sensitivity to routes of paradoxical embolism outside of the heart, and the fully alert and cooperative state of the patient during the study, allowing a vigorous Valsalva maneuver to be performed during bubble injection.

Though strong empirical evidence is lacking, it is intuitively compelling that the risk of paradoxical embolism with any recurrence of venous thromboembolism will be greater with a PFO that is larger and that carries a larger right-to-left shunt, present at rest as well as with Valsalva. Features of a large right-to-left shunt and shunting present at rest are often taken as reasons to more strongly consider endovascular PFO closure. In the patient in this case, with strong suspicion for an ongoing risk of venous thromboembolism, and a PFO with prominent right-to-left shunting at rest and with Valsalva maneuver, a recommendation for endovascular closure of the PFO seemed prudent. The device placed was an atrial septal occluder, FDA-approved for closure of atrial septal defects with shunting at rest.

Tip

In a young patient with stroke that is truly cryptogenic, particularly when suspicion of venous thrombosis is high, it is advisable to extend the search for potential right-to-left shunting beyond echocardiography to performance of TCD – bubble studies, often detecting a PFO missed by echocardiography.

Case 4. Stroke-like symptoms, and paradoxical emboli, can come from more than one source

Case description

A 25-year-old woman initially presented with an episode of sudden numbness of both hands lasting 10 minutes, followed by persisting right hand numbness and difficulty writing. Brain MRI revealed only a developmental venous anomaly. Seven months later, while smoking, she noted sudden nausea, right hand and leg numbness, and difficulty speaking, without headache, and presented to another medical center. A brain scan reportedly documented a stroke, and symptoms resolved over several days. The work-up was negative save for demonstration of a "small" PFO on TEE, which was promptly closed with an Amplatzer septal occluder device, followed by treatment with aspirin and clopidogrel. Nevertheless, one week later she had recurrent symptoms consisting of bilateral hand numbness lasting for 10 minutes, with a headache following 10 minutes later. Repeat TEE was reportedly negative for interatrial shunting, and migraine was diagnosed. However, cerebral angiography showed filling defects in distal branches of the left MCA, suggestive of cerebral embolism.

Four months later she presented to our center for a second neurovascular opinion. A repeated brain MRI scan showed suggestion of additional chronic small lesions in the left parietal, frontal, and opercular cortical areas, new in comparison to prior brain MRI scans, and thought to possibly represent post-inflammatory change, versus atypical ischemic lesions (Figure 10.8). Lumbar puncture was done, with cerebrospinal fluid (CSF) studies normal, and negative for oligoclonal bands. Hypercoagulable testing was negative. She was continued on aspirin and clopidogrel for several months, then on aspirin alone, and did well except for occasional unilateral headaches.

One year later, repeat TEE at another medical center showed evidence for persistent shunting into the left atrium, without any specific atrial septal defect identified. Soon thereafter, she experienced an episode of left-sided numbness involving left face, arm, leg and foot, lasting for 6 hours. Brain MRI reportedly was "normal." Review of the TEE images showed that the bubbles appeared in the left atrium after three to four cardiac cycles, suggesting an extracardiac right-to-left shunt. A chest CT angiogram revealed a pulmonary arteriovenous malformation (Figure 10.9), which was closed percutaneously. No other vascular malformations were observed, and there was no personal or family history of unexplained bleeding episodes.

Over the following year anxiety and frequent migraine-like headaches persisted, with occasional recurrent episodes of left-sided numbness lasting for hours. Migraine prophylactics were attempted but were not tolerated. She did well with occasional ibuprofen for headaches and alprazolam for anxiety. Repeat brain MRI after a 3-year interval showed no new lesions.

Discussion

Establishing the diagnosis of embolic stroke in a young person is often not straightforward. Stroke mimics, including migraine, seizure, inflammatory or demyelinating diseases, and psychogenic symptoms, can often confound the picture, and even when brain ischemia is established, uncommon mechanisms of ischemia such as angiitis or vasoconstriction must be considered. If the appearance of lesions on brain imaging is equivocal, lumbar puncture and analysis for immunoglobulins and oligoclonal bands may be indicated to evaluate for inflammatory conditions and multiple sclerosis. Migraine- and anxiety-driven events must be recognized and treated as best as possible. Even in retrospect, as in this case, it often remains unclear whether individual symptomatic events were ischemic or due to other mechanisms. In light of such uncertainty, the significance of the finding of a PFO can be quite unclear. This uncertainty must be acknowledged in discussions with the patient, and a rush to procedural "fixes" resisted. In this case, in which the PFO was not accompanied by any high-risk anatomical features, in retrospect it does not appear that device closure of the PFO was strongly indicated.

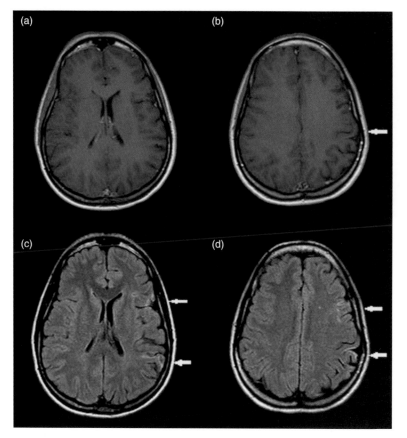

Figure 10.8 Selected brain MRI T1-weighted (a, b) and FLAIR (c, d) images obtained 4 months after the second event. There were areas of subtle gyral hyperintensity in left frontal and parietal cortical areas (b, c, d, arrows) and punctate areas of hyperintensity on FLAIR imaging in some deep left hemispheric and juxtacortical white matter areas.

In cases with definitive evidence for embolic stroke, and suggestion of venous thromboembolism as the source, a pulmonary arteriovenous malformation can sometimes be the route of paradoxical embolism, rather than a septal defect in the heart. Often the characteristic timing of appearance of bubbles on an echocardiographic study, with bubble appearing in the left atrium only after three to four cardiac cycles, offers evidence for the presence of an extracardiac site of shunting. A small pulmonary arteriovenous malformation is often well-tolerated, but such malformations carry ongoing risks of hemoptysis, hemothorax, and cerebral abscess formation, as well as of stroke. Malformations with larger feeding artery diameters of 3 mm or more, or those that grow over time, are thought to carry higher risks, and percutaneous embolic occlusion can be considered, although high-level evidence from prospective controlled trials is not available. Again, a tendency to attribute all symptomatic events to an identified anatomic anomaly can mislead patients and doctors alike into expecting that further symptoms can be prevented with a simple procedure. There should be a careful weighing of whether symptomatic events are truly embolic in nature, and attempt at appropriate medical therapy, as decisions regarding procedural treatment options are made. In this case, with a pulmonary arteriovenous malformation with a large feeding artery diameter, it seems possible that this was a more likely source for paradoxical embolism than was the PFO. Although detailed results of the initial echocardiogram are not available for review, it may be that careful assessment of the timing of bubble appearance in the left atrium in this study would have suggested the presence of the pulmonary arteriovenous malformation from the start.

Tip

When the PFO is small, without prominent right-to-left shunting, and without associated atrial septal aneurysm, the possibility of its role in causing stroke should be regarded with heightened skepticism, and other more pertinent etiological risk factors should be sought.

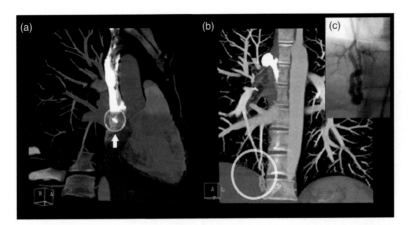

Figure 10.9 Planar reconstruction images from chest CT angiogram showing atrial septal occluder device in place in the interatrial septum (a) and identifying a large pulmonary arteriovenous malformation (b, circle). The pulmonary arteriovenous malformation was confirmed in pulmonary angiography (c, inset) and embolized endovascularly.

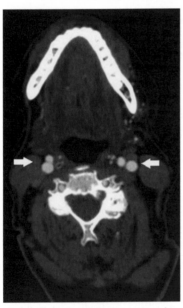

Figure 10.10 Representative section of neck CT angiogram and the level of carotid bifurcations (arrows), showing absence of any evidence of vascular wall changes suggestive of atherosclerotic plaque.

Case 5. Closure for the young at heart?

Case description

A 66-year-old man, with prior history only of treated prostate cancer, presented with sudden inability to speak after bending down to pick up a paper in his office at work. His colleagues reported that he kept saying "I don't know." There were no other symptoms. He had no history of smoking and no risk factors for vascular disease. At a local hospital, a stroke was diagnosed, with work-up unrevealing of any atherosclerotic disease or cardiac arrhythmia, but with transthoracic echocardiogram showing PFO with atrial septal aneurysm. Speaking improved over the next 24 hours. He was treated with warfarin, later switched to dabigatran, and referred for second opinion.

In neurological assessment, a subtle global aphasia was detected, but the examination was otherwise normal. Review of the outside work-up found brain MRI showing an area of restricted diffusion in the left frontotemporal cortex, CT angiogram of head and neck showing normal findings, with no signs of stenosis or early plaque in cervical carotid arteries (Figure 10.10), and lipid panel showing low-density lipoprotein (LDL) cholesterol of 61 mg/dL. The stroke was considered cryptogenic. The lack of a strong evidence base favoring PFO device closure for stroke prevention was presented to the patient, and closure was deferred. He was advised to continue on anticoagulation for 3 months, followed by a transition to aspirin therapy.

Eighteen months later an elective brain MRI, done to investigate chronic hearing loss, showed an incidental small acute to early subacute infarction in the left cerebellum, as well as the chronic left peri-Sylvian cortical infarction (Figure 10.11). The only possible recent symptom he could relate was that he had inexplicably fallen several days earlier while walking his dogs. His neurological examination was fully normal. A 30-day ambulatory cardiac monitor was placed, and showed no evidence for atrial arrhythmias or atrial fibrillation. In light of the recurrence of cryptogenic infarction, in this patient with PFO accompanied by atrial septal aneurysm, endovascular device PFO closure was recommended. He underwent placement of a 30 mm cribriform atrial septal occluder without complications.

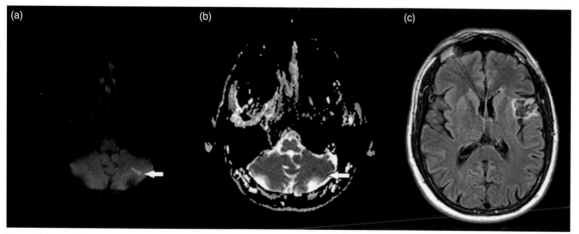

Figure 10.11 Diffusion-weighted (a) and absolute diffusion coefficient map (b) images showing a small early subacute cerebellar infarction (arrows). A chronic cortical infarction in left frontotemporal peri-Sylvian cortex could be seen on FLAIR images (c).

He was subsequently treated with antiplatelet therapy, and was doing well at the last visit 6 months later.

Discussion

In older patients with cryptogenic stroke, particular attention must be paid to investigation for early atherosclerosis or paroxysmal atrial fibrillation as cause. Merely ruling out major vascular stenosis is not sufficient to eliminate the possibility of atherosclerosis as the most likely cause of stroke; review of vessel wall images in carotid ultrasound or CT angiogram studies can often reveal identifiable atherosclerotic plaque, culpable as a source for thromboembolism, even though not causing significant stenosis. If vascular risk factors and vascular pathology is absent, concerns are increased for paroxysmal atrial fibrillation as cause for embolic stroke. Extended cardiac monitoring, for 30 days or longer, will reveal paroxysmal atrial fibrillation in 10–20% of cases, even when short-term cardiac monitoring has been negative. Discovery of non-stenotic atherosclerotic plaque in an appropriate vessel or of paroxysmal atrial fibrillation makes these more likely sources for thromboembolism than the PFO, which can be expected to be present as a purely incidental finding in some 25–30% of patients. In cases where a conventional risk for stroke is documented, this should be considered the presumed etiology for the stroke, rather than the PFO.

Even in a truly cryptogenic stroke, in a patient of the typical age range for stroke (over 60 years), early atherosclerosis can be present without overt vascular risk factors, and the finding of a PFO should be regarded as most likely incidental. Treatment aimed at conventional risk factors should be applied for secondary prevention [7]. Thus, conventional secondary prevention with antiplatelet therapy would be selected over anticoagulation therapy in most such cases, high-intensity statin therapy should generally be recommended, and blood pressure treatment instituted.

When cryptogenic stroke patients have recurrent stroke despite appropriate medical therapy, there is usually a strong desire on the part of both patient and physician to search for a better means of preventing further stroke. Substitution of one antiplatelet agent for another, or of anticoagulation for antiplatelet therapy, is sometimes chosen, without strong evidence demonstrating the efficacy of such an approach [12]. When a PFO is present, especially when accompanied by higher risk anatomical features such as atrial septal aneurysm, recurrent stroke can also be a reason to consider moving to device closure of PFO. Here, repeated failure of antiplatelet therapy was deemed sufficient in this patient to recommend PFO closure; the alternative offered to him was a recommendation of lifelong anticoagulation. Some guidelines, however, may require failure of anticoagulation therapy with stroke recurrence before allowing for consideration of device placement. In practice, it is usually not a comfort to patients to tell them that they need to wait until another stroke occurs before getting PFO closure; often the patient will seek out and readily find another physician willing to perform the procedure.

Finding a PFO in the work-up of a stroke patient is an opportunity for the neurologist to contribute specialized knowledge and careful reasoning to the correct interpretation of the clinical data. Discipline in clinical reasoning is required to avoid the facile but incorrect inferences that finding a PFO necessarily indicates an etiological role for it, or that suspecting paradoxical embolism as the etiology of stroke is reason enough to recommend PFO closure. It is the neurologist's privilege and responsibility to assess in each case the most likely etiology of stroke, and the value of alternative treatment choices, and to appropriately guide treatment decisions in light of this assessment [13].

Tip

In older patients, the finding of PFO should generally be regarded as incidental. Exceptionally strong evidence for an anatomically high-risk PFO, and for risk of recurrent paradoxical embolism, should be required before considering PFO device closure.

References

1. Hagen PT, Scholz DG, Edwards WD. Incidence and size of patent foramen ovale during the first 10 decades of life: an autopsy study of 965 normal hearts. *Mayo Clin Proc* 1984;59:17–20.

2. Lechat P, Mas JL, Lascault G, et al. Prevalence of patent foramen ovale in patients with stroke. *N Engl J Med* 1988;38:1148–52.

3. Mas J-L, Arquizan C, Lamy C, et al. Recurrent cerebrovascular events associated with patent foramen ovale, atrial septal aneurysm, or both. *N Engl J Med* 2001;345:1740–6.

4. Homma S, Di Tullio MR, Sacco RL, et al. Characteristics of patent foramen ovale associated with cryptogenic stroke: a biplane transesophageal echocardiographic study. *Stroke* 1994;25:582–6.

5. Furlan AJ, Reisman M, Massaro J, et al. Closure of medical therapy for cryptogenic stroke with patent foramen ovale. *N Engl J Med* 2012;366:991–9.

6. Carroll JD, Saver JL, Thaler DE, et al. Closure of patent foramen ovale after cryptogenic stroke. *N Engl J Med* 2013;368:1092–100.

7. Kernan WN, Ovbiagele B, Black HR, et al. Guidelines for the prevention of stroke in patients with stroke and transient ischemic attack: a guideline for healthcare professionals from the American Heart Association/American Stroke Association. *Stroke* 2014;45:2160–236.

8. Kearon C, Kahn SR, Agnelli G, et al. Antithrombotic therapy for venous thromboembolic disease. American College of Chest Physicians Evidence-based clinical practice guidelines (8th Edition). *Chest* 2008;133:454S–545S.

9. Johnston SC, Rothwell PM, Nguyen-Huynh MN, et al. Validation and refinement of scores to predict very early stroke risk after transient ischaemic attack. *Lancet* 2007;369(9558):283–92.

10. Giardini A, Donti A, Formigari R, et al. Comparison of results of percutaneous closure of patent foramen ovale for paradoxical embolism in patients with versus without thrombophilia. *Am J Cardiol* 2004;94:1012–16.

11. Rajamani K, Chaturvedi S, Jin Z, et al. Patent foramen ovale, cardiac valve thickening, and antiphospholipid antibodies as risk factors for subsequent vascular events. The PICSS-APASS Study. *Stroke* 2009;40:2337–42.

12. Homma S, Sacco RL, Di Tullio MR, et al. Effect of medical treatment in stroke patients with patent foramen ovale: patent foramen ovale in cryptogenic stroke study. *Circulation* 2002;105:2625–31.

13. Meissner I, Khandheria BK, Heit JA, et al. Patent foramen ovale: innocent or guilty? Evidence from a prospective population-based study. *J Am Coll Cardiol* 2006;47:440–5.

Chapter 11

The diagnosis and overdiagnosis of cerebral vasculitis

Ruth Geraldes

Introduction

Neurologists are often asked to determine if a patient with stroke or other multifocal cerebral dysfunction has "cerebral vasculitis." However, several challenging problems arise with this frequently asked question: "Does this patient have cerebral vasculitis?"

The first one is that the term "vasculitis" is not a disease but a pathological appearance [1] that implies that there is inflammation within the vessel wall [2]. The classic core histopathological change comprises an inflammatory infiltrate within (not just around) the vessel wall, associated with destructive mural changes ("fibrinoid necrosis"), precipitating vascular occlusion and/or vessel dilatation/aneurysm formation. The inflammatory infiltrate may have specific characteristics such as the presence of granulomata or of eosinophils [3,4]. Also the type of vessel involved may vary from arteries to veins and capillaries, from small to medium and/or large vessels. Though biopsy of central nervous system (CNS) tissue showing vasculitis is the only definitive test, having access to pathological examination of CNS vessels is not always easy or possible and the assumption of cerebral vasculitis is sometimes considered based on the clinical setting and results from complementary evaluation. However, neurological manifestations are not pathognomonic and paraclinical tests are not specific.

After demonstrating cerebral vasculitis there are several causes that should be considered.

Primary central nervous system vasculitis (PCNSV), also known as primary angiitis of the central nervous system (PACNS), is an uncommon disease in which lesions are limited to the brain and spinal cord. Proposed diagnostic criteria [5] are: (1) presence of a neurological or psychiatric dysfunction not explained otherwise; (2) classical angiographic or

histopathological changes; and (3) exclusion of other disorder that may mimic the angiographic or pathological changes. In fact, most patients with the initial suspicion of PCNSV have alternative diagnoses [5].

In the present chapter several real life clinical scenarios will guide us through different steps of the diagnosis of cerebral vasculitis, namely PCNSV. Initially we will focus on separating disorders that mimic cerebral vessel dysfunction but do not actually involve the cerebral vessel wall itself and on distinguishing inflammatory from noninflammatory disorders affecting the cerebral vessels. Also, the importance of excluding infection as cause of cerebral vasculitis will be reinforced. Finally, to make the diagnosis of PCNSV, systemic vasculitis, involving the CNS vessels, has to be excluded. Pitfalls regarding complementary diagnostic procedures in PCNSV and its subtypes will also be illustrated.

Distinguishing cerebral vasculitis from noninflammatory vasculopathies and intravascular disorders

Case 1. Does this young woman with headache, visual impairment, and multiple arterial stenoses have cerebral vasculitis? A case of reversible cerebral vasoconstriction syndrome

Case description

A 47-year-old woman, with a previous history of a pineal cyst, depression treated with sertraline 100 mg/

Common Pitfalls in Cerebrovascular Disease: Case-Based Learning, ed. José Biller and José M. Ferro. Published by Cambridge University Press. © Cambridge University Press 2015.

day, trazodone and olanzapine, and smoking habits (10 units/day), frequently complained of dizziness associated with hypotension and was recently on etilefrine 10 mg three times a day (a sympathomimetic amine of the 3-hydroxy-phenylethanolamine series used in treating orthostatic hypotension). She was admitted to a community hospital due to a sudden onset bifrontal headache with occipital propagation, associated with nausea, sonophobia, and photophobia. Headache was so intense that she resisted to every head/neck movement and neurological examination was unremarkable though there were doubts regarding possible terminal neck stiffness. Brain CT (within 12 hours after headache onset) only disclosed the already known pineal cyst. A lumbar puncture (LP) was performed but cerebrospinal fluid (CSF) was not xanthochromic after centrifugation, had elevated protein content (70 mg/dL), normal glucose, an increased leukocyte (300 μL) count, and no quantification of erythrocytes. On blood tests there was a slight leukocytosis (14.0×10^9/L) with negative C-reactive protein (CRP). CSF changes were attributable to an LP but antibiotics to community-acquired bacterial meningitis (ceftriaxone, vancomycin), with

dexamethasone, were prescribed. As the patient had persistent episodes of thunderclap headache, despite analgesia with paracetamol (acetaminophen), clonixine (nonsteroidal anti-inflammatory used to treat pain in many countries in Europe and South America), and tramadol, she was transferred to a tertiary hospital center. Neurological examination was unremarkable and brain MRI disclosed bilateral parieto-occipital hyperintensities on FLAIR sequence, with normal diffusion-weighted images, and no signs of hemorrhage on T2* sequences (Figure 11.1a). There was an increase in flow velocities on transcranial Doppler (TCD) in both middle cerebral arteries (MCAs) (systolic velocity [sV] 225 cm/s), and distal vertebral and basilar arteries (sV 155 cm/s). A repeated CSF analysis was normal. Initial CSF cultures were negative and antibiotics were discontinued. The diagnosis of posterior reversible encephalopathy syndrome (PRES) associated with cerebral vasoconstriction was made. Normal saline (2000 mL/day) and oral nimodipine 60 mg every 4 hours was started. Two days after admission she developed cortical blindness and left hemiparesis associated with hypotensive profile. On a repeat brain MRI there

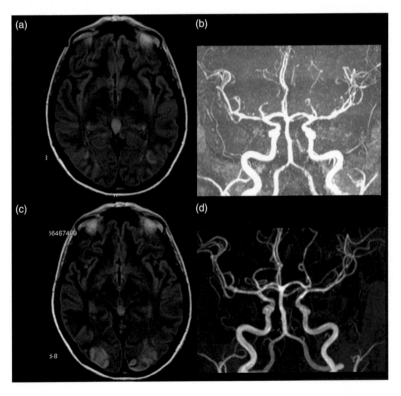

(a) (b) (c) (d)

Figure 11.1 Reversible cerebral vasoconstriction syndrome. (a) First brain MRI FLAIR axial section showing subcortical parieto-occipital hyperintensities. (b) Angio-MRI showing segmental narrowing of both middle, left anterior and posterior cerebral arteries, and vertebral arteries. (c) Second brain MRI FLAIR axial section, after clinical neurological worsening showing extension of the occipital hyperintensities. (d) Three-month follow-up angio-MRI showing complete resolution of vasoconstriction.

was an extension of FLAIR hyperintensities and a new right precentral gyrus ischemic lesion (Figure 11.1b). Angio-MRI revealed several stenoses in the cerebral arteries: left vertebral artery, initial segment of the MCAs and left anterior artery (ACA) (Figure 11.1c). Normal saline was increased to 3000 mL. There was a gradual improvement of the headache and complete resolution of the neurological deficit, in parallel with normalization of flow velocities on TCD at 1-month follow-up and partial resolution of the parieto-occipital lesions on brain MRI. At 3 months brain MRI with angio-MRI only disclosed a small precentral hyperintensity in FLAIR sequence and complete normalization of the parieto-occipital changes and no cerebral vessel changes (Figure 11.1d). A definite diagnosis of reversible cerebral vasoconstriction syndrome (RCVS) was made.

Discussion

This is an illustrative case of a patient with a thunderclap headache where subarachnoid hemorrhage (SAH) had to be excluded. At the community hospital there were doubts regarding neck stiffness and a traumatic LP was not helpful in excluding bacterial meningitis, so antibiotics were started. Since locally it was not possible to investigate other causes of thunderclap headache (e.g., cerebral venous thrombosis, cervical arterial dissection) the patient was referred to a tertiary hospital.

Headache is one of the most common clinical manifestations of cerebral vasculitis, occurring in up to 63% of patients with PCNSV [6,7]. Altered cognition, hemiparesis, and visual symptoms are also frequently reported. Typically headaches in PCNSV are progressive [5,8,9]. A significant number of patients with suspected PCNSV will have headache and other focal neurological signs caused by vasospasm instead of vasculitis of the cerebral vessels [8]. In fact, some of the earliest series of PCNSV included a subgroup named benign angiopathy of the CNS, which is currently considered to be a vasoconstriction syndrome [10,11]. Distinguishing RCVS from PCNSV is crucial, since treatment options are completely different. However, misdiagnosis is not infrequent and leads to unnecessary invasive diagnostic procedures or exposure of patients to immunosuppressive treatments [12]. Patients with RCVS usually present with sudden (peaking in <1 minute) onset of severe headache (thunderclap headache) that, as in the present case, warrants exclusion of

SAH. When there are several typical episodes of thunderclap headache, as in this patient, RCVS is a most probable diagnosis [13].

CSF is usually unremarkable in RCVS whereas it is abnormal in 80–90% of patients with cerebral vasculitis [14]. In the present case a traumatic LP initially confused the diagnosis. In patients with PCNSV, CSF pleocytosis rarely exceeds 250 cells/μL and the presence of CSF leukocytosis greater than 250 cells/μL, along with a white blood cell differential showing increased polymorphonuclear rather than lymphocytic cell count, should be a red flag leading to an aggressive search for infection [8].

Several conditions and substances have been associated to RCVS. Therefore it is very important to review all the medications that the patient is using, including over-the-counter substances [13,15]. Typically the patient has been exposed to vasoactive substances, such as etilefrine, the sympathomimetic recently prescribed to this patient, immunosuppressant or blood products, etc. RCVS may be associated with posterior reversible encephalopathy syndrome (PRES) [16]. Acute headache, confusion, seizures, and cortical blindness associated with a characteristic MR imaging pattern with FLAIR bilateral symmetrical hemispheric junctional/boundary high signal in the cortex, subcortical and deep white matter, particularly in the parietal and occipital regions but that may also involve the frontal areas as in our patient [17]. Segmental vasoconstriction of cerebral arteries demonstrated by angiography (magnetic resonance angiography (MRA), computed tomography angiography (CTA), or catheter angiography) is the key feature of RCVS and is at times difficult to distinguish from PCNSV. However, irregular and asymmetrical arterial stenosis and multiple occlusions suggest PCNSV rather than RCVS [11,13,18]. Finally, to make a definite diagnosis it is crucial to demonstrate the reversibility of the angiographic changes in a follow-up angiogram [14]. TCD is also very useful for monitoring temporal evolution of cerebral vasoconstriction [19].

RCVS treatment with fluids and nimodipine is still empirical. Avoiding exposure to predisposing substances is very important. Cerebral ischemia can occur in 6–9% of the patients, usually in the second week. Long-term recurrences are rare [14].

Pitfall and tips

Both RCVS and PCNSV are associated with headache, focal neurological signs, and segmental cerebral vessel constriction. Headache pattern, predisposing causes, and typical imaging features help to distinguish RCVS from PCNSV. Headache is usually acute (not progressive) and intense ("the worst headache ever") in RCVS. Thorough review of exposure to medications or drugs that may cause vasoconstriction is very important. RCVS may be associated with typical features of PRES on brain MRI.

Case 2. Does this young woman with multifocal ischemic strokes have cerebral vasculitis? A case of non-infectious endocarditis

Case description

A 41-year-old woman, with smoking habits and a previous history, 4 months before admission, of right lower limb deep vein thrombosis (DVT), was admitted due to sudden onset of left facial and left arm weakness. She had recent weight loss (8 kg in 3 months) and typical features of Raynaud syndrome. One month prior to admission she complained of fever, thoracic pain, and myalgia and after common infections were excluded, she was referred to the Rheumatology outpatient clinic. Examination disclosed a subungual purpuric lesion of the second digit of the left hand, a central left facial paresis, and a slight drift of the left upper limb. Brain MRI showed acute ischemic lesions in the right MCA, left MCA, the left posterior cerebral artery (PCA) territory, and

the left anterior-inferior cerebellar artery (AICA) territory, as well as multiple subacute bihemispheric ischemic lesions (Figure 11.2). On angio-MRI there was no flow in the distal cortical right MCA branches and in the P3 and P4 segments of the left PCA, and a distal small left internal carotid artery aneurysmatic dilatation.

Cerebral infarcts in different territories and signs and symptoms of systemic disease indicate the following diagnostic hypotheses: (1) autoimmune connective tissue disorder (e.g., systemic lupus erythematosus (SLE); primary systemic vasculitis) with cerebral involvement (associated with vasculitis or prothrombotic autoantibodies); or (2) cardioembolism from infective endocarditis/non-infective endocarditis/atrial myxoma.

Laboratory work-up revealed leukocytosis (13 800 leukocytes and 78% neutrophils with normal CRP and procalcitonin). Antinuclear (ANA) antibodies, anti-double-stranded (ds-DNA) antibodies, anti-Sjögren's syndrome-related antigen A (anti-Ro/SSA) and anti-Sjögren's-syndrome-related antigen B (anti-La/SSB) antibodies, anti-neutrophil cytoplasmic antibody (ANCA) antibodies, lupus anticoagulant (LA), and antiphospholipid (AP) antibodies and cryoglobulins were negative. Blood cultures and comprehensive infection screening were negative. CSF examination was unremarkable. Dermatological evaluation of the finger lesion pointed to a nailfold small infarct and biopsy only showed nonspecific changes (no signs of vasculitis). Retinal angiography was unremarkable. She had a normal ECG. Transesophageal echocardiogram (TEE)

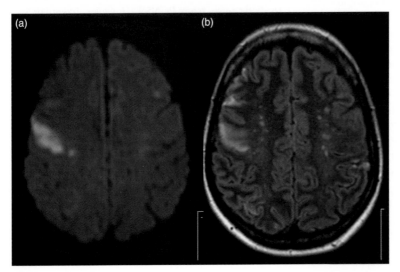

(a)   (b)

Figure 11.2 Non-infective endocarditis. Brain MRI, axial sections. (a) Diffusion-weighted image and (b) FLAIR showing right prefrontal (with correspondent hypointensity in the apparent diffusion coefficient (ADC) map) and left frontal hyperintensities (isointense in the ADC map) suggesting, respectively, acute and non-recent ischemic lesions in the territory of both middle cerebral arteries.

disclosed mitral valve vegetations with moderate mitral valve regurgitation and an aortic valve vegetation. A thoraco-abdominal-pelvic CT disclosed distal bilateral pulmonary embolism. Initial empirical treatment for infective endocarditis with intravenous ceftriaxone 2 g/day was started, until infectious work-up was completed. At this point the diagnosis of non-infective endocarditis was made and full dose anticoagulation started.

Discussion

One important differential diagnosis of cerebral vasculitis is endocarditis, particularly infective endocarditis, because both conditions may present with similar clinical (multiple strokes, encephalopathy) and ancillary findings (multivessel narrowing and aneurysmatic dilations) [20]. Differentiating these two entities is extremely important because treatment is completely different and exposing a patient with infective endocarditis to immunosuppressive agents, such as cyclophosphamide, may have catastrophic consequences.

Cerebral ischemia in several arterial territories, which was documented in this patient, is a frequent finding in patients with cerebral vasculitis [6,21]. Our patient had a small carotid artery aneurysmatic dilation and multiple vessel occlusions. This pattern, though not typical, could occur in a patient with cerebral vasculitis. However, multifocal cerebral ischemia is also a key feature of cardioembolic stroke and of prothrombotic disorders such as the antiphospholipid syndrome and others.

In this patient there were clear symptoms and signs (fever, myalgias, skin lesions, weight loss) pointing to a systemic disease with CNS involvement. The main question was whether the cerebral ischemia was related to secondary cerebral vasculitis (related to a systemic disease) or to cardioembolism.

Infective endocarditis and cerebral vasculitis (primary or secondary) are associated with elevated inflammatory markers (erythrocyte sedimentation rate (ESR), CRP). CSF is usually abnormal in cerebral vasculitis (elevated CSF protein content, positive oligoclonal bands, elevated leukocyte count) [8]. In contrast, CSF examination is less frequently abnormal in infective endocarditis, but some cases with CSF pleocytosis have been reported [20]. Thus, these markers are not really helpful in distinguishing these two conditions. TEE is essential for the diagnosis of endocarditis. TEE disclosed valvular vegetations in our patient. The occurrence of a previous DVT and negative inflammatory markers, such and CRP and procalcitonin, as

well as complete negative infectious work-up, pointed to a non-bacterial thrombotic endocarditis (NBTE), associated with either an autoimmune disorder (e.g., Libman–Sacks endocarditis in SLE) or, as in our patient, a tumor.

Pitfalls and tip

Cerebral vasculitis (primary or secondary) and endocarditis (infective or non-infective) may present with multifocal cerebral ischemia. Also, bacterial endocarditis can be associated with cerebral vessel changes with multifocal stenosis and aneurysmatic dilations. TEE should be included in the diagnostic work-up of patients with suspected cerebral vasculitis, whenever a cardioembolic source of embolism has to be excluded.

Case 3. Does this young woman with seizures, raised inflammatory serological markers, and multifocal CNS white matter changes have cerebral vasculitis? A case of cerebral lymphoma

Case description

A 47-year-old previously healthy woman was admitted to the internal medicine ward because of unremitting fever, anemia, and raised inflammatory markers (ESR 110 mm/s, CRP 23 mg/dL). An extensive work-up had excluded infection. Thoraco-abdomino-pelvic CT, PET-CT, and myelogram were unremarkable. Neurological consultation was requested due to complex partial seizures. After recovering from the seizures, her physical examination was unremarkable. Brain MRI showed multiple subcortical fuzzy hyperintense lesions on FLAIR sequences, the largest one with slight contrast enhancement in the right temporal lobe suggesting demyelinating areas. No changes in cerebral angio-MRI were found (Figure 11.3a). CSF examination showed a protein content of 117 mg/mL and six normal lymphocytic cells. Infectious work-up was unremarkable. At this point, the hypothesis of cerebral vasculitis was raised. Brain biopsy was proposed but the patient refused this procedure. Seizures resolved with antiepileptic medication and there was an improvement of white matter changes with high dose corticosteroids. However, one week later, she had persistent fevers, new spleen enlargement, and serum

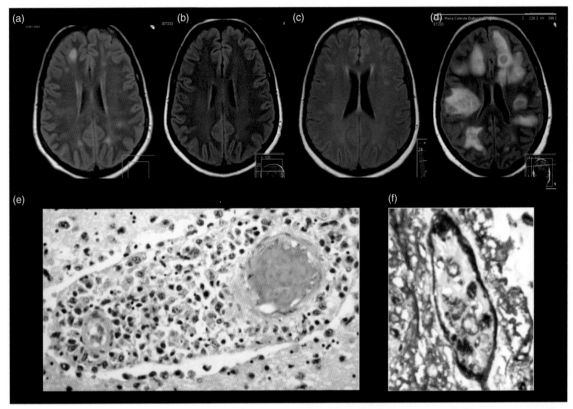

Figure 11.3 Brain lymphoma. (a) The first brain MRI showed multiple subcortical fuzzy lesions hyperintense in FLAIR sequence, suggesting demyelinating areas. (b) Brain MRI 1 week and (c) 3 months after steroid treatment showing disappearance of some previously observed lesions and fading of others. (d) Brain MRI after clinical worsening showing multiple hyperintense white matter lesions. (e) Brain pathological examination (hematoxylin and eosin 200×) showing a monoclonal large and immature B-lymphocytic infiltrate. (f) Lung pathological examination (immunohistochemistry anti CD-20) – showing a perivascular and intravascular monoclonal B-lymphocyte infiltrate.

ferritin elevation (>10 000 ng/mL). Spleen biopsy was performed and pathological examination demonstrated hemophagocytosis. The diagnosis of acquired adult hemophagocytic lymphohistiocytosis with CNS involvement was made and the HLH-94 chemotherapy protocol was started together with steroids. Her symptoms improved as did the white matter lesions after one week (Figure 11.3b) and at 3-month follow-up with brain MRI studies (Figure 11.3c). Two months after completion of the HLH-94 protocol induction phase she was readmitted with somnolence, disorientation, and visual hallucinations. Brain MRI showed a severe recrudescence of supratentorial white matter lesions (Figure 11.3d). Her clinical status rapidly deteriorated with coma and death related to diffuse brain edema. Postmortem pathology was consistent with an intravascular lymphoma identified in the kidney and lungs and CNS diffuse large B-cell monoclonal lymphoma (Figure 11.3e and f).

Discussion

Cerebral lymphomas should be included in the differential diagnosis of PCNSV. Intravascular lymphoma can mimic both clinical and radiological features of PCNSV. Constitutional symptoms such as fever, malaise, weight loss, and arthralgias are common in intravascular lymphoma and other lymphomas but are less common in PCNSV. Acute-phase reactants are typically markedly elevated in intravascular lymphoma, but these tend to be normal in PCNSV; and the CSF is usually abnormal in PCNSV but cannot really differentiate it from intravascular lymphoma. Cerebral angiography can be normal in PCNSV, particularly if only small vessels are affected [22]. Hodgkin lymphoma has been associated with granulomatous angiitis of the CNS. Rarely cerebral vasculitis can be the first manifestation of Hodgkin lymphoma [23–25].

CNS biopsy is very important in the diagnosis of PCNSV, since alternative diagnoses can be made in 39% of cases of suspected PCNSV [26]. The sensitivity of brain biopsy for diagnosing PCNSV varies between 50% and 80%, and in most reports brain biopsy has had a morbidity of about 2%, with a negligible mortality when done by an experienced neurosurgeon [27,28]. Cerebral biopsy is particularly important in the differential diagnosis of cerebral vasculitis involving the small cerebral vessels, usually presenting with brain MRI abnormalities and normal cerebral angiograms. Intravascular lymphoma is an extremely rare B-cell lymphoma with a dismal prognosis, involving the CNS in around 34% of the cases and with a known association with hemophagocytic lymphohistiocytosis [29]. Demonstrating a monoclonal B-cell cerebral/vessel infiltration by a cerebral biopsy is the only way to make a definitive diagnosis, in patients presenting initially only with CNS symptoms and no evidence of systemic involvement.

Pitfall and tip

Intravascular lymphoma and other lymphomas with CNS involvement may mimic PCNSV. Cerebral biopsy is crucial to make an early diagnosis.

Case 4. Does this 63-year-old man with headaches, memory loss, and photopsias have cerebral vasculitis? A case of cerebral inflammatory amyloid angiopathy

Case description

A 63-year-old hypertensive and diabetic man, with a past medical history of myocardial infarction on antiplatelet treatment, had a 2-month history of left parietal headaches and mild memory deficits, and complained of photopsias in the previous week. On examination blood pressure was 200/100 mmHg. There was a slight dysmetria in the right upper limb. Brain MRI disclosed cortico-subcortical bilateral temporo-occipital FLAIR hyperintensities (Figure 11.4a), suggestive of vasogenic edema, multiple microbleeds on T2* sequence (Figure 11.4b), and discrete left cortical occipital enhancement after gadolinium injection. Laboratory work-up, including CSF analysis, transthoracic echocardiogram (TTE), cervical vessel ultrasonography, and TCD were unremarkable. No epileptiform discharges

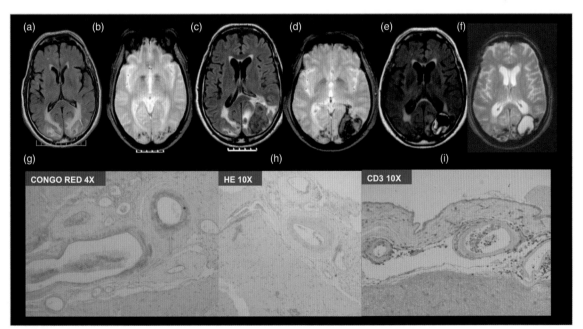

Figure 11.4 Inflammatory cerebral amyloid angiopathy. (a) The first brain MRI showing parieto-occipital FLAIR hyperintensities suggestive of vasogenic edema and (b) T2* microbleeds. (c) Second brain MRI, after clinical worsening, showing a left occipital lobar hematoma in FLAIR, and (d) T* sequences. (e) Follow-up FLAIR and (f) T2* brain MRI showing the sequelae of the left occipital hematoma but no new lesions. On pathological examination there was (g) leptomeningeal thickening with amyloid deposition in meningeal vessels in Congo Red, (h) hematoxylin–eosin colorations, and (i) perivascular lymphocytic infiltrate, with CD3 predominance in immunohistochemistry studies.

were detected on EEG. Blood pressure was controlled, valproic acid was started, and the patient was discharged home with no further symptoms. However, 3 days later the patient was readmitted due to headache recurrence, psychomotor slowing, and disorientation. On neurologic examination there was a right homonymous hemianopsia and optic ataxia in the right visual field. Brain CT disclosed a left temporo-occipital hematoma. On a repeat brain MRI, in addition to the lobar hematoma and vasogenic edema, no new lesions were identified (Figure 11.4c and d). Conventional cerebral angiography was unremarkable. At this point the diagnosis of a possible inflammatory type of cerebral amyloid angiopathy (ICAA) was raised and a brain biopsy was performed. On pathological examination there was leptomeningeal thickening with amyloid deposition in meningeal vessels and a perivascular lymphocytic infiltrate, with CD3 predominance, supporting ICAA diagnosis (Figure 11.4g, h, and i). In this context intravenous methylprednisolone 1 g/day for 5 days, followed by prednisone 1 mg/kg per day was prescribed with clear clinical improvement. Two months later, after an attempt at lowering the steroid dose, there was a clinical worsening with cognitive impairment and aggressive behavior and agitation. Intravenous cyclophosphamide (0.6 g/m^2, monthly for 6 months) was prescribed and the patient stabilized with residual memory deficits. On 6-month follow-up brain MRI no new lesions were found (Figure 11.4e and f).

Discussion

Lobar intracerebral hemorrhage is the most frequently recognized clinical manifestation of CAA. In a subset of patients with amyloid beta (Ab) vascular deposition, vascular inflammation is also present. Such patients often present with findings of subacute cognitive decline, seizures, headaches, and T2-hyperintense lesions, and respond to immunosuppressive treatment [30,31]. Two pathologic subtypes have been described: one with a perivascular non-destructive inflammatory infiltration, so-called CAA-related inflammation (CAA-RI), and the second with a vasculitic transmural, often granulomatous, inflammatory infiltrate (Ab-related angiitis or ABRA) [30,32–34]. It has been proposed that ABRA is more closely related to PCNSV than to CAA without inflammatory infiltrates. Thus ABRA would be a definable subset of PCNSV characterized by older age, high frequency of cognitive dysfunction and seizures/spells, increased spinal fluid protein levels, high frequency of enhancing leptomeningeal lesions,

and favorable response to glucocorticoids alone or in combination with cyclophosphamide [30,34]. In our patient focal seizures have preceded the lobar hematoma, as already described in patients with CAA [35]. Also in this age group CAA would be the most probable diagnosis, rather than PCNSV. Notwithstanding, intracranial hemorrhage was reported in 12.2% of patients with PCNSV [36], intracerebral hemorrhage being more frequent than SAH. In our patient the diagnosis of CAA-RI was made. It is possible that CAA-RI and ABRA are part of the same pathologic spectrum and imaging abnormalities suggestive of vasogenic edema/mass effect have been reported in a significant number of patients with ABRA or CAA-RI [37]. Our patient had a clear response to steroids, clinical worsening as steroids were tapered, and stabilization with cyclophosphamide, which suggested that inflammation was responsible for the clinical symptoms.

Pitfall and tip

PCNSV may present with lobar hematomas. ABRA is possibly a subset of PCNSV. This diagnosis should be considered in older patients, with lobar hematomas or a history of rapidly progressive cognitive deterioration, since it responds to immunosuppressive treatment.

Documenting cerebral vessel inflammation

Case 5. Does this middle-aged woman with recurrent strokes, dementia, elevated ESR, and several cerebral artery stenoses have cerebral vasculitis? A case of angiography positive PCNSV

Case description

A 58-year-old hypertensive black woman had (3 months before admission) a posterior circulation ischemic stroke, with mild left hemiparesis and gait ataxia. She was readmitted due to sudden onset of right hemichorea. The patient had worked as an accountant and was independent until 6 months before admission. Since then, her family had noticed progressive behavioral changes with lack of initiative, memory loss, and lack of insight that clearly interfered with her daily life activities. She also complained of constant headaches. General examination was unremarkable. On neurological examination she was disoriented in time and space, had verbal memory impairment, low verbal output, and a grade 4 right hemiparesis and right hemibody choreic movements. Brain MRI disclosed a recent ischemic lesion in the left caudate nucleus and anterior limb of the internal capsule and several non-recent ischemic lesions, extensive leukoaraiosis and gadolinium enhancement of both ACAs, left MCA (Figure 11.5a and b), and basilar artery (Figure 11.5c and d), without leptomeningeal enhancement. Conventional cerebral angiography showed multiple stenoses of the proximal segments of intracranial arteries (particularly segmental stenosis with poststenotic dilation of the distal M1 segment and M2 right MCA), right posterior communicating artery aneurysm,

left intracranial internal carotid artery stenosis with marked poststenotic dilatation, irregularities of the A1 segment of the left ACA, and irregularities of the basilar artery (especially middle third) (Figure 11.5e, f, and g).

The ESR was 97 mm/h and the CRP was 2.9 mg/dL. On CSF analysis there were 5 cells/mm^3 with a predominance of lymphocytes, high protein content of 94.5 mg/dL, and high CSF/serum IgG index. CSF cultures were negative. Anti-dsDNA, ANAs, and AP antibodies were negative as was infection screening (Venereal Disease Research Laboratory (VDRL) test, varicella zoster, hepatitis, HIV). Cardiac evaluation, including TTE, was unremarkable. Also thoracic-abdominal-pelvic CT was unrevealing. At this point the main working diagnoses were (1) systemic vasculitis involving the cerebral vessels, namely giant cell arteritis (new onset headache in a patient older

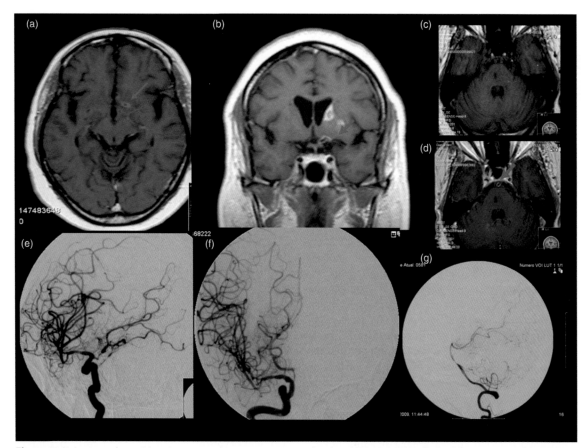

Figure 11.5 Angiography positive primary central nervous system vasculitis. (a and b) Brain MRI (T1 after gadolinium injection) disclosed a recent ischemic lesion in the left caudate nucleus and anterior capsule and gadolinium enhancement of left middle cerebral artery and (c) basilar artery (c before and d after gadolinium injection) (arrows), without leptomeningeal enhancement. Conventional cerebral angiography revealed (e) left intracranial internal carotid stenosis with marked poststenotic dilatation, (f) irregularities of the A1 segment of left anterior cerebral artery, and (g) irregularity of the basilar artery.

than 50, elevated ESR) or (2) PCNSV. Temporal artery biopsy and whole body PET-CT showed no signs of vasculitis. A brain biopsy only showed nonspecific changes, scarce inflammatory infiltrate, and no amyloid deposition. However, because the patient had multiple ischemic strokes with documented angiographic stenosis and dilations in several cerebral vessels that showed gadolinium enhancement of the vessel wall on brain MRI, and an inflammatory CSF pattern, and after excluding other possible causes, the diagnosis of PCNSV was made and prednisone 1 mg/kg/day was started. The patient had a clear clinical and imaging improvement, although she was left with memory deficits. Steroids were slowly tapered over the course of 2 years. On the fourth year of clinical follow-up the patient still had short-term memory loss but there were no recurrent strokes or other new neurological symptoms.

Discussion

This is a typical case of angiography positive PCNSV. This patient presented with headaches, recurrent ischemic strokes and cognitive decline, and an inflammatory CSF pattern with an increase of protein content and particularly elevated IgG CSF/serum index. In this patient the ESR was increased. Although acute phase reactants are usually reported as normal in PCNSV, there may be an increase of ESR in 30% of biopsy confirmed PCNSV patients [38]. However, in a patient older than 50, with headaches and an elevated ESR, temporal artery biopsy was requested since, although temporal artery ultrasonography may be very helpful in the diagnosis of giant cell arteritis (GCA) [39], pathological evaluation still remains the gold diagnostic standard complementary test [40]. In fact, a similar non-invasive evaluation of the intracranial vessels, capable of demonstrating vessel wall inflammation, would be most welcome in the diagnosis of PCNSV. Küker et al. [41] studied the value of contrast-enhanced MRI, proven to be sensitive to extradural arteritis, for the identification of intracranial vessel wall inflammation and found that wall thickening and intramural contrast uptake are frequent findings in patients with active cerebral vasculitis affecting large brain arteries. In this patient the MRI scan protocol suggested by Küker et al. was performed and vessel wall gadolinium enhancement at the sites of arterial stenosis was detected, supporting the diagnosis of vasculitis. However, the exact specificity or sensitivity of contrast-enhanced MRI in the diagnosis of PCNSV is still not well established.

In this patient a definite diagnosis was attempted through a cerebral biopsy but this invasive examination was not conclusive. One of the main reasons to perform a brain biopsy in patients that will probably be submitted to immunosuppression is that it may reveal an alternative diagnosis[8,26], particularly infection or neoplasms. Vasculitis affects vessels in a skipped and segmental pattern and this may account for negative findings in biopsy specimens because of sampling error [8]. As previously mentioned, sensitivity of brain biopsy is variable among series, from 50% to 80% [27,28], and reported studies have many possible biases. In this case, since there was a good clinical response to steroids, cyclophosphamide was not prescribed and the patient did not have any relapses. Patients with PCNSV treated with immunosuppression (mainly steroids and cyclophosphamide) were found to have a low mortality on long-term follow-up [21].

Pitfall and tip

Although cerebral biopsy is the only test that can definitely document intramural vessel inflammation in PCNSV and is very important in excluding alternative diagnoses, it may be negative. Contrast-enhanced MRI may be useful in documenting vessel wall inflammation in PCNSV.

Case 6. Does this elderly man with rapidly progressive dementia have cerebral vasculitis? A case of biopsy proven PCNSV

Case description

A 70-year-old man with history of depression was admitted with a 2-week progressive course of cognitive impairment. On neurological examination he was disoriented, had difficulties in naming, and severe memory deficits, scoring 3 on the Mini Mental State Examination (MMSE). Brain MRI showed confluent hyperintense areas in T2/FLAIR sequences in the periventricular and subcortical white matter, extending to the right parietal cortex and basal ganglia (Figure 11.6a). Laboratory investigation disclosed a raised ESR (80 mm/h). On CSF examination there were 121 leukocytes/mm^3 and increased protein content (154.2 mg/dL). Serologies and cultures were negative. Conventional cerebral angiography was unremarkable. A targeted stereotactic brain biopsy was performed,

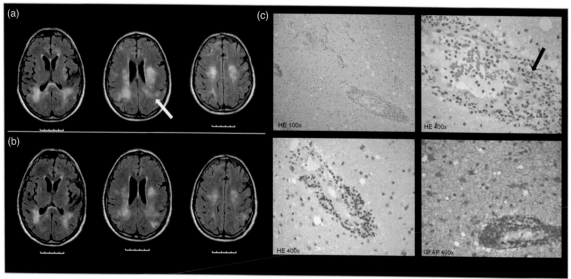

Figure 11.6 Biopsy positive primary central nervous system vasculitis. (a) First brain MRI, FLAIR showing confluent hyperintense areas in T2/FLAIR in the periventricular and subcortical white matter, extending to the right parietal cortex and basal ganglia (stereotactic biopsy site, arrow). (b) Brain MRI, FLAIR one week after treatment. (c) Pathological examination showing transmural and perivascular small vessel inflammatory infiltrate and fragmented neutrophils (arrow). Microglia activation, gliosis, and sparse lymphocytes and neutrophils in the brain parenchyma are also observed. GFAP, glial fibrillary acidic protein; HE hematoxylin and eosin.

which disclosed a perivascular and transmural small vessel inflammatory infiltrate composed mainly of neutrophils, compatible with a leukocytoclastic vasculitis. There was also microglia activation, gliosis, and sparse lymphocytes and neutrophils in the brain parenchyma. No fibrinoid necrosis, granulomas, or giant cells were found (Figure 11.6b). Further laboratory investigation and body imaging excluded associated systemic inflammatory disease, vasculitis, infection, or neoplasm. The patient was treated with oral prednisolone (1 mg/kg). After 12 days on treatment, cognitive function improved, with an MMSE score of 14. ESR decreased to 38 mm/h. A repeat lumbar puncture revealed 28 lymphocytes/mm^3 and a protein content of 121.4 mg/dL. MRI images also improved, showing less extensive signal changes (Figure 11.6c). Due to frequent urinary tract infections it was not possible to start cyclophosphamide. The patient was continued on oral prednisolone, showing no cognitive decline after a 6-month follow-up period.

Discussion

In this patient the diagnosis of small vessel PCNSV was based on a CNS biopsy specimen showing vasculitis, normal cerebral angiography, and exclusion of systemic involvement [42]. Three main histopathologic patterns have been reported in PCNSV [43,44].

Granulomatous inflammation was the most common (58%) with nearly half of the cases associated with deposition of β-A4 amyloid in the vessel wall. Pure lymphocytic infiltration was described in 28% of the cases, and acute necrotizing was seen in 14% of cases. No statistically significant differences in outcome were noted among the three histopathologic groups. Leukocytoclastic vasculitis with CNS involvement is occasionally described in systemic vasculitis, such as in hypersensitivity vasculitis, microscopic polyangiitis, Behçet's disease, Sjögren's syndrome, systemic lupus erythematosus, and *Mycoplasma pneumoniae* infection. In this patient, the diagnosis of small vessel PACNS was considered, as there were no additional features of systemic vasculitis.

Stereotactic biopsy is mainly recommended for mass lesions, but in this case it was performed in a region that was clearly affected on brain MRI and there were no complications of the procedure. When lesions are not easily accessible, for reasons of safety and optimal yield, a biopsy should be performed at the non-dominant temporal tip. Owing to frequent involvement of the leptomeningeal vessels, the leptomeninges should be included to enhance diagnostic yield, though there is conflicting data as to whether sampling regions of leptomeningeal enhancement increases sensitivity [8]. Brain biopsy is not a trivial procedure and has an estimated morbidity of 0.5–2% [1,27]. However, the benefit of making a correct diagnosis, which avoids empirical treatments, should always be considered [5,8].

Pitfall and tip

PCNSV may be a treatable cause of rapidly progressive dementia. In small vessel PCNSV, intra-arterial angiography is unremarkable and the diagnosis can only be made through a properly targeted brain biopsy.

Secondary or primary cerebral vasculitis? Excluding infection

Case 7. Does this man with transient ischemic attacks and a middle cerebral artery stenosis have cerebral vasculitis? A case of varicella zoster virus (VZV) cerebral vasculitis

Case description

A 62-year-old man without vascular risk factors had Waldenström macroglobulinemia since 2010. In February 2013, while on chemotherapy, he developed a left Ramsay Hunt syndrome, treated with acyclovir. In August 2013, he presented with repeated transient episodes of right hemiparesis over 2 weeks. Brain diffusion weighted image (DWI) MRI revealed several acute ischemic lesions in the left middle cerebral artery (MCA) territory (small cortical frontal and parietal lesions, lenticular and caudate nucleus); angio-MRI showed a severe proximal left MCA stenosis. Blood analysis, cervical vessel ultrasonography, 24 h Holter, TTE, and HIV, hepatitis and syphilis serologies were normal; CSF revealed 6 cells/mm^3 and polymerase chain reaction (PCR) for varicella zoster virus (VZV) was positive. The patient was treated with acyclovir (10 mg/kg/day) for 21 days and prednisolone (1 mg/kg/day) for 5 days. He had no new focal signs during admission. He was discharged on valacyclovir, and had no further symptoms during the follow-up. Serial assessments with TCD and repeated angio-MRI showed maintenance of MCA stenosis. Repeated CSF analysis showed 2 cells/mm^3 and PCR for VZV was negative.

Discussion

If this patient had vascular risk factors and was not immunocompromised, transient ischemic attacks could easily be attributed to intracranial large vessel atherosclerosis. In adults atherosclerosis commonly mimics the vasculitis angiographic pattern [45]. Though atherosclerotic plaques preferentially affect the branching points of large vessels, and in vasculitis more distal segmental stenoses are observed, it is often difficult to distinguish between the two disorders.

VZV is a frequent cause of cerebral vasculitis affecting mainly large cerebral vessels. Often the intracranial carotid artery bifurcation and the M1 segment of the MCA, as in this patient, are affected, but the posterior circulation can also be affected [46]. The clinical diagnosis of VZV vasculopathy is usually based on a history of recent zoster followed by neurologic symptoms and signs, imaging abnormalities indicating cerebral ischemia, infarction, or hemorrhage, angiographic evidence of narrowing or beading in cerebral arteries, and a CSF pleocytosis [47]. VZV vasculopathy can be unifocal, usually following ophthalmic zoster in elderly adults or childhood chickenpox, affecting large arteries of the anterior or posterior circulation, or multifocal, usually affecting branches of large cerebral arteries or small cerebral arteries, mostly in immunocompromised individuals. In the present case there was a history of Ramsay Hunt syndrome and VZV DNA was positive in the CSF. However, in up to 40% of patients with confirmed VZV vasculopathy there is no history of rash or other evidence of viral infection. The detection of anti-VZV IgG antibody in the CSF is more sensitive than VZV DNA detection. Actually in a serial CSF analysis of a patient with VZV vasculopathy, viral DNA would be undetected 2 weeks after the rash, when the viral antibody could still be detected [46]. There is often a delay between viral infection and cerebral vasculopathy that can be up to several months.

In this patient there was a unifocal large artery involvement; however, in one of the largest series of VZV vasculopathy [46], combined brain imaging and vascular studies showed that involvement of both large and small arteries in the same patient was most common (50%), followed by exclusive small artery involvement (37%).

There are no randomized clinical trials on VZV vasculopathy treatments and most centers treat patients with intravenous acyclovir alone or combined with steroids. A higher percentage of patients treated with both acyclovir and steroids seem to have improved or stabilized [46].

Tip

CSF PCR for VZV DNA and anti-VZV antibodies should be routinely requested in all patients with a suspicion of cerebral vasculitis, particularly in patients with unifocal vessel involvement.

When cerebral vasculitis is not isolated: excluding primary systemic vasculitis

Case 8. Does this man with vertebrobasilar territory transient ischemic attacks and elevated ESR have cerebral vasculitis? A case of giant cell arteritis (GCA)

Case description

A 74-year-old man with history of atrial fibrillation (AF) and dyslipidemia, on clopidogrel and amiodarone, was admitted due to paroxysmal episodes of vertigo lasting a few minutes. Five days later, he had a 6-hour episode of dysarthria and left hemiparesis. He also had weight loss of 10 kg in 3 months, associated with malaise, myalgias, and bilateral temporal headaches that got worse with local pressure, jaw claudication, and dysphagia. Neurologic examination on admission was normal. Brain MRI with angio-MRI showed remote left cerebellar and thalamic ischemic lesions, moderate leukoaraiosis (Figure 11.7a1–4), and no flow signal in the vertebral arteries (VA), basilar trunk, and PCAs (Figure 11.7b). ESR was 74 mm/h. Superficial temporal artery (STA) pulses were diminished. Cervical vessel ultrasonography showed VA stenosis associated with hypoechoic image along the vessel wall, suggestive of an inflammatory halo (Figure 11.7c). The STA halo was also observed by color echo Doppler (Figure 11.7d). The ECG showed atrial fibrillation. TTE examination was normal. Ocular vasculitis was excluded. Pathological examination of the right STA showed marked lymphocytic inflammatory infiltration across the wall of the vessel with Langhans-type and foreign-body-type multinucleated giant cells and focal destruction of the internal elastic lamina, according with a diagnosis of GCA (Figure 11.7e1–4). High dose steroid therapy was started with clinical improvement and ESR normalization. Though initially on aspirin, the patient was discharged on oral anticoagulation due to AF. At 1-year follow-up, after slow tapering of steroids, no more ischemic events were detected and a Doppler ultrasound control study showed improvement of arterial stenosis and of the inflammatory halo.

Discussion

GCA is one of the most common primary systemic vasculitides [48], predominantly affecting large arteries, usually the aorta and its major branches, with a predilection for the branches of the carotid and the vertebral arteries [49]. GCA typically involves the STAs, but also other branches of the external carotid artery. Ischemic stroke/transient ischemic attacks rarely occur as the first manifestation of GCA [50], but are one of the most feared complications after optic nerve ischemia [51]. GCA is often associated with polymyalgia rheumatica (PMR).

The present case reinforces that in elderly patients with cerebral ischemia, even with other possible etiologies, the presence of headache, systemic complaints, and/or increased inflammatory parameters should prompt investigation for GCA. Actually this patient fulfills all the diagnostic criteria for GCA: (1) age of onset >50 years; (2) new onset headache; (3) jaw claudication; (4) painful STA arteries/diminished pulses; (5) ESR >50 mm/h; (6) STA biopsy documenting vasculitis.

Diagnosing GCA implies a different therapeutical management that includes immunosuppression. Low dose aspirin is recommended for secondary ischemic stroke prevention in patients with stroke and GCA [52]. However, in our patient, the presence of AF led to anticoagulation. Though there are a few case reports [53] of oral anticoagulants in VB territory associated with GCA, their role in this context is unknown.

In our case, ultrasonography was very important since the identification of a hypoechoic halo along the VA and STA walls suggested the diagnosis of GCA, later confirmed by pathological examination of the right STA. Temporal artery biopsy remains the gold standard for diagnosis of GCA [39]. However, it can give false negative results, since GCA can involve some arterial segments and spare others. Cervical vessels and STA color echo Doppler ultrasound seems to be very useful in this context [38], since it is a non-invasive method that can depict both the vessel lumen and the vessel wall, of several different vessels. Excluding extracranial vessel involvement is crucial to make the diagnosis

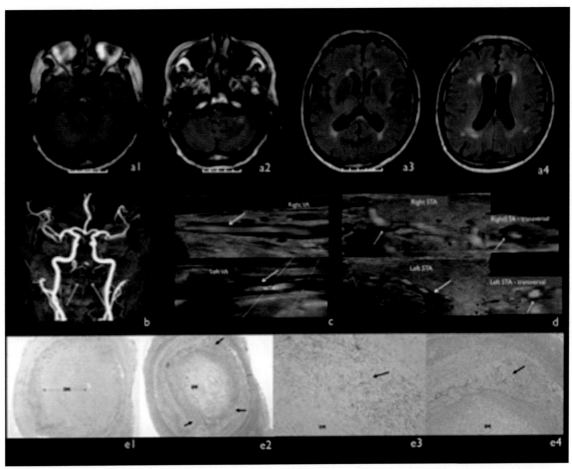

Figure 11.7 Giant cell arteritis. (a) Brain MRI-FLAIR showed remote cerebellar (a1 and a2) and thalamic (a3) ischemic lesions and moderate leukoaraiosis (a4). (b) Angio-MRI: no flow signal in the vertebral arteries, basilar trunk, and posterior cerebral arteries. (c) Cervical vessels (vertebral arteries) color echo Doppler and (d) superficial temporal arteries color echo Doppler: hypoechoic image along the vessel wall, suggestive of an inflammatory halo. (e) Pathological examination (right STA); e1 (hematoxylin–eosin) marked intimal (IM) thickening and lumen reduction; inflammatory infiltration across the wall of the vessel; e2 (Verhoeff's stain) focal fragmentation and disappearance of internal elastic lamina (arrows); e3 (hematoxylin–eosin); and e4 (Verhoeff): predominantly lymphocytic inflammatory infiltrate with Langhans-type and foreign-body-type multinucleated giant cells (e3, arrow) with focal destruction of the internal elastic lamina (e4, arrow).

of PCNSV. A complete physical observation, including all palpable pulses, should always complement neurological evaluation in patients with suspected PCNSV and guide complementary imaging evaluation.

Tip

To make the diagnosis of PCNSV vasculitis involvement of extracranial vessels should be excluded. GCA may involve intracranial vessels and cause ischemic stroke. STA color echo Doppler may document the inflammatory halo in the vessel wall in large artery vasculitis.

Acknowledgments

Professor José Ferro for the critical review of this chapter; Dr. Carolina Pires and Dr. Candida Barroso for sharing Case 6; Dr. Cristiana Silva, Dr. Ana Castro Caldas and Professor José Pimentel for sharing Case 4; Dr. Valter Fonseca for his collaboration in Case 3; Dr. Luis Abreu for sharing Case 7.

References

1. Scolding NJ. Central nervous system vasculitis. *Semin Immunopathol* 2009;31:527–36.

2. Watts RA, Scott DG. Classification and epidemiology of the vasculitides. *Baillieres Clin Rheumatol* 1997;11:191–217.

3. Jennette JC, Falk RJ, Andrassy K, et al. Nomenclature of systemic vasculitis. The proposal of an international consensus conference. *Arthritis Rheum* 1994;37:187–92.

4. Schmidley JW (2000) *Central Nervous System Angiitis.* Oxford: Butterworth-Heinemann.

5. Calabrese LH, Mallek JA. Primary angiitis of the central nervous system. Report of 8 new cases, review of the literature, and proposal for diagnostic criteria. *Medicine (Baltimore)* 1988;67:20–39.

6. Salvarani C, Brown RD Jr., Calamia KT, et al. Primary central nervous system vasculitis: analysis of 101 patients. *Ann Neurol* 2007;62(5):442–51.

7. Kraemer M, Berlit P. Primary central nervous system vasculitis: clinical experiences with 21 new European cases. *Rheumatol Int* 2011;31(4):463–72.

8. Birnbaum J, Hellmann DB. Primary angiitis of the central nervous system. *Arch Neurol* 2009;66:704–9.

9. Moore PM. Diagnosis and management of isolated angiitis of the central nervous system. *Neurology* 1989;39(2, pt 1):167–73.

10. Hajj-Ali RA, Furlan A, Abou-Chebel A, Calabrese LH. Benign angiopathy of the central nervous system: cohort of 16 patients with clinical course and long-term follow-up. *Arthritis Rheum* 2002;47(6):662–9.

11. Calabrese LH, Dodick DW, Schwedt TJ, Singhal AB. Narrative review: reversible cerebral vasoconstriction syndromes. *Ann Intern Med* 2007;146(1):34–44.

12. Koopman K, Uyttenbogaart M, Luijckx GJ, Keyser J, Vroomen P. Pitfalls in the diagnosis of reversible cerebral vasoconstriction syndrome and primary angiitis of the central nervous system. *Eur J Neurol* 2007;14:1085–7.

13. Ducros A, Bousser MG. Reversible vasoconstriction syndrome. *Pract Neurol* 2009; 9: 256–67.

14. Crane R, Kerr LD, Spiera H. Clinical analysis of isolated angiitis of the central nervous system: a report of 11 cases. *Arch Intern Med* 1991;151(11):2290–4.

15. Ducros A, Boukobza M, Porcher R, et al. The clinical and radiological spectrum of reversible cerebral vasoconstriction syndrome. A prospective series of 67 patients. *Brain* 2007;130:3091–101.

16. Lee VH, Wijdicks EF, Manno EM, et al. Clinical spectrum of reversible posterior leukoencephalopathy syndrome. *Arch Neurol* 2008;65:205–10.

17. Bartynski WS. Posterior reversible encephalopathy syndrome, part 1: fundamental imaging and clinical features. *AJNR Am J Neuroradiol* 2008;29:1036–42.

18. Calabrese LH, Furlan AJ, Gragg LA, et al. Primary angiitis of the central nervous system: diagnostic criteria and clinical approach. *Cleve Clin J Med* 1992;59:293–306.

19. Chen SP, Fuh JL, Chang FC, et al. Transcranial color Doppler study for reversible cerebral vasoconstriction syndromes. *Ann Neurol* 2008;63:751–7.

20. Berlit P. Isolated angiitis of the CNS and bacterial endocarditis: similarities and differences. *J Neurol* 2009; 256:792–5.

21. Boysson H, Zuber M, Naggara O, et al. Primary angiitis of the central nervous system. Description of the first fifty-two adults enrolled in the French cohort of patients with primary vasculitis of the central nervous system. *Arthritis Rheumatol* 2014;66(5):1315–26.

22. Haroon M, Molloy E, Farrell M, Alraqi S. Central nervous system vasculitis: all that glitters is not gold. *J Rheumatol* 2012;39:662–3.

23. Guennec L, Roos-Weil D, Mokhtari K, et al. Granulomatous angiitis of the CNS revealing a Hodgkin lymphoma. *Neurology* 2013;80:323–4.

24. Rosen CL, DePalma L, Morita A. Primary angiitis of the central nervous system as a first presentation in Hodgkin's disease: a case report and review of the literature. *Neurosurgery* 2000;46:1504–8.

25. Morotti A, Malagola M, Cancelli V, et al. Central nervous system angiitis in Hodgkin's disease. *J Neurol* 2013;260(11):2897–9.

26. Alrawi A, Trobe JD, Blaivas M, Musch DC. Brain biopsy in primary angiitis of the central nervous system. *Neurology* 1999;53:858–60.

27. Parisi JE, Moore PM. The role of biopsy in vasculitis of the central nervous system. *Semin Neurol* 1994;14:341–8.

28. Lie JT. Primary (granulomatous) angiitis of the central nervous system: a clinicopathologic analysis of 15 new cases and a review of the literature. *Hum Pathol* 1992;23(2):164–71.

29. Ferreri A, Dognini G, Campo E, et al. On behalf of the International Extranodal Lymphoma Study Group. Variations in clinical presentation, frequency of hemophagocytosis and clinical behavior of intravascular lymphoma diagnosed in different geographical regions. *Haematologica* 2007;92:486–92.

30. Salvarani C, Hunder GG, Jonathan MM, et al. Ab-related angiitis. Comparison with CAA without inflammation and primary CNS vasculitis. *Neurology* 2013;81:1–8.

31. Eng JA, Frosch MP, Choi K, et al. Clinical manifestations of cerebral amyloid angiopathy-related inflammation. *Ann Neurol* 2004;55:250–6.

32. Scolding NJ, Joseph F, Kirby PA, et al. Ab-related angiitis: primary angiitis of the central nervous system associated with cerebral amyloid angiopathy. *Brain* 2005;128:500–15.

33. Kinnecom C, Lev MH, Wendell L, et al. Course of cerebral amyloid angiopathy-related inflammation. *Neurology* 2007;68:1411–16.

34. Salvarani C, Brown RD Jr., Calamia KT, et al. Primary central nervous system vasculitis: comparison of patients with and without cerebral amyloid angiopathy. *Rheumatology* 2008;47:1671–7.

35. Charidimou A, Baron JC, Werring DJ. Transient focal neurological episodes, cerebral amyloid angiopathy, and intracerebral hemorrhage risk: looking beyond TIAs. *Int J Stroke* 2013;8(2):105–8.

36. Salvarani C, Brown RD Jr., Calamia KT, et al. Primary central nervous system vasculitis presenting with intracranial hemorrhage. *Arthritis Rheum* 2011;63:3598–606.

37. Oh U, Gupta R, Krakauer JW, et al. Reversible leukoencephalopathy associated with cerebral amyloid angiopathy. *Neurology* 2004;62:494–7.

38. Hankey GJ. Isolated angiitis/angiopathy of the central nervous system. *Cerebrovasc Dis* 1991;1:2–15

39. Houtman PM, Doorenbos BM, Dol J, Bruyn GA. Doppler ultrasonography to diagnose temporal arteritis in the setting of a large community hospital. *Scand J Rheumatol* 2008;37(4):316–8.

40. Salvarani C, Cantini F, Boiardi L, Hunder GG. Polymyalgia rheumatica and giant-cell arteritis. *N Engl J Med* 2002; 347(4): 261–71.

41. Küker A, Gaertner S, Nägele T, et al. Vessel wall contrast enhancement: a diagnostic sign of cerebral vasculitis. *Cerebrovasc Dis* 2008;26:23–9.

42. Pires C, Foreid H, Barroso C, Ferro JM. Rapidly progressive dementia due to leukocytoclastic vasculitis of the central nervous system. *BMJ Case Rep* 2011; doi:10.1136/bcr.08.2011.4619.

43. Miller DV, Salvarani C, Hunder GG, et al. Biopsy findings in primary angiitis of the central nervous system. *Am J Surg Pathol* 2009;33:35–43.

44. Giannini C, Salvarani C, Hunder G, Brown R. Primary central nervous system vasculitis: pathology and mechanisms. *Acta Neuropathol* 2012;123(6):759–72.

45. Kueker W. Cerebral vasculitis: imaging signs revisited. *Neuroradiology* 2007;49:471–9.

46. Wengenroth M, Jacobi C, Wildemann B. Cerebral vasculitis. In: Hähnel S, ed. *Inflammatory Diseases of the Brain, Medical Radiology. Diagnostic Imaging.* Berlin, Heidelberg:Springer-Verlag; 2013: 19–38.

47. Nagel MA, Cohors RJ, Mahalingam R, et al. The varicella zoster virus vasculopathies. Clinical, CSF, imaging, and virologic features. *Neurology* 2008;70: 853–60.

48. Liu NH, LaBree LD, Feldon SE, et al. The epidemiology of giant cell arteritis. *Ophthalmology* 2001;108:1145–9.

49. Jennette JC, Falk JR, Bacon PAF, et al. 2012 revised international Chapel Hill Consensus Conference Nomenclatures of vasculitides. *Arthritis Rheum* 2013;65(1):1–11.

50. Wiszniewska M, Devuyst G, Bougousslavsky J. Giant cell arteritis as a cause of first-ever stroke. *Cerebrosvasc Dis* 2007;24:226–30.

51. Gonzalez MA, Blanco R, Rodriguez-Valverde V, et al. Permanent visual loss and cerebrovascular accidents in giant cell arteritis: predictors and response to treatment. *Arthritis Rheum* 1998;41:1497–504.

52. Dasgupta B. Concise guidance: diagnosis and management of giant cell arteritis. *Clin Med* 2010;10(4):381–6.

53. Boettinger M, Sebastian S, Gamulescu MA, et al. Bilateral vertebral artery occlusion with retrograde basilary flow in three cases of giant cell arteritis. *BMJ Case Rep* 2009; doi: 10.1136/bcr.07.2008.0488.

Chapter 12

Recognizing cerebrovascular etiologies of "thunderclap" headaches

Raquel Gil-Gouveia

Introduction

Thunderclap headache (TCH) is a sudden onset severe headache, named as such due to its explosive and unpredictable quality, much like a "clap of thunder" [1]. Primary thunderclap headache is defined as a severe pain of abrupt onset that reaches maximum intensity in less than one minute, lasts at least 5 minutes and where an underlying cause was promptly and exhaustively excluded [2]. The imperative of excluding secondary TCH is revealing of the high frequency (from 1/4 in the community to up to 2/3 in hospital setting [3]) of pathological processes that can underlie this symptom, even in patients with a completely normal neurological examination (Figure 12.1). Nowadays, most physicians recognize that TCH is a medical emergency, and it has become almost a synonym of probable subarachnoid hemorrhage (SAH). However, there are many other relevant disorders that can cause secondary TCH, so the investigation of these patients cannot be limited to a brain CT and lumbar puncture (LP). The most important take-home message of this chapter is that sudden headache must always be considered a major red flag in the evaluation of a headache patient. The importance of a thorough history, complemented by detailed observation and rigorous ancillary investigations of these patients cannot be overemphasized.

The pathological mechanisms involved in the production of thunderclap headache include direct arterial vessel damage by rupture, inflammation or rapid change in vessel caliber, processes that stimulate periadventitial nociceptive fibers [4]. This can happen in SAH, arterial dissection, cerebral vasoconstriction, sentinel headache, and acute hypertensive crisis. Similar pain may be reproduced during cerebral angiography and endovascular procedures, in response to specific maneuvers that increase intra-arterial pressure and/or to the contact of substances (contrast dye, glue, coils, balloons) with the vessel wall. Pain location elicited in these procedures usually reflects the anatomical distribution of nociceptive arterial nerve fibers of the manipulated vessel [4], although such topographic correlation is not as clear in vascular disease. Sudden, intense sharp head pain may also be a consequence of increased intracranial pressure or meningeal stimulation, as occurs in cerebral venous thrombosis (CVT), ischemic or hemorrhagic stroke, pituitary apoplexy, meningitis, colloid cyst of the third ventricle, hydrocephalus, or subdural hematoma. Surprisingly, spontaneous intracranial hypotension can also present as TCH [5].

There are no clinical characteristics of the headache itself that allow differentiation between primary and secondary TCH [3]. A thorough history will help the clinician in the identification of the sudden onset and/or excruciating "worst of their life" intensity characteristics of the headaches. Any of these features is enough to warrant full etiological investigation. Accompanying symptoms that have been found to increase the likelihood of a secondary cause include nausea, impaired consciousness, seizures, and diplopia [3,6]. Vomiting, transient loss of consciousness, and focal neurologic symptoms are slightly more frequent in symptomatic (secondary) TCH [3]. Female sex, neck stiffness, and abnormalities in neurological examination are also more likely in symptomatic TCH [3,6].

Ancillary evaluation of TCH may be directed to the most probable underlying cause, given the patient's history. This may require CT scan, LP, MRI, angiographic arterial and/or venous intracranial imaging (by CT or MRI), transcranial Doppler (TCD) or even digital subtraction angiography (DSA).

Common Pitfalls in Cerebrovascular Disease: Case-Based Learning, ed. José Biller and José M. Ferro. Published by Cambridge University Press. © Cambridge University Press 2015.

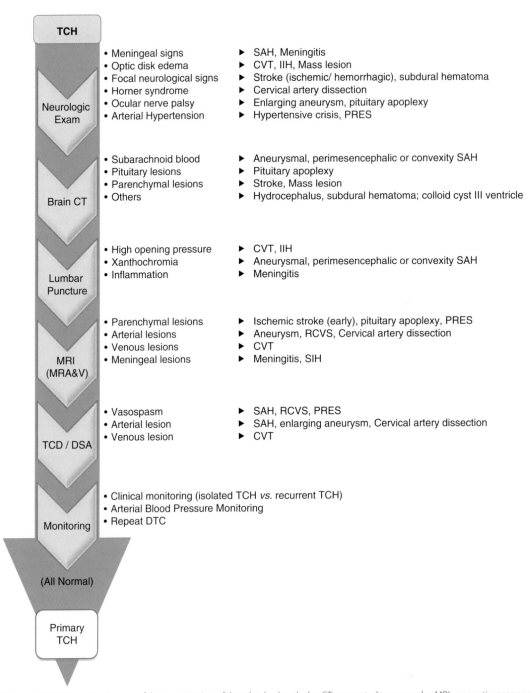

Figure 12.1 Schematic diagram of the investigation of thunderclap headache. CT, computed tomography; MRI, magnetic resonance imaging; MRA, magnetic resonance angiography; MRV, magnetic resonance venography; TCD, transcranial Doppler; DSA, digital subtraction angiography; SAH, subarachnoid hemorrhage; CVT, cerebral venous thrombosis; IIH, idiopathic intracranial hypertension; RCVS, reversible cerebral vasoconstriction syndrome; PRES, posterior reversible encephalopathy syndrome; SIH, spontaneous intracranial hypotension.

This chapter will review the most relevant cerebrovascular etiologies of TCH focusing on the worst diagnostic challenge of TCH – the approach to patients with isolated TCH, i.e., TCH with normal neurological examination.

Case 1. Focal neurological signs 3 weeks after non-remitting TCH

Case description

A 38-year-old hairdresser presented to the emergency room (ER) with an intense non-remitting headache that awakened her from sleep with immediate vomiting, five nights before. The bilateral pain had occipital location, radiated to the neck, always accompanied by nausea and frequent vomiting, photophobia, phonophobia. Headache worsened with head and neck movement and physical effort. She had a previous history of migraine without aura, cigarette smoking (23 pack-years), and oral contraceptive use (desogestrel 0.15 mg plus ethinylestradiol 0.02 mg). Her migraines had started at the age of 16, current attack frequency was four episodes monthly, lasting 2 to 3 days. Her attacks were severe and each month she had at least one to two days of work absenteeism on account of her migraine. She had never been on migraine preventive treatment and treated her attacks with ibuprofen and domperidone. She noted some differences of this headache to her usual migraine: it was stronger than usual, bilateral and posterior in location, resistant to usual analgesics and lasted longer. Her vital signs and neurological examination were normal. A CT scan performed at the ER was also normal. She was discharged after partial improvement of her pain with intravenous analgesics and metoclopramide. She was prescribed amitriptyline 25 mg daily, naproxen 500 mg with metoclopramide three times daily for 5 days, and zolmitriptan 5 mg, as rescue medication.

Over the next 2 weeks she noticed progressive improvement of the intensity of her headaches. Vomiting stopped but the pain was still disrupting enough to prevent her from returning to work. She was using zolmitriptan once or twice daily. Around 20 days after the beginning of her headache, the pain suddenly became more intense, without nausea and vomiting, and a couple of hours later she noticed weakness of her left arm and was brought to the ER. She was somnolent and her speech was slurred. She was unable to walk without assistance due to left-sided hemiparesis (central facial palsy, arm strength 2/5, leg strength 3/5). Her blood pressure was 150/85 mmHg, pulse 64 with normal rhythm.

Brain CT and magnetic resonance imaging (MRI) revealed subarachnoid blood and a recent infarct of the deep territory of the right middle cerebral artery (MCA) (Figure 12.2). Magnetic resonance angiography (MRA) identified narrowing of the right internal carotid and middle cerebral arteries. TCD showed a marked increase in blood flow velocities in the right MCA (systolic velocity 370 cm/second, diastolic velocity 200 cm/second) compatible with vasospasm and mild increases in the left anterior cerebral (ACA) and basilar arteries (systolic speed 290, diastolic speed

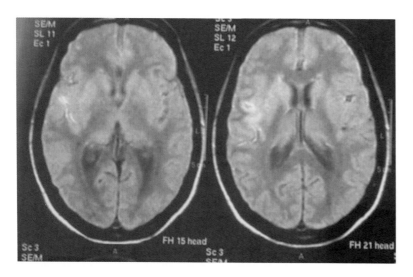

Figure 12.2 Case 1: brain MRI. Axial T2 FLAIR sequences showing a subarachnoid hemorrhage of the supra-cisternal and right Sylvian fissure and an acute ischemic stroke of the deep territory of the right middle cerebral artery (MCA) and insular cortex.

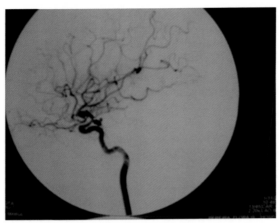

Figure 12.3 Case 1: digital subtraction angiography. Saccular aneurysm of the right posterior communicating artery.

160). Angiography confirmed marked (>50%) vessel caliber reduction in the right internal carotid and middle cerebral arteries, moderate (25–50%) spasm of the anterior cerebral arteries, and identified a single saccular aneurysm (8 × 4 mm) with wall irregularity of the right posterior communicating artery (Figure 12.3).

She was started on oral nimodipine, euvolemia was restored with crystalloid fluids and blood pressure was controlled, keeping her systolic values between 130 and 170 mmHg. There was rapid clinical and TCD improvement. She underwent aneurysm treatment by microsurgical clipping within 72 hours of admission. Control angiography confirmed aneurysm exclusion. She showed progressive improvement of her symptoms and was discharged with no further complications after 2 weeks, with residual left hemiparesis (modified Rankin scale 2).

Discussion

SAH is the most frequent cause of symptomatic TCH. Misdiagnosis still occurs in around 12% of cases, either due to lack of recognition of its importance (by patients and/or physicians) or to not performing a comprehensive complementary evaluation [7,8].

The most common misdiagnoses of SAH are tension-type headache and/or migraine. The risk of misdiagnosis is increased in patients who are fully conscious and without focal neurological signs (Hunt and Hess grades 1 or 2), and with previous history of migraine of hypertension. Low physician suspicion [8,9] and consequently delayed diagnosis increases the likelihood of death or disability fourfold [7].

The mode of onset of the headache is the most important feature in TCH characterization that typically occurs during or after strenuous tasks or exercise, especially in patients aged over 60 [10]. Nevertheless, the majority occur during effortless everyday routines or even during sleep, the latter often preventing both patient and doctor from identifying its sudden onset. The pain may be severe and unremitting, but also brief and self-limited, which is typically the case of the "sentinel" headache occurring in warning leaks, in 10–40% of patients [7]. Up to 20% of patients have milder headaches, isolated neck pain, or no headache at all [7]. When the headache's onset is unclear, the high-intensity "worst of a lifetime" pain is the second clinical characteristic that mandates immediate complementary investigation. Although a normal neurological examination does not exclude any serious underlying disorder in a patient with TCH, it is important to screen for subtle neurological signs that may bring further clues to the diagnosis, such as a unilateral dilated and hyporesponsive pupil, mild nuchal rigidity, or ophthalmoscopic changes (including papilledema or peripapillar hemorrhages). These may elude the less trained general practitioner or ER doctor. The presence of focal neurological signs and changes in consciousness at presentation increase diagnostic accuracy [7,8].

The most sensitive test for the diagnosis of acute SAH is non-contrast CT scan, with sensitivity similar to MRI FLAIR, of almost 100% in the first 3 days of SAH. The sensitivity of CT decreases to around 85% by the fifth day and 30% after 2 weeks, MRI being superior to CT in this time frame. In the evaluation of TCH, a normal CT or MRI in the first 2 weeks makes it mandatory to perform a lumbar puncture to search for CSF xanthochromia. Traumatic, very early (<6 to 12 hours) or late (> 2 weeks) taps can be falsely negative [7,11]. Small (< 3 mm) aneurysms may fail detection by CT or MR angiography [7], but may be revealed by intra-arterial digital subtraction angiography (DSA). In non-perimesencephalic SAH, some patients have falsely negative findings on initial DSA, either due to technical reasons, concomitant vasospasm, thrombosis, or obliteration of the aneurysm by adjacent hematoma. Repeating DSA within 2 to 6 weeks if initial findings are inconclusive has a diagnostic yield of around 12% and is a current recommendation [11].

The inadvertent use of triptans in SAH has been described; the few cases reported documented an anti-nociceptive effect of triptans in headache due to SAH, as has happened in our patient [12,13]. The use of triptans in SAH-related headache increases both the risk of misdiagnosis and of arterial vasospasm, as triptans carry the potential of arterial vasoconstriction. Nevertheless, in the few cases described, vasospasm occurrence seemed unrelated to triptan use. In our patient, despite daily use of an oral triptan, vasospasm occurrence was delayed in relation to its most frequent timing [14].

Pitfall

This case illustrates the two major difficulties in the identification of TCH when taking the history – the typical sudden onset of the headache was missed due to headache onset during sleep and severity of pain was devalued due to a previous history of severe migraine. A normal initial neurological examination does not exclude SAH, but remember – it increases the odds for misdiagnosis.

Tip

Keep in mind the limitations of the complementary investigation in suspected SAH. In this patient, an LP was mandatory to exclude SAH due to lack of sensitivity of the CT scan on the fifth day after headache onset.

Case 2. Recurring excruciating TCH

Case description

A 60-year-old secretary presented in the emergency room (ER) due to headache episodes that had started 10 days before. The first episode was of a progressive bilateral frontal pressure-like pain, without accompanying symptoms that persisted through the day but suddenly worsened acutely, without any precipitating factor. This excruciating pain was predominantly over the left temple, lasted around half an hour, and was accompanied by nausea and vomiting. There was no photophobia, phonophobia, worsening with Valsalva's or with physical effort. A mild bilateral frontal pain persisted, yet she was able to function normally. Repeated and identical exacerbation episodes occurred suddenly at rest, the second time 48 hours after the first and the third 72 hours after the second, always with mild persistent pain between these episodes. She often took paracetamol (acetaminophen) and reported mild relief from baseline pain. On the ninth day, she woke up from her night sleep with the fourth sudden excruciating pain episode, accompanied by persistent vomiting, which lasted longer than one hour. She then decided to

seek medical attention. Her past medical history was remarkable for mild essential hypertension controlled with bisoprolol 5 mg daily, and nephrolithiasis. She had no previous history of migraine or other primary headaches. She denied any contact with other pharmacological or toxic agents, including selective serotonin reuptake inhibitors (SSRIs), cannabis, or nasal decongestants. She had no previous complaints of fever, joint pain, skin rashes, oral ulcers, or ocular disorders except mild presbyopia in the last couple of years.

Upon admission to the ER her vital signs and neurological examination were completely normal, yet she was very uncomfortable with headache graded 10 out of 10 on a visual analog scale and was still vomiting. A CT scan and routine blood work-up were normal. An LP revealed a normal CSF without xanthochromia. Serologic (neurotropic viruses, *Borrelia* species) and vasculitis screen revealed a positive ANA titer of 1/320 without any other abnormalities.

Brain MRI revealed multiple T2 non-enhancing hyperintense subcortical white matter lesions, with highest expression in the right frontal area. MRA identified multiple narrowing of the distal branches of both MCAs and of the posterior circulation. TCD on the tenth day failed to disclose changes in blood flow velocities in proximal MCAs, ACAs, or basilar arteries (Figure 12.4).

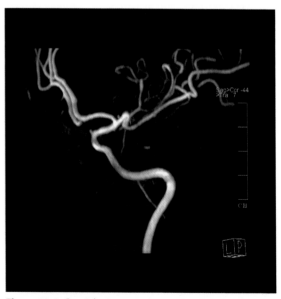

Figure 12.4 Case 2: brain magnetic resonance angiography. MRI 3D time-of-flight maximum intensity projection (MIP) showing string of beads appearance of M2 branches of left MCA.

Her headache was treated with metamizole, tramadol, and metoclopramide. Oral nimodipine 60 mg every 6 hours was started, with improvement of baseline pain and no further recurrence of TCH episodes. Control MRA after 4 weeks had complete normalization of all previous changes; nimodipine was stopped after 8 weeks.

Discussion

Repeated episodes of TCH are very characteristic of reversible cerebral vasoconstriction syndrome (RCVS), an entity described since the 1970s, known to be associated with diverse conditions. RCVS causes characteristic diffuse cerebral arterial stenosis; when no cause or association is identified, common terms include idiopathic reversible cerebral segmental vasoconstriction or Call–Fleming syndrome [15,16].

One of the most important clues to the diagnosis is the epidemiological context. RCVS is more frequent in middle-aged female patients and in up to 60% of cases is precipitated by specific conditions such as the postpartum period or by vasoactive substances, including therapeutic agents (such as selective serotonin reuptake inhibitors, nasal decongestants, triptans, ergot alkaloid derivatives, intravenous immunoglobulin, red-blood-cell transfusion, or interferon alfa) but also over-the-counter or recreational substances such as ginseng and other herbal medicines, alcohol (binge drinking), cannabis, cocaine, methylenedioxymethamphetamine, amphetamines, and lysergic acid diethylamide [15].

In the case presented, the headache had two red flags for a secondary etiology: onset after the age of 50 and thunderclap-like pain. RCVS can be responsible for up to 9% of TCH cases without changes in general or neurologic examination [17], especially when repeated episodes of TCH are reported; indeed, the second important clue for the diagnosis is the temporal profile of pain. Over a background of mild to moderate persistent pain, a set of TCH exacerbations usually occur within a limited time window of 1 to 4 weeks. Seizures can occur in up to 20% of patients. The neurological examination is usually normal, unless RCVS is complicated by stroke, which produces persistent focal deficits. Meningeal signs are rare, unless concomitant convexity SAH occurs. Convexity SAH is very suggestive of RCVS in young individuals [15,16].

Differential diagnosis of recurrent TCH includes sentinel headache from SAH, CVT or other conditions that induce intracranial hypertension, primary angiitis of the central nervous system (PACNS), and several primary headache syndromes such as migraine, primary cough headache, primary headache associated with sexual activity, primary exercise headache, and primary thunderclap headache [2]. The clinical distinction between these primary or idiopathic headache syndromes and RCVS can be very challenging, as RCVS-related TCH is triggered, in 80% of patients, by sexual activity, Valsalva's maneuver, stressful situations, physical exertion, coughing, sneezing, or other situations. Migraine-like features (nausea, vomiting, photophobia, and phonophobia) are very often present in RCVS headache and previous headache history of migraine is present in up to 40% of patients. The two important clues not to miss to the diagnosis of RCVS are the sudden onset of the attacks and the perception of the patient that the headache is different from their usual migraine attacks [15]. Mistaking RCVS headache for migraine is dangerous, as it may result in the prescription of triptans for pain control with a consequent increase in risk of brain ischemia [15].

The diagnosis of RCVS requires identification of cerebral arterial vasoconstriction by MRA, computed tomography angiography (CTA) or TCD, or catheter cerebral angiography. However, results can be normal depending on the timing of the examination, as spasm is a dynamic process that is thought to begin in small distal arteries and then progress toward medium- and large-sized vessels [18]. Vasospasm is usually only detectable by MRA after 8 to 10 days and usually peaks after 3 weeks [17]. The sensitivity of these non-invasive techniques in detecting arterial spasm is also important, as vasospasm involving distal cerebral arterial branches is not detected by TCD and sometimes not even by MRA, the gold standard being digital subtraction angiography [16]. One-fifth of patients have early MRI changes such as distal hyperintense vessels (HVs) on fluid-attenuated inversion recovery (FLAIR) imaging that are hypothesized to represent engorged distal vessels, an observation that could point to the diagnosis.

In summary, a high index of suspicion is necessary to identify RCVS in the first or second TCH episode. If all the initial ancillary evaluations are negative, follow-up is mandatory to try to document vasospasm later. At this point, it is important to decide whether or not nimodipine should be started – on one hand, symptomatic control is necessary as the headaches of RCVS are usually resistant to analgesics; on the other hand, initiating vasodilator drugs may influence future TCD results and further delay the diagnosis. It is still debatable if nimodipine provides any treatment effect except symptomatic control [15].

In the present case, it was possible to identify early distal vasoconstriction and after starting treatment with nimodipine a clear symptomatic improvement occurred, resolution was complete and uneventful, supporting the diagnosis of RCVS. RCVS has to be distinguished from PACNS, in which headache is usually accompanied by cortical symptoms (e.g.,. cognitive dysfunction), CSF analysis shows lymphocytic pleocytosis (rare in RCVS), and clinical course is progressive. The outcome of RCVS is usually benign, the course is self-limited, and most patients (70–95%) have complete resolution without residual symptoms [16]. Persistent neurologic deficits may occur with RCVS-associated stroke. Very severe cases resulting in death or dependency are rare (less than 5%), as is recurrence [16,17].

Treatment options are empirical and based on vasodilator drugs such as nimodipine, as used to treat vasospasm associated with SAH. Response to treatment is very good (up to 80%) in terms of headache resolution. The effect of nimodipine on vasospasm and stroke prevention in RCSV is less obvious. Treatment with steroids may be harmful. Treatment regimens are continued for 4 to 8 weeks, which is the time in which spontaneous resolution eventually happens. Avoidance of the offending situation in the future is recommended, as the rare recurrences described were related to re-exposures [15,16].

Pitfall

RCVS may be very difficult to diagnose because the arterial changes are dynamic (progress from small distal to medium and then proximal large-sized arteries over days to weeks), so serial evaluations are mandatory for diagnosis and monitoring.

Tip

Remember that primary cough headache, primary headache associated with sexual activity, primary exercise headache, and primary thunderclap headache require exclusion of any secondary cause, including RCVS. A single arterial evaluation is not enough to exclude RCVS.

Case 3. TCH during viral Infection

Case description

A 29-year-old woman described a one-week history of nausea, abdominal pain, diarrhea, and low-grade fever starting in her summer holidays. Three days later she had a sudden onset intense headache occurring while at rest in bed, lasting around 5 minutes and improving to a moderate tightening band-like pain, with mild photophobia and neck pain which increased upon neck movement. She visited her primary care physician (PCP), who prescribed loperamide 2 mg twice daily, paracetamol 1 g every 8 hours, and ibuprofen 600 mg as needed, for headache. Her diarrhea and abdominal pain resolved within the next week, but the headache intensity worsened and she needed to alternate paracetamol with ibuprofen every 4 hours, even at night. Pain was not worse with effort or with Valsalva. She had mild photophobia and anorexia. Pain persisted without improvement for another week so she was referred by the PCP to the ER. She had always been healthy and had no previous headache history; she was taking oral contraception (drospirenone 3 mg plus ethinylestradiol 0.03 mg).

Her neurological examination revealed prostration and mild nuchal rigidity but she had no fever nor any changes of her vital signs. Brain CT was normal. Routine blood work-up revealed a normal white blood cell (WBC) count with a relative lymphocytosis of 53%, a positive C-reactive protein (CRP) of 3.56 mg/dL (normal < 0.60), and three- to four-fold increase on liver function tests. CSF analysis revealed mild lymphocytic pleocytosis (18 cells/μL) with normal glucose and protein levels. Gram staining was negative and cultures were sterile. Opening pressure was not measured. A diagnosis of probable viral meningitis was made. Serological testing for human immunodeficiency virus, for the Herpesviridae family (herpes simplex, varicella-zoster, Epstein–Barr, and cytomegalovirus) and for Coxsackie and Echovirus was negative. The headache improved in the first 48 hours after admission. On the third day after admission, she had a sudden episode of tingling and numbness of the right hand that progressed to the arm, then neck and right side of the face over around 5 minutes; she then noticed difficulties in her speech and had some paraphasias that lasted 3 minutes. Her neurological examination after this event was completely normal, including normal funduscopic examination.

A brain MRI and magnetic resonance venography (MRV) identified a superior longitudinal sinus thrombosis (Figure 12.5) with bilateral parietal cortical lesions compatible with small venous infarcts. She was started on subcutaneous low-molecular-weight heparin (LMWH) and had complete resolution of her headache after 24 hours. She maintained oral

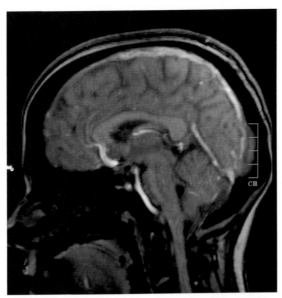

Figure 12.5 Case 3: brain magnetic resonance imaging. Sagittal T1 MRI showing thrombosis of the superior sagittal sinus.

anticoagulation for 6 months. Screening for thrombophilia was negative.

Discussion

This young woman initially presented with a viral infection with gastrointestinal symptoms, during which a TCH occurred, that persisted for 2 weeks. At this point she had mild nuchal rigidity, changes in blood inflammatory parameters and in liver function tests, thus, the hypothesis of viral meningitis was considered. CSF analysis presented lymphocytic pleocytosis that was perhaps too mild for viral meningitis. The CSF opening pressure measurement could have helped in establishing the correct diagnosis at this point although an increase in intracranial pressure can also be identified in aseptic meningitis. Her headache improved in the first 48 hours after admission, reinforcing the working diagnosis of probable self-limited aseptic meningitis. However, unexpected new symptoms led to diagnostic revision: a transient neurological deficit that progressed in one hemisphere sequentially over the sensory and language cortices, was self-limited and lasted 8 minutes. Differential diagnosis of this phenomenon included migrainous aura, transient ischemic attack (which was unlikely due to topographic progression), and focal seizures.

Taking the duration and progression of the observed phenomena, it fulfilled the International Classification of Headache Disorders, 3rd edition (beta version) criteria for migraine aura. However, there were a few caveats – no previous history of migraine; no visual symptoms (which happen in 99% of aura patients); shorter duration than average (usually 20 to 30 minutes) [2,19]; and no headache aggravation (only 10% of patients have isolated auras). Brain MRI was crucial in establishing the diagnosis of cerebral venous thrombosis (CVT) and the transient neurological phenomena were interpreted as a symptomatic seizure secondary to a parietal cortical venous infarct.

The most frequent initial symptom of CVT is headache, occurring in up to 80% of patients, either isolated, within an intracranial hypertension syndrome, or accompanied by focal neurological signs, seizures, or encephalopathy [20,21].

CVT can present as isolated headache in up to 14% of cases, without intracranial hypertension or parenchymal lesions. Headache onset is usually progressive, but TCH was documented to occur in 17% of isolated headache cases in one series [22]. Pain is usually continuous, but no changes in neurological examination, CT scan, or CSF analysis are identified in this group of patients. Isolated headache is usually associated with thrombosis of the lateral sinus, is usually unilateral and on the same side of the occluded sinus and the majority of these cases have an excellent prognosis, although cases with early diagnosis are more likely to present with neurological deterioration [22,23].

The presence of multiple etiologies for CVT in any patient is the rule in up to 44% of cases, so the identification of a cause should not discourage the search for others; if no cause is found, a long follow-up with repeated investigations is mandatory [20]. Besides infection, other factors predisposing to CVT in this patient included dehydration after diarrhea, the use of oral contraceptives, and lumbar puncture – CVT has been described after a dural puncture, either for epidural or spinal anesthesia, myelography, intrathecal administration of drugs or diagnostic. LP is not mandatory for the diagnosis of CVT, but is often performed in this context for differential diagnosis. Current evidence does not support a deleterious effect of LP in patients with CVT either in the development of new brain lesions or in long-term prognosis [24].

CVT recommended treatment in the acute phase includes body weight-adjusted subcutaneous LMWH or continuous intravenous heparin. After the acute phase, anticoagulation should be switched to oral agents for a variable period. Severe or complicated CVT might require intravenous or local thrombolysis or decompressive craniectomy [25]. Prognosis is favorable in the vast majority of patients. Poor prognostic factors include male sex, age over 37, coma, mental status change or brain hemorrhage upon admission, thrombosis of the deep venous system, and additional severe underlying disorders such as CNS infection or systemic malignancy [21].

Pitfall

There is no evidence that lumbar punctures are deleterious in CVT patients when performed to exclude other diagnostic hypotheses. However, there is an increasing recognition that lumbar punctures by themselves are risk factors for developing CVT and should not be performed in CVT patients with previously established diagnosis. Caution is warranted in other patients with additional risk factors for CVT (known thrombophilias and/or concomitant use of drugs with prothrombotic effect).

Tip

The imaging diagnosis of CVT requires specifically a CT or MRI venography; do not settle for conventional brain imaging when the clinical suspicion is high or you might miss lateral sinus thrombosis and only diagnose CVT later, after thrombus extension to the superior longitudinal sinus (SLS) or the occurrence of parenchymal complications.

Case 4. TCH with minor neck trauma

Case description

A 41-year-old healthy female violinist had a sudden left-sided frontal headache during a concert, while playing as the concertmaster. She was able to finish her performance adequately, although the pain was intense and did not subside. She attributed the pain to a sudden neck movement while playing and thought of it as a probable muscle strain, as her neck felt tender. She started self-medicating with analgesics and nonsteroidal anti-inflammatory agents, which resulted in transient pain improvement but not in pain remission. On the sixth day after the concert she felt a sudden episode lasting around one hour of difficulty in articulating her speech and right-sided paresthesia of the face and arm, for which she came into the emergency department. At admission she had a left-sided Horner's syndrome and her vital signs revealed mild hypertension (175/95 mmHg) with heart rate of 96.

A brain MRI and MRA (Figure 12.6) identified a left carotid artery dissection with recent left distal small frontal and insular areas of cortical ischemia. CT angiography showed a long-segment and irregular postbulbar carotid artery high-grade stenosis (sting sign; Figure 12.6b).

She was started on LMWH and monitored closely in the stroke unit. General measures and blood pressure control were applied according to the guidelines [26,27]. The intensity of her headaches improved after 24 h of anticoagulation associated with symptomatic treatment. The remaining cardiovascular investigation was normal. She was discharged 5 days after admission with a modified Rankin scale score of zero.

Discussion

Cervical artery dissection (CAD) is a rare disease, with an estimated incidence of 2.6 to 3 per 100 000 individuals per year for carotid dissections and 1.0 to 1.5 per 100 000 per year for vertebral disease [28]. The risk of

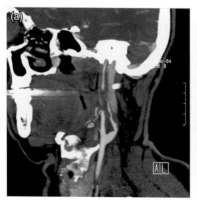
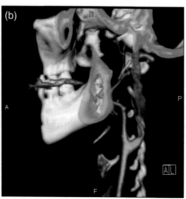

Figure 12.6 Case 4: computed tomography angiography. (a) 3D maximum intensity projection. (b) 3D volume rendering. Initial CTA showing a long-segment and irregular postbulbar carotid artery high-grade stenosis (sting sign).

stroke after cervical artery dissection is around 70% in carotid artery and 85% in vertebral artery dissections, being one of the most frequent causes of stroke in young adults (15–20% of cases). Most often stroke occurs due to distal atheroembolism from intraluminal thrombi forming at the site of the intimal tear, but it can also be a consequence of distal hemodynamic compromise caused by severe stenosis or arterial occlusion [28,29]. In almost half the cases (47%), the risk of stroke may be prevented by starting antithrombotic treatment as soon as the initial symptoms occur, so the challenge is to establish the diagnosis before the advent of ischemic complications, which occur after a median delay of 4 days [30].

Ipsilateral headache is the most frequent symptom of CAD, occurring in up to 75% of patients; it is the initial symptom in 30–50% of patients and its onset is most often gradual (72% of patients) but in 22% it presents as TCH. Neck pain often accompanies headache from CAD, more frequently in vertebral (46%) than in carotid artery dissections (26%). It is most often a constant pain, projecting to the anterior part of the head in carotid disease and to the occipital region in vertebral disease [30].

The epidemiological context is an important aid to diagnosis, CAD occurring in 1–2% of patients with major blunt trauma such as motor vehicle accidents, direct hit to the neck, or strangulation. In around 40% of cases, it occurs in the context of minor trauma or movements that involve hyperextension or sudden neck rotation, such as coughing or vomiting, during sports or leisure activities (e.g., golf, running, scuba diving, roller coaster rides), neck chiropractic manipulation or iatrogenic (e.g., neck hyperextension for anesthesia intubation, catheter placement, needle aspiration biopsy of the neck) [31]. Host characteristics also influence CAD occurrence, as it is more frequent in migraine patients, in patients with connective tissue diseases (e.g., Ehlers–Danlos syndrome, Marfan's syndrome, osteogenesis imperfecta), and fibromuscular dysplasia.

Besides pain of CAD, which is thought to result from distension of the artery wall by mural hematoma, other symptoms may accompany or follow dissection before ischemia; in carotid disease the typical ipsilateral Horner's syndrome results from damage to pericarotid sympathetic fibers (painful Horner – classic sign of CAD) and more rarely, lower cranial nerve palsies [31]. TIA or classic transient monocular blindness (amaurosis fugax) may precede established stroke in carotid CAD in up to one in four patients; around

15% of vertebral CAD patients have a previous TIA presenting with vertigo, nausea and vomiting, facial numbness, ataxia, and visual symptoms [29,31]. In any patient with a TIA, especially young patients with headache, noninvasive imaging of the cervical vessels should be performed routinely and within 24 h of symptoms [26]. Investigation using duplex ultrasonography is recommended as it is less expensive than other sorts of imaging, and is fast and readily available; its sensitivity is higher for carotid (up to 96%) than for vertebral dissections (up to 86%) but the false negative rate rises when dissections do not cause arterial stenosis [31]. In high suspicion cases CT or MR angiography should be performed, having over 90% sensitivity for these diagnoses, CTA being slightly superior in vertebral artery disease [29,31]. Cervical MRI with T1-weighted fat-suppressed sequences is the gold standard for the diagnosis of intramural carotid hematomas [31]; the current role of catheter-based angiography in CAD diagnosis is now reserved for complex or inconclusive cases [29].

Antithrombotic treatment is recommended for CAD, either with antiplatelet therapy or anticoagulation [29]; the superiority of either treatment option is still debated [32,33].

Pitfall

It is frequent for CAD pain to be misinterpreted as a muscle condition, especially when it is accompanied by neck pain.

Tip

Persistent de novo head and/or neck pain in a young patient after minor head or neck trauma should be enough to raise suspicion of CAD, even in the absence of other neurological signs.

Case 5. Exercise recurrent TCH

Case description

A 15-year-old healthy high-school student self-referred to the headache outpatient clinic for recurrent headaches. He had had a bout of similar headaches at the age of 13 that persisted over a period of around 6 months, in winter months, and spontaneously subsided for a full year. He had become symptomatic again 8 months before the appointment; his headaches would only occur during physical effort, but not every time he exercised. His usual training habits included swimming one hour per week and two periods of 90 minutes of school gymnastics, in which he would play group sports or do athletics; this pattern had not changed in the last years.

He related the headache onset with the intensity of the exercise – if the warm-up was slow and he did not do high-intensity cardiovascular exercise, he could maintain most or all of his training without headache. If he decided to do push-ups or pull-ups, he would have a sudden occipital intense throbbing headache with dizziness and malaise, lasting a few minutes but then persisting at lower intensity for about 2 hours. There were no other accompanying symptoms, such as photophobia, phonophobia, nausea, or visual changes. There was also no shortness of breath, fainting, chest pain or leg pain with exercise. The same type of sudden attacks would happen immediately with any exercise if he was not able to warm up before, or even with a simple fast run to catch the bus. He had already been evaluated by his pediatrician, who had ordered a brain CT, 24 h Holter monitoring, and a treadmill test, all reported back as normal.

His height was 1.73 m (75th percentile) and weight was 78 kg (90th percentile), having a body mass index of 26 kg/m². His blood pressure (right arm) was 130/75 mmHg (90th percentile for his height), and heart rate was 80 beats per minute. Pulses of the four limbs were not explored. His neurological examination was normal. MRI with MRA/MRV was normal and an ambulatory pressure monitoring was requested with the specific instruction that he should exercise during that day. The monitoring was positive for severe systo-diastolic diurnal and systolic nocturnal hypertension (Figure 12.7).

Complete routine blood analysis revealed normal results, including thyroid and parathyroid levels, lipid profile, estimated glomerular filtration rate, toxicological screening, and 24 h urinary metanephrine, normetanephrine, and aldosterone. A chest and renal CT angiography identified an aortic coarctation as the cause of his hypertension; he was admitted to the

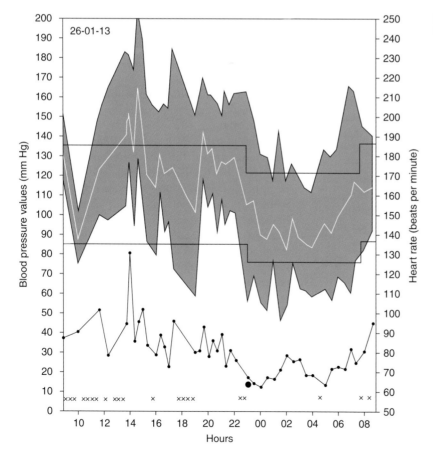

Figure 12.7 Case 5: ambulatory arterial blood pressure monitoring.

cardiology department and treated with balloon angioplasty. After recovery, he showed marked improvement in his exercise tolerability. At the 6-month follow-up he was able to exercise freely but still needed daily antihypertensive treatment.

Discussion

This boy's headache could be classified as primary exercise headache because he had more than two episodes of headache occurring exclusively during or after strenuous exercise and subsiding within 48 hours [2]. Exercise headache occurs in around 10% of the population and 80% of exertional headache is primary [34]. It is mandatory to exclude secondary causes of TCH and even of progressive exercise headache but the degree of suspicion lowers in reverse proportion to the length of the headache history.

Understanding the physiology of exercise may bring some clues to the eventual cause or trigger of the headache and even in benign exercise-related headaches it is helpful to assist the patient to adapt his exercise profile and avoid triggering headaches. Initial or rapid effort imposes the major workload in fast or glycolytic muscle fibers (anaerobic metabolism) and depends on a fast increase of cardiac output above 85% of the maximal heart rate (triggered sympathetic activation), especially in lower-trained individuals; this type of effort may result in acute onset short-lasting headaches, as it did in our patient. Progressive higher effort or prolonged low-intensity exercise are mainly aerobic and cardiac output is maintained mainly by blood flow redistribution, allowing lower (40–85% of maximal) heart rates and steady increases in systolic blood pressure. In this setting, a progressive "effort associated" headache can occur, which is believed to be related to dehydration, heat, and fatigue [35]. Exercise can also be a precipitant of migraine attacks, in migraine patients.

In static exercise, muscle contraction increases peripheral arterial resistance which results in an increase of the diastolic blood pressure, which usually does not happen with dynamic exercise. In static arm exercises the increase in blood pressure is up to 10% higher than with static leg exercises, because the muscle mass and vasculature of the arms is smaller [36]. Static arm exercises were exactly the kind of exercise our patient could not tolerate, suggesting that a blood pressure increase could be contributing to this patient's headaches. Although there was a previous evaluation by a

pediatrician, the borderline value of his resting systolic blood pressure measured in office could easily have been interpreted as a "white coat syndrome." The patient had a treadmill test with completely normal results but the Bruce Protocol stress test reproduces precisely the type of exercise our patient tolerated perfectly well– a progressive low-intensity exercise always monitoring for heart rates below 85% of the maximum. When asked, the patient mentioned having had no problem whatsoever in performing the treadmill, he did not feel tired nor did he have headache during the test.

Exercise headaches are usually throbbing and bilateral but most often frontal and last less than 1 hour in over 80% of patients [37], although no typical exercise headache pattern is required in the classification [2]. Concomitant nausea can occur but dizziness or visual symptoms are usually not described. The alternative diagnosis, headache attributed to hypertensive crisis without hypertensive encephalopathy, is also bilateral throbbing headache that can be precipitated by physical activity and resolves within 1 hour of normalization of blood pressure, being often occipital in location, a pattern that is more in line with our patient's headache description [2]. In severe hypertension, symptoms of end-organ damage may also occur; the most frequent central nervous system manifestations are headache and dizziness, but nausea, confusion or weakness can also occur. In this case, idiopathic intracranial hypertension or RCVS were important differentials.

Serial blood pressure measurement or continuous monitoring of the blood pressure in an active day establishes the diagnosis; the identification of the cause of the hypertension required an extended complementary evaluation. Although pulses of the four limbs were not explored in the appointment, there were no other clinical clues for the diagnosis, such as asymmetries in limb development, changes or delays in growth pattern, nor other symptoms of coarctation of the aorta.

Pitfall

The long remission period of this boy's headaches had no clear justification (there were no major changes in exercise patterns in the previous two years and his weight gain was in line with his previous growth pattern) but it caused his pediatrician to believe mistakenly that he had primary thunderclap headache.

Tip

Emphasize monitoring blood pressure measurements in the outpatient clinic. If a "white coat syndrome" is suspected, do serial evaluations or request a continuous monitoring of blood pressure in an active day.

In summary, recognizing TCH is pivotal and requires only being able to ask properly about headache onset and to listen to the patient. A secondary cause of TCH is more likely to be identified if the neurological examination is abnormal and some etiologies of TCH rarely occur without focal neurological symptoms (e.g. ischemic or hemorrhagic stroke, meningitis, hydrocephalus, or subdural hematoma). The cases presented illustrate most of the serious pathologies that frequently present with completely normal observations. Complementary investigation is mandatory but the clinician must decide not only the appropriate test but also test limitations according to the time frame in which the test is being done. Primary thunderclap headache requires adequate exclusion of all secondary causes, often only possible with repeated testing.

Acknowledgments

The author thanks Dr. Pedro Vilela for his precious help in selecting the images to illustrate the presented cases.

References

1. Ferrante E, Tassorelli C, Rossi P, Lisotto C, Nappi G. Focus on the management of thunderclap headache: from nosography to treatment. *J Headache Pain* 2011;12:251–8.

2. (IHS) HCCotIHS. The international classification of headache disorders, 3rd edition (beta version). *Cephalalgia* 2013;33:629–808.

3. Linn FH, Rinkel GJ, Algra A, van Gijn J. Headache characteristics in subarachnoid haemorrhage and benign thunderclap headache. *J Neurol Neurosurg Psychiatry* 1998;65:791–3.

4. Gil-Gouveia R, Fernandes Sousa R, Lopes L, Campos J, Pavo Martins I. Headaches during angiography and endovascular procedures. *J Neurol* 2007;254:591–6.

5. Schwedt TJ. Thunderclap headaches: a focus on etiology and diagnostic evaluation. *Headache* 2013;53:563–9.

6. Landtblom AM, Fridriksson S, Boivie J, Hillman J, Johansson G, Johansson I. Sudden onset headache: a prospective study of features, incidence and causes. *Cephalalgia* 2002;22:354–60.

7. Connolly ES, Rabinstein AA, Carhuapoma JR, Derdeyn CP, Dion J, Higashida RT, et al. Guidelines for the management of aneurysmal subarachnoid hemorrhage: a guideline for healthcare professionals from the American Heart Association/American Stroke Association. *Stroke* 2012;43:1711–37.

8. Ferro J, Lopes J, Melo T, Oliveira V, Crespo M, Campos J, et al. Investigation into the causes of delayed diagnosis of subarachnoid hemorrhage. *Cerebrovasc Dis* 1991;1(3):160–4.

9. Edlow JA, Caplan LR. Avoiding pitfalls in the diagnosis of subarachnoid hemorrhage. *N Engl J Med* 2000;342:29–36.

10. Vlak MH, Rinkel GJ, Greebe P, van der Bom JG, Algra A. Trigger factors for rupture of intracranial aneurysms in relation to patient and aneurysm characteristics. *J Neurol* 2012;259:1298–302.

11. Steiner T, Juvela S, Unterberg A, Jung C, Forsting M, Rinkel G, et al. European Stroke Organization guidelines for the management of intracranial aneurysms and subarachnoid haemorrhage. *Cerebrovasc Dis* 2013;35:93–112.

12. Rosenberg JH, Silberstein SD. The headache of SAH responds to sumatriptan. *Headache* 2005;45:597–8.

13. Pfadenhauer K, Schönsteiner T, Keller H. The risks of sumatriptan administration in patients with unrecognized subarachnoid haemorrhage (SAH). *Cephalalgia* 2006;26:320–3.

14. Bauer AM, Rasmussen PA. Treatment of intracranial vasospasm following subarachnoid hemorrhage. *Front Neurol* 2014;5:72.

15. Ducros A. Reversible cerebral vasoconstriction syndrome. *Handb Clin Neurol* 2014;121:1725–41.

16. Sattar A, Manousakis G, Jensen MB. Systematic review of reversible cerebral vasoconstriction syndrome. *Expert Rev Cardiovasc Ther* 2010;8:1417–21.

17. Grooters GS, Sluzewski M, Tijssen CC. How often is thunderclap headache caused by the reversible cerebral vasoconstriction syndrome? *Headache* 2014;54:732–5.

18. Chen SP, Wang SJ. Hyperintense vessels: an early MRI marker of reversible cerebral vasoconstriction syndrome? *Cephalalgia* 2014;34(13):1038–9.

19. Russell MB, Olesen J. A nosographic analysis of the migraine aura in a general population. *Brain* 1996;119 (Pt 2):355–61.

20. Bousser MG, Ferro JM. Cerebral venous thrombosis: an update. *Lancet Neurol* 2007;6:162–70.

21. Ferro JM, Canhão P, Stam J, Bousser MG, Barinagarrementeria F – for the ISCVT Investigators. Prognosis of cerebral vein and dural sinus thrombosis: results of the international study on cerebral vein and dural sinus thrombosis (ISCVT). *Stroke* 2004;35:664–70.

22. Cumurciuc R, Crassard I, Sarov M, Valade D, Bousser MG. Headache as the only neurological sign of cerebral venous thrombosis: a series of 17 cases. *J Neurol Neurosurg Psychiatry* 2005;76:1084–7.

23. Gameiro J, Ferro JM, Canhão P, Stam J, Barinagarrementeria F, Lindgren A, et al. Prognosis of cerebral vein thrombosis presenting as isolated headache: early vs. late diagnosis. *Cephalalgia* 2012;32:407–12.

24. Canhão P, Abreu LF, Ferro JM, Stam J, Bousser MG, Barinagarrementeria F, et al. Safety of lumbar puncture in patients with cerebral venous thrombosis. *Eur J Neurol* 2013;20:1075–80.

25. Einhäupl K, Stam J, Bousser MG, De Bruijn SF, Ferro JM, Martinelli I, et al. EFNS guideline on the treatment of cerebral venous and sinus thrombosis in adult patients. *Eur J Neurol* 2010;17:1229–35.

26. Jauch EC, Saver JL, Adams HP, Bruno A, Connors JJ, Demaerschalk BM, et al. Guidelines for the early management of patients with acute ischemic stroke: a guideline for healthcare professionals from the American Heart Association/American Stroke Association. *Stroke* 2013;44:870–947.

27. Committee ESOEE, Committee EW. Guidelines for management of ischaemic stroke and transient ischaemic attack 2008. *Cerebrovasc Dis* 2008;25:457–507.

28. Medel R, Starke RM, Valle-Giler EP, Martin-Schild S, El Khoury R, Dumont AS. Diagnosis and treatment of arterial dissections. *Curr Neurol Neurosci Rep* 2014;14:419.

29. Brott TG, Halperin JL, Abbara S, Bacharach JM, Barr JD, Bush RL, et al. 2011 ASA/ACCF/AHA/AANN/AANS/ACR/ASNR/CNS/SAIP/SCAI/SIR/SNIS/SVM/SVS guideline on the management of patients with extracranial carotid and vertebral artery disease. Executive summary: A report of the American College of Cardiology Foundation/American Heart Association Task Force on Practice Guidelines, and the American Stroke Association, American Association of Neuroscience Nurses, American Association of Neurological Surgeons, American College of Radiology, American Society of Neuroradiology, Congress of Neurological Surgeons, Society of Atherosclerosis Imaging and Prevention, Society for Cardiovascular Angiography and Interventions, Society of Interventional Radiology, Society of Neurointerventional Surgery, Society for Vascular Medicine, and Society for Vascular Surgery. Developed in collaboration with the American Academy of Neurology and Society of Cardiovascular Computed Tomography. *Catheter Cardiovasc Interv* 2013;81:E76–123.

30. Silbert PL, Mokri B, Schievink WI. Headache and neck pain in spontaneous internal carotid and vertebral artery dissections. *Neurology* 1995;45:1517–22.

31. Debette S, Leys D. Cervical-artery dissections: predisposing factors, diagnosis, and outcome. *Lancet Neurol* 2009;8:668–78.

32. Kennedy F, Lanfranconi S, Hicks C, Reid J, Gompertz P, Price C, et al. Antiplatelets vs anticoagulation for dissection: CADISS nonrandomized arm and meta-analysis. *Neurology* 2012;79:686–9.

33. Sarikaya H, da Costa BR, Baumgartner RW, Duclos K, Touzé E, de Bray JM, et al. Antiplatelets versus anticoagulants for the treatment of cervical artery dissection: Bayesian meta-analysis. *PLoS One* 2013;8:e72697.

34. Halker RB, Vargas BB. Primary exertional headache: updates in the literature. *Curr Pain Headache Rep* 2013;17:337.

35. Williams SJ, Nukada H. Sport and exercise headache: Part 2. Diagnosis and classification. *Br J Sports Med* 1994;28:96–100.

36. Rivera-Brown AM, Frontera WR. Principles of exercise physiology: Responses to acute exercise and long-term adaptations to training. *PMR* 2012;4:797–804.

37. Chen SP, Fuh JL, Lu SR, Wang SJ. Exertional headache–a survey of 1963 adolescents. *Cephalalgia* 2009;29:401–7.

Chapter 13

Underdiagnosis of reversible cerebral vasoconstriction syndromes

Arash Salardini, Aneesh B. Singhal, and José Biller

What are the reversible cerebral vasoconstriction syndromes?

Reversible cerebral vasoconstriction syndromes (RCVS) are a group of conditions characterized by reversible segmental narrowing of the cerebral arteries. Most patients develop recurrent sudden, severe ("thunderclap") headaches at onset. Approximately one-third to one-half develop ischemic or hemorrhagic strokes, or brain edema. Recent publications describing stereotypical clinical-imaging features, including the usually dramatic onset with thunderclap headaches and benign outcomes, have made RCVS recognizable to the experienced clinician. However, RCVS can be difficult to diagnose due to the absence of validated diagnostic criteria; moreover, the diagnosis cannot be confirmed until the reversibility of arterial narrowing is established, which can take up to 3 months. Further complicating the diagnosis is that until recently, patients with RCVS were reported under a variety of terms and eponyms, each reflecting the associated clinical setting (Table 13.1). The unifying term "cerebral vasoconstriction syndrome" was proposed in 2002 [1,2], but the syndrome became widely recognized only after the 2007 publication by a multidisciplinary group of authors [3] listing the key elements for diagnosis (Table 13.2).

RCVS is more common in women than in men (approximately 2:1 to 4:1). It typically occurs between the ages of 20 and 60 years, though children can be affected. One-third of cases are considered idiopathic and may overlap with certain "primary" headaches including primary cough headache, benign sexual headache, and benign exertional headache. The other two-thirds are associated with hormonal influences (e.g., obstetric delivery), vasoactive substances (such as medications or blood products), or mechanical forces

Table 13.1 Selected conditions included under RCVS

- Postpartum angiopathy
- Eclampsia-associated vasoconstriction
- Drug-induced angiitis ("angiitis" is a misnomer as there is no vessel inflammation)
- Migraine "angiitis" (again, a misnomer)
- Thunderclap headache with reversible vasospasm
- CNS pseudovasculitis
- Benign angiopathy of the central nervous system (CNS)
- Call's syndrome, or Call–Fleming syndrome

Table 13.2 Key elements for diagnosis [3]

- Transfemoral angiography or indirect computed tomography angiography (CTA) or magnetic resonance angiography (MRA) documenting multifocal segmental cerebral artery vasoconstriction
- No evidence for aneurysmal subarachnoid hemorrhage (SAH)
- Normal or near-normal cerebrospinal fluid (CSF) analysis (protein level <80 mg%, leukocytes <10 mm³, normal glucose level)
- Severe, acute headaches, with or without additional neurologic signs or symptoms
- Reversibility of angiographic abnormalities within 12 weeks after onset. If death occurs before the follow-up studies are completed, autopsy rules out such conditions as vasculitis, intracranial atherosclerosis, and aneurysmal SAH, which can also manifest with headache and stroke

(such as surgery or trauma). Due to distinct yet overlapping clinical, laboratory, and imaging findings, primary angiitis of the CNS (PACNS) remains on the list of differential diagnoses. Imaging in RCVS typically shows reversible but prolonged multifocal segmental vasoconstriction, which probably progresses distally to proximally, and is predominantly intracranial. The time course of imaging changes does not always correlate with symptoms, such as thunderclap headaches or focal neurological signs [4]. Management can be a combination of symptomatic (pain and

Table 13.3 Management of RCVS [6]

Supportive and symptomatic measures
- Observation
- Discontinue vasoconstrictive medications
- Seizure prophylaxis (long-term antiepileptic drugs unnecessary)
- Intravenous fluids, analgesics, laxatives
- Pharmacological blood pressure control is controversial

Specific pharmacotherapy
- Calcium channel blockers (e.g., nimodipine or verapamil) – duration 4–8 weeks or until headaches subside
- Intravenous magnesium

Interventions
- Balloon angioplasty or intra-arterial vasodilators (nicardipine, milrinone, prostacyclin) may be attempted if progressive clinical decline

anxiety), supportive (blood pressure control), and disease-specific (calcium channel blockers) treatments (Table 13.3). Intravascular intervention may be indicated in more severe and clinically progressive cases, as progression to death has been documented in exceptional cases. Headaches may recur for a few weeks. Most patients recover completely although visual deficits and mild hemiparesis can persist in a minority. Relapses are rare. It seems logical to discontinue potentially contributing medications such as selective serotonin uptake inhibitors (SSRIs), triptans, ergot derivatives, and over-the-counter sympathomimetics used as decongestants or diet medications [5].

Idiopathic RCVS

Case 1. Post-coital headache (source: Calabrese et al. [3])

A 46-year-old man with a history of common migraine with vascular risk factors of hypertension and hyperlipidemia presented with severe post-coital thunderclap headache. There was a recurrence of the headache on day 3, this time with coexistent cortical blindness and mild left hemiparesis. An emergent computed tomography angiography (CTA) showed the presence of multifocal segmental stenosis affecting multiple vessels including the basilar, posterior cerebral artery (PCAs) and superior cerebellar arteries (SCAs) as well as middle cerebral arteries (MCAs) bilaterally. Diffusion-weighted magnetic resonance imaging (MRI) showed symmetrical bilateral occipital lobe and

small cerebellar and right frontal infarcts (Figure 13.1). CSF examination and laboratory testing was inconsistent with vasculitis or subarachnoid hemorrhage (SAH). The patient was treated with analgesia and verapamil. His symptoms abated in the following 3 weeks and magnetic resonance angiography (MRA) documented the resolution of the vasoconstriction.

Discussion

Here we detail a patient who presented with thunderclap headaches which may have been diagnosed as primary post-coital headaches except for the recurrence of pain, followed by the development of cortical visual symptoms in the presence of widespread multifocal cerebral arterial narrowing. No hormonal, medication, or traumatic triggers were identified in this case. The patient did not have recurrences of RCVS during prolonged follow-up [6].

Primary and secondary headaches as mimics of RCVS

RCVS overlaps with a number of primary headaches including post-coital headaches, migraines, cough-induced headaches, and primary thunderclap headaches [4,7,8]. The distinction between these conditions and RCVS is the presence of prolonged reversible intracranial arterial narrowing. Whether the pathophysiologies of these idiopathic headaches are similar to RCVS or not requires further investigation.

Imaging in suspected RCVS

New onset thunderclap headaches merit urgent brain imaging to exclude several life-threatening conditions (Table 13.4)[9]. A recent small series suggests that the rate of RCVS in patients with thunderclap headaches (without evidence of hemorrhage) could be as high as 8.8% [10]. Imaging may demonstrate complications such as convexity SAH or brain edema (Table 13.5). Convexity SAH has a broad differential diagnosis (Table 13.6), but RCVS is the most common cause in young individuals below age 60 years, or in the setting of recurrent thunderclap headache. Magnetic resonance venography (MRV) or CT venography (CTV) is indicated when cerebral venous sinus thrombosis (CVST) is suspected.

It is important to note that initial brain parenchymal as well as vascular imaging may be normal in patients with RCVS. If the index of suspicion is high, imaging should be repeated in a few days. Common findings include the presence of intracranial blood including intracranial hemorrhage, subarachnoid

(a)

(b)

(c)

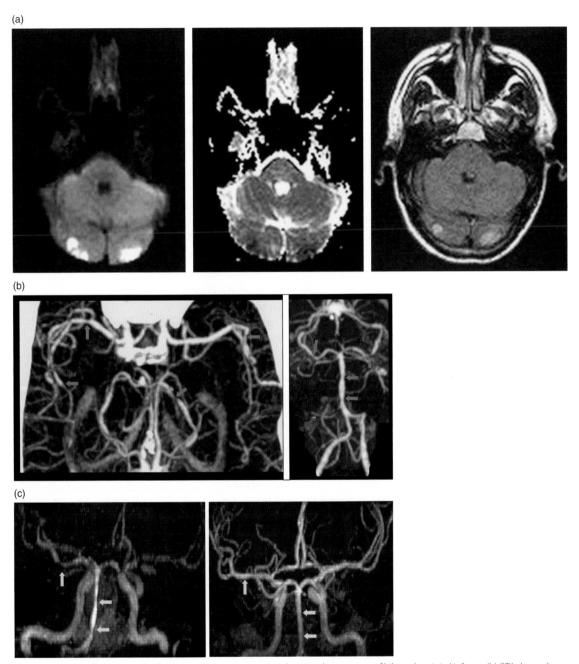

Figure 13.1 (a) Diffusion-weighted magnetic resonance imaging showing the presence of bilateral occipital infarcts. (b) CTA shows the presence of multifocal segmental stenosis in both MCAs bilaterally, the basilar artery, PCAs and SCAs. (c) The reversal of stenosis (the image on the right) compared to initial imaging (left). (Source: Calabrese et al., *Ann Intern Med* 2007; 146(1): 34–44.)

Table 13.4 Differential diagnosis of thunderclap headache

With neck rigidity

-Subarachnoid hemorrhage (SAH)

-Meningitis, encephalitis

Without neck rigidity

-Cervical artery dissections

-Acute ischemic stroke (PCA embolus)

-Intracranial hematoma including pituitary apoplexy

-Cerebral venous sinus thrombosis (CVST)

-Intracranial hypotension syndrome

-Hypertensive crises/pressor responses (e.g.,
   pheochromocytoma)

-Posterior reversible encephalopathy syndrome (PRES)

-Reversible cerebral vasoconstriction syndrome (RCVS)

-Sphenoid sinusitis (complicated sinusitis)

-*Primary thunderclap headaches*

Table 13.5 Complications of RCVS

Convexity (non-aneurysmal) SAH

Brain edema

Parenchymal hemorrhage

Cerebral infarction

Seizures

Table 13.6 Causes of non-traumatic cortical SAH [11]

Vascular anomalies

- Pial arteriovenous malformation
- Dural arteriovenous fistula
- Cavernous malformations
- Infectious (mycotic) aneurysms
- Cervical arterial dissections

Obstructive and hemodynamic causes

- Dural and cortical venous sinus thrombosis
- Moyamoya
- Severe atherosclerotic carotid artery disease
- Posterior reversible encephalopathy syndrome (PRES)

Increased risk of bleeding

- Coagulopathy
- Cerebral amyloid angiopathy (CAA)

Destructive lesions

- Tumors

Inflammatory causes

- Infective endocarditis

Reversible cerebral vasoconstriction syndrome

blood, brain edema, watershed infarcts, and multiple areas of vascular narrowing (beading).

RCVS in the obstetric population

Case 2. Late prepartum

A 27-year-old right-handed G1P0 woman in her 35th week of pregnancy was referred to the neurology service for acute severe headache and transient neurologic symptoms. She had been hospitalized for a high-risk pregnancy due to the presence of gestational diabetes and "mild" pre-eclampsia. During a prenatal clinical visit the patient was found to have raised blood pressure and proteinuria. Her hepatic, renal, and hematological status were stable. The patient was admitted to be monitored on the obstetrics ward as the date of delivery approached. She was treated with intravenous hydralazine and magnesium sulfate. She was also started on steroids to accelerate fetal lung maturity. During the hospitalization the patient had an acute onset of left face numbness which over the next 5 minutes spread to her left hand. The staff also noted the presence of mild slurring of speech. She complained of severe occipital headache. She had no visual symptoms: no scintillation, no blurring of vision, diplopia, or transient visual loss.

On examination, the patient's blood pressure was 160/101 mmHg. General examination was normal except for bilateral pitting edema. She had no neck stiffness. Neurologic examination failed to show the presence of objective hypoesthesia or cerebellar signs. There was no hyperreflexia. A non-contrasted cerebral CT showed the presence of a small non-traumatic SAH in the right hemispheric high convexity (Figure 13.2a). The patient was transferred for an urgent CTA study, after her obstetric team deemed the risks acceptable in the third trimester, which confirmed the presence of the subarachnoid blood and additionally revealed the widespread presence of segmental intracranial vasoconstriction worse in the right anterior circulation (Figure 13.2d).

The patient was transferred to the high dependency unit for blood pressure monitoring. An extra loading dose of magnesium sulfate was given intravenously under the supervision of her obstetrician and oral nimodipine was instituted. Anxiolytics and pain relief were administered. An MRI was performed after she was stabilized. It showed a subjacent area of FLAIR signal hyperintensities consistent with vasogenic edema. Extensive work-up for vasculitis was found to be

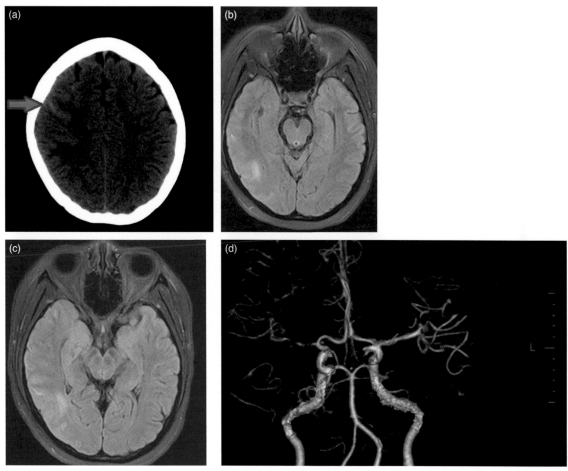

Figure 13.2 (a) Non-contrast brain CT with the arrow pointing to the presence of blood in the right hemispheric convexity. (b and c) Two cross-sections of FLAIR imaging which confirm the presence of blood and additionally show some subcortical edema. (d) A three-dimensional image reconstructed from CT angiography data which shows widespread areas of alternating narrowing and dilatation.

negative. She was transferred for a cesarean section as soon as she was stable and gave birth to a healthy child. She was kept in for observation for 10 days postpartum by which time her headaches had abated. Serial transcranial Doppler (TCD) documented the resolution of "vasospasm" over the period of her hospitalization.

Case 3. Early postpartum

A 34-year-old woman, G5P3, 1 week postpartum presented acutely with severe head pain with concomitant photophobia and abdominal pain. Her symptoms started acutely at 1 a.m. when she was awoken from her sleep with the worst headache of her life. She ignored the symptoms and the headache temporarily abated with time but recurred the afternoon of the following day. She went to a local hospital in the afternoon where

she had an emergent CT which showed the presence of right-frontal intraparenchymal hemorrhage and bilateral frontal SAH with blood along the falx cerebri. She was taken emergently to the angiography suite where a catheter angiogram showed significant reduction in blood flow into the right middle cerebral artery secondary to severe M1 vasospasm. The patient was treated with intra-arterial calcium channel blocker which caused a reversal of the intracranial vasoconstriction (Figures 13.3a, b, and c). She was transferred to the intensive care unit (ICU) for close monitoring.

Discussion

The first case represents transient neurologic symptoms and the presence of convexity SAH in a late prepartum woman due to RCVS. The second case shows intracranial

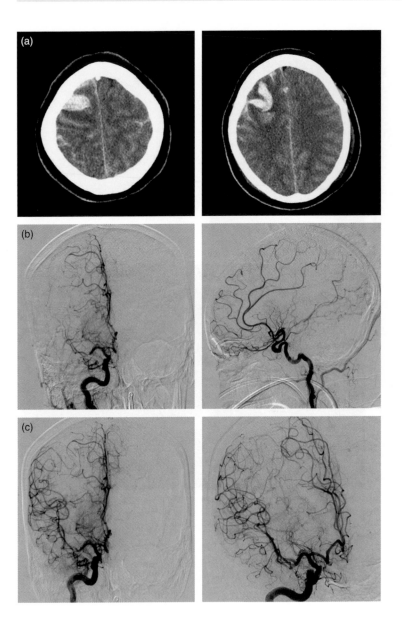

Figure 13.3 (a) Unenhanced head CT shows the presence of intraparenchymal and subarachnoid blood. (b) Catheter angiogram shows the presence of severe M1 vasoconstriction. (c) The same patient after intra-arterial calcium channel blockers.

hemorrhagic complications and intracranial vasoconstriction associated with severe preeclampsia.

Association of pregnancy and RCVS

The association between RCVS and pregnancy is well known. The risk of RCVS is highest in the first few days (up to 6 weeks) postpartum and in this context it is also referred to as postpartum cerebral angiopathy or PCA. While most cases of PCA occur postpartum, presumably because of exposure to vasoactive drugs during delivery or because of sudden hormonal changes which occur after birth, RCVS can rarely occur in late prepartum. There is some overlap, both in terms of pathophysiology and symptomatology, with eclampsia and preeclampsia. RCVS has also been associated with the hemolysis, elevated liver enzymes, low platelet count (HELLP) syndrome. The majority of cases, however, occur in patients who have completed a normal pregnancy. In common with other forms of RCVS, PCA presents with thunderclap headaches, with or without neurologic symptoms or

Table 13.7 Types and causes of postpartum headaches

Primary headache disorders

-Migraine, tension-type headache, other primary headaches

Secondary headaches

-Post-dural puncture

-Embolic stroke

-Cervical artery dissection

-Aneurysmal SAH

-Intracranial hemorrhage

-CVST

-Pituitary apoplexy or Sheehan syndrome

-Postpartum preeclampsia or eclampsia

-Coincidental conditions (brain tumor)

-PRES

-RCVS

Table 13.8 Postpartum headache red flags

Nature of the headache

-Thunderclap headache

-Presence of neurological symptoms

-Neck stiffness

-Prolonged headache (>24 hours)

-"New kind of headache"

Patient red flag

-Systolic blood pressure >160 mmHg

-Hereditary connective tissue disease

-Proteinuria, eclampsia, preeclampsia, HELLP

-Patients with coagulopathies

-Patients on vasoactive medications or recreational drugs

seizures. The patient will have nausea and vomiting, and sometimes photophobia. These symptoms may initially be misinterpreted as migraines. However, in patients with a history of migraines, the PCA head pain is quite unlike the pain they have experienced previously both qualitatively and in terms of severity. Hypertension is common at presentation. In the majority of cases the course of the disease is relatively benign with spontaneous resolution of symptoms with supportive care. However, ischemic stroke, intracerebral hemorrhage, or SAH can and do occur in PCA and in a small but significant subset there is rapid progression of neurological decline due to progressive ischemia and/or hemorrhage and the resultant brain edema [12].

Relationship with other peripartum headaches

Headaches are somewhat common in the peripartum period. A list of the differential diagnoses is presented in Table 13.7.

The risks of complications depend both on patient factors and characteristics of the headaches. A low-risk headache is one that is consistent with the patient's "usual" headaches, which is short-lived (<24 hours) and is unaccompanied by neurological symptoms or neck stiffness. Headaches that require investigation include thunderclap headaches, headaches that last for more than a day, ones associated with neurological symptoms or neck stiffness, and those seen in patients with "red flags" in their history (Table 13.8) [13]. These red flags include patients with risk factors for thrombosis, those who have symptoms of preeclampsia, and those who have other risk factors for strokes [12].

Management consideration

Treatment of PCA is largely supportive and involves the management of hypertension, pain, and anxiety and treatment of acute seizures. Medications used in pregnancy for blood pressure control include hydralazine, methyldopa, labetalol, or nifedipine [14]. Case 3 (early puerperium) received intra-arterial treatment; however, it should be noted that most patients do well with simple observation, and intra-arterial therapies can precipitate reperfusion injury which itself can prove fatal. Hence intra-arterial therapies should be reserved for patients with progressive clinical decline and not simply to treat the imaging appearance of severe vasoconstriction. For pain relief, nonsteroidal anti-inflammatories (NSAIDs) present an acceptable risk. The resolution of vasoconstriction may be monitored by repeat CTA or MRA, or digital subtraction angiography (DSA). In centers where TCDs are available, the technique allows for repeated examination of the cerebral vasculature. Most patients do very well when treated in a timely fashion. Of note, the time course of vasoconstriction differs from the time course of headache or resolution of focal neurologic deficits.

Clinical pearl

Peripartum headaches are common and can be benign or clinically significant. A headache out of character for a particular patient, one that persists for more than 24 hours or one associated with focal neurological symptoms, should prompt further neuroimaging in every case. The index of suspicion should be higher if the patient has evidence of proteinuria, preeclampsia, or high blood pressure. The treatment of peripartum RCVS should be done in conjunction with obstetricians, especially in the prepartum period.

Mechanically triggered RCVS

Case 4. Postsurgical RCVS

A 51-year-old right-handed woman presented with severe right-sided temporal headaches associated with blurring of the left eye, intermittent left hand weakness, and slurring of speech. The patient had had surgery for a right-sided acoustic neuroma via a translabyrinthine/retrosigmoid approach. Since hospital discharge 2 weeks earlier, the patient had been having recurrent severe headaches (which peaked in seconds) associated with neurological symptoms. All previous episodes had resolved on their own. However, the last episode was still present 24 hours after the onset for which the patient presented to the emergency department. On examination the patient had a left superior homonymous quadrantanopsia and mild left arm drift. She also had dysprosodia, worse for comprehension of emotional content of speech. She had mild proposagnosia for famous faces. She also had decreased acuity of hearing on the right, decreased right corneal reflex, and anesthesia of the external acoustic meatus (Hitzelberger sign). An urgent MRI showed the presence of cytotoxic edema in the right posterior watershed area (Figure 13.4a). MRA showed the presence of multiple intracranial vessel narrowing worse in the anterior circulation and on the right (Figure 13.4b). The patient was treated with calcium channel blockers and magnesium, and had only minimal residual symptoms after rehabilitation. During the 6-month follow-up there was a resolution of the vasoconstriction on the MRA (Figure 13.4c), although the stroke was still visible on the FLAIR imaging.

Discussion

Here we present a case of a patient with postsurgical RCVS. The recovery was fairly good on rehabilitation but likely represented compensatory mechanisms as the FLAIR signal abnormalities persisted in the follow-up period.

Association of RCVS with mechanical etiologies

The risk of vasospasm is increased when abnormal mechanical forces act on cerebral vessels (Table 13.9).

During surgical operations, vasoactive medications and blood products may be administered which increase the risk of vasospasm. In this case the resection of a cerebello-pontine angle schwannoma seems to have triggered RCVS. RCVS is also seen after carotid endarterectomy. Head trauma, cervical artery dissection, and even unruptured aneurysms have been associated with RCVS. Finally intracranial hypotension causing downward forces on the brain, especially in the posterior fossa, may precipitate RCVS [6].

Clinical pearls

Post-craniotomy headache is common due to local wound and skull pain, nerve regeneration, and presence of inflammation. However, the risk of RCVS is also increased during this same period and the presence of rapidly accentuating headache (thunderclap) should prompt more detailed imaging.

Case 5. "Migraine angiitis" (source: Singhal et al. [2])

A woman 46 years of age presented with sudden onset headache associated with blurring of vision and nausea. She had past medical history of migraines but this episode was described by her as the "worst ever" headache of her life. She also had a history of depression and asthma. The patient's medications included sertraline, trazodone, thioridazine, clonazepam, albuterol, and for the previous 48 hours also dextromethorphan-guaifenesin for colds. The patient had normal vitals, clinical examination, CSF examination, and non-contrast CT. On day 5 she had worsening of her headache and visual problems which on further investigation turned out to be due to Balint's syndrome. She also had some dysarthria. The patient had a repeat lumbar puncture (LP) and was re-imaged with MRI which was normal acutely, but the next day showed the presence of a left parieto-occipital ischemic stroke on diffusion-weighted imaging (DWI) (Figure 13.5). Four-vessel catheter cerebral angiogram showed the presence of a left vertebral artery stenosis (70%) and a 5 mm left internal carotid artery aneurysm. Testing for hypercoagulability and a rheumatological screen did not show the presence of any abnormalities. On day 16 the patient had another exacerbation of her headache, as well as a left homonymous hemianopsia, and a repeat DWI showed the presence of additional infarcts. A right frontal lobe biopsy did not

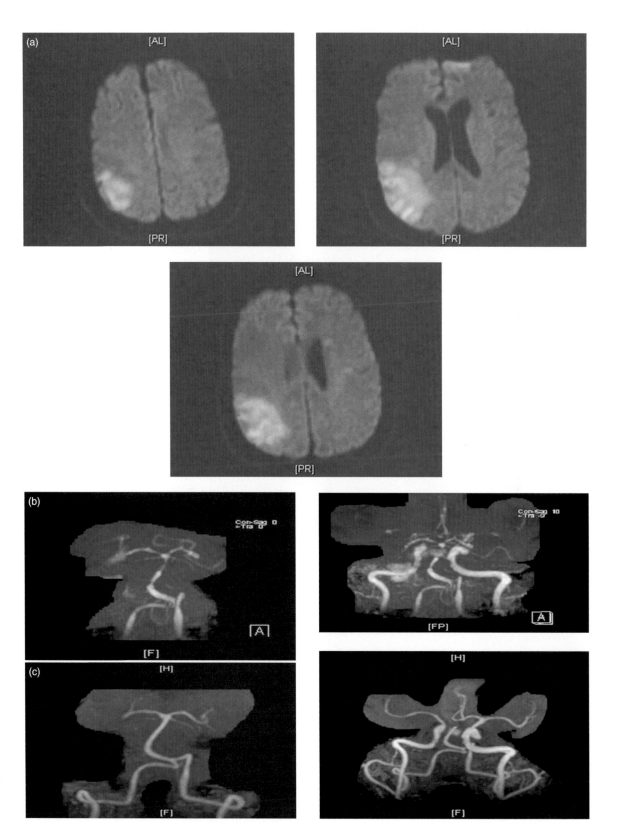

Figure 13.4 (a) Diffusion-weighted images showing an infarct in the territory of the right middle cerebral artery. (b) Initial MRA showing multiple segments of vasoconstriction. (c) Resolution of the vasospasm documented by MRA.

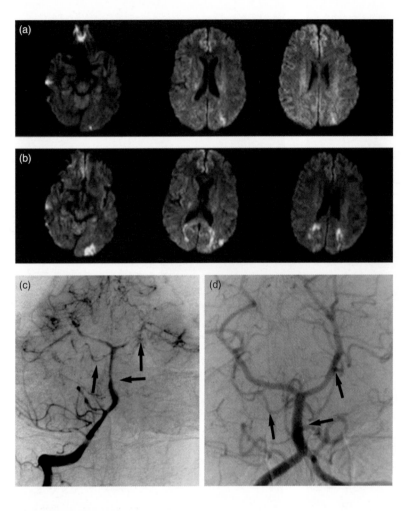

Figure 13.5 (a) Set of diffusion-weighted images scanned on day 2 showing infarcts in the occipito-parietal area on the left. (b) Bilateral occipito-parietal infarcts demonstrated on diffusion-weighted imaging on day 16. (c) Initial angiogram showing multiple areas of arterial narrowing in the posterior circulation. (d) Angiogram demonstrating the resolution of reversible arterial narrowing. (Source: Singhal AB et al. Cerebral vasoconstriction and stroke after use of serotonergic drugs. *Neurology* 2002;58:130–3.)

Table 13.9 Mechanical causes of RCVS

Head trauma
Open neurosurgical procedures
Post carotid endarterectomy
Cervical artery dissections
Unruptured intracranial aneurysm
Intracranial hypotension

show vasculitis. RCVS was diagnosed and the patient was taken off sertraline and the cold medications. The symptoms improved over the following week and the basilar artery peak systolic velocities began to normalize in the subsequent 3 months.

Discussion

In this case we present a young woman who has a history of migraine and a combination of serotonergic medications, who presented with new onset thunderclap headaches. Both migraine and serotonergic medications have been implicated as risk factors for RCVS.

Migraine as a risk factor for RCVS

Migraine is an important risk factor for RCVS as are anti-migraine medications. The patient with a history of migraine and new onset thunderclap headache may present with a history of the worst migraine headache of their life. However, on further questioning the patient reveals that the headache was sudden, reached its peak in less than a minute, and that there was no prodrome or aura. Making the distinction is an extremely important one because the medications used to treat migraine can exacerbate or worsen the symptoms of RCVS and lead to complications. Migraine patients who have a history of RCVS should be discouraged from using vasoconstrictive medications to treat their migraine.

Iatrogenic and endogenous vasoactive agents can trigger RCVS

Vasoactive substances have logically been implicated in the etiology and pathophysiology of RCVS. These vasoactive substances may be endogenous as is the case in pheochromocytoma and other neuroendocrine syndromes, or be exogenous. Table 13.10 presents the common vasoactive substances implicated in RCVS. Hypercalcemia can cause vasoconstriction and this is easy to remember when one notes that calcium channel blockers are used as vasodilators. Blood products and certain immuno-modulators are the third large group of substances that cause vasoconstriction [6].

Clinical pearls

A history of chronic headaches does not preclude the occurrence of RCVS. Special heed needs to be paid to the symptomatology and severity of the headache if out of character for the recurrent headaches.

RCVS or primary angiitis of the CNS?

Case 6. RCVS or PACNS

A 43-year-old woman presented to our neurology clinic for a second opinion. The patient was admitted the previous year to an outside hospital with an acute onset of severe holocephalic headaches and seizures. At that time, the patient had an MRI of the brain which showed patchy FLAIR changes in the posterior and internal watershed zones. The differential diagnosis at that time was between PRES and CNS vasculitis (Figure 13.6a). A catheter cerebral angiogram showed multiple areas of intracranial arterial vessel narrowing (Figure 13.6b). The patient was diagnosed with presumed PACNS as no evidence of systemic vasculitis was present. The index of suspicion was high enough not to motivate a brain biopsy at that time. The patient was then started on high dose prednisone and cyclophosphamide. In the interim, the patient started to have side effects from the medications and developed striking cushingoid features. Our repeat history revealed acute onset of the original headache, which was no longer present. The headaches had continued for a few weeks after the start of the medication but had since abated. She had no further seizures and throughout the course of her disease the patient had no other obvious focal neurologic signs or symptoms. Her background history included migraines as well as asthma, lower back pain, obstructive sleep apnea, and fatty liver disease. She had a 9 pack-years of smoking history but no history of illicit drug use. On examination the patient had a subtle left superior homonymous quadrantanopsia and subtle left appendicular ataxia. Examination was otherwise normal. The patient was now diagnosed as having RCVS. Catheter cerebral angiogram showed resolution of the previously documented multiple cerebral arterial narrowing (Figure 13.6c). The patient was slowly weaned off the prednisone and the cyclophosphamide therapy was discontinued. The patient was seen on follow-up, feeling less depressed and regaining her baseline appearance. She had not had any recurrence of headaches or seizures.

Discussion

PACNS and RCVS

PACNS is a type of vasculitis that affects the small- to medium-sized vessels of the CNS and is not associated with systemic involvement. PACNS is a mimic for RCVS and can present with headaches, strokes, cognitive changes, and seizures. They are both associated with multiple vascular narrowings and infarcts or white matter lesions. In contrast to RCVS, the headache of PACNS is insidious in onset and continuous in its time course. The CSF in RCVS is usually bland. In PACNS, the CSF examination usually shows pleocytosis and raised protein levels. The MR imaging also differs in that the infarcts of PACNS are scattered and widespread (and not necessarily in watershed areas). The segmental narrowings are longer on angiography in RCVS giving the appearance of "sausage on a string," whereas in vasculitis they can be notched (Table 13.11). MRI is very sensitive to the presence of PACNS (90–100%) but not very specific. Angiography has a sensitivity of about 60% (40–90%), and a specificity of 30% for PACNS. Leptomeningeal biopsy, though fairly specific, has a sensitivity of 75% (due to sampling error) and is invasive. Thus, the diagnosis of PACNS is a difficult task. PACNS is confirmed by biopsy and the diagnosis is made when alternative explanations are discounted. When lymphocytic infiltration is seen on biopsy, infectious and malignant causes need to be excluded by staining and immuno-phenotyping. Treatment for PACNS consists of a combination of high dose steroids and cyclophosphamide. Steroids can exacerbate RCVS [15].

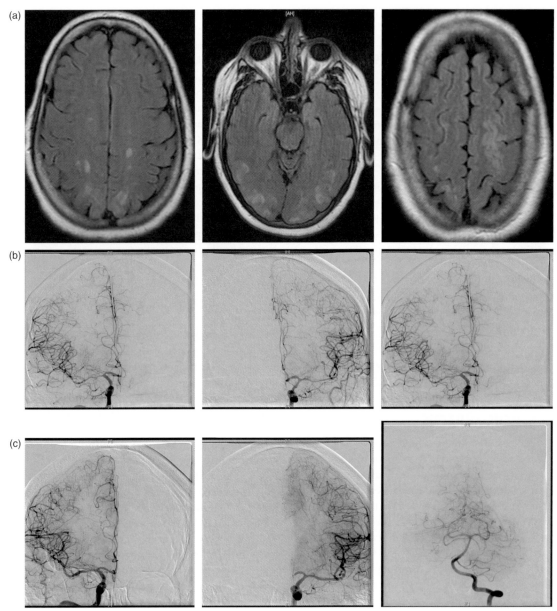

Figure 13.6 (a) FLAIR images show the presence of patchy vasogenic edema in the posterior and internal water shed areas. (b) Catheter cerebral angiogram at the outset shows the presence of multiple areas of narrowing. (c) Repeat catheter angiogram shows the resolution of the intracranial angiographic abnormalities.

Clinical pearl

PACNS is often higher on neurologists' differential diagnoses (for historical reasons) than is warranted by its prevalence. In fact, whenever PACNS is suspected, RCVS is the more likely diagnosis in almost every case.

RCVS or subarachnoid hemorrhage?

Case 7. RCVS or SAH

A 50-year-old woman with a history of rheumatoid arthritis and migraines without aura presented to

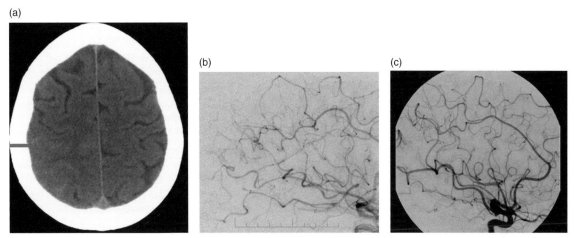

Figure 13.7 (a) A non-contrast head CT shows the presence of blood in the right lateral high convexities. (b) A catheter angiogram at the outset shows the presence of multiple areas of narrowing. (c) The repeat catheter angiogram shows the resolution of the angiographic anomalies.

Table 13.10 RCVS: associated conditions and triggers

- Endogenous
- Pheochromocytoma
- Carcinoid syndrome
- Glomus tumor
- Exogenous
- Phenylpropanolamine
- Pseudoephedrine
- Ephedrine
- Ergotamine tartrate
- Methylergonovine
- Bromocriptine
- Lisuride
- Triptans
- Isometheptene
- Cocaine
- SSRIs
- Methylenedioxymethamphetamine (Ecstasy)
- Amphetamines
- LSD

Blood products and immuno-modulators
- Immuno-modulators
- Tacrolimus
- Cyclophosphamide
- Interferon alpha
- Blood-related products
- Erythropoietin
- IVIG
- RBC transfusions
- Porphyria

Other
- Binge drinking
- Ginseng
- Nicotine patches
- Marijuana
- Hypercalcemia

Table 13.11 Diagnostic criteria for PACNS

- Neurological and psychiatric deficit not explained by other diagnosis
- Presence of either classic angiographic or histological features
- No evidence of other mimics including systemic vasculitis or RCVS

our clinic for a second opinion after being diagnosed with SAH (Figure 13.7a). Several days previously the patient had had a sudden onset of severe headache and had presented to the emergency department of her local hospital. She was initially discharged with no further work-up as the headache was thought to be a recurrence of her migraines. When she returned to the emergency department with similar symptoms she was given analgesics and again sent home. She returned for a third visit with protracted headaches and was admitted to the hospital. MRI scan showed the presence of blood products in the right parietal high convexity. CSF findings were consistent with subarachnoid blood. A CTA showed a suspicious anomaly of the left supra-clinoid left ICA. However, a catheter cerebral angiogram ruled this out and instead showed narrowing of the distal ACA and MCA branches but no evidence of aneurysms Figure 13.7b). She was nevertheless treated with nimodipine. As her headaches improved she was discharged home. She was told by the hospital that she had a "vein rupture at the back of the head." By the time the patient presented to the clinic she was symptom free and had a normal neurologic examination. Follow-up catheter cerebral angiography documented the resolution of the intracranial vasoconstriction (Figure 13.7c).

Discussion

As mentioned previously, the presence of chronic headaches should not distract from a headache which is qualitatively and quantitatively different from the patient's habitual headache. In this case the patient was treated with nimodipine to prevent presumed vasospasm secondary to SAH. It is in fact much more likely that RCVS was the primary event. This is because primary high convexity SAH (traumatic or non-traumatic) has far less probability of being complicated by vasospasm. Conversely, RCVS is commonly complicated by SAH often in the high lateral convexities. In both cases the treatment involves mitigation of vasospasm. Resolution of the vasospasm should be documented before discharge.

References

1. Singhal AB. Cerebral vasoconstriction syndromes. *Top Stroke Rehabil* 2004;11(2):1–6.

2. Singhal, AB, Caviness VS, Begleiter AF, Mark EJ, Rordorf G, Koroshetz WJ. Cerebral vasoconstriction and stroke after use of serotonergic drugs. *Neurology* 2002;58(1):130–3.

3. Calabrese, LH, Dodick DW, Schwedt TJ, Singhal AB. Narrative review: reversible cerebral vasoconstriction syndromes. *Ann Intern Med* 2007;146(1):34–44.

4. Ducros A, Boukobza M, Porcher R, Sarov M, Valade D, Bousser MG. The clinical and radiological spectrum of reversible cerebral vasoconstriction syndrome. A prospective series of 67 patients. *Brain* 2007;130(Pt 12):3091–101.

5. Singhal AB, Hajj-Ali RA, Topcuoglu MA, et al. Reversible cerebral vasoconstriction syndromes: analysis of 139 cases. *Arch Neurol* 2011;68(8):1005–12.

6. Ducros A. Reversible cerebral vasoconstriction syndrome. *Lancet Neurol* 2012;11(10):906–17.

7. Chen SP, Fuh JL, Lirng JF, Chang FC, Wang SJ. Recurrent primary thunderclap headache and benign CNS angiopathy: spectra of the same disorder? *Neurology* 2006;67(12):2164–9.

8. Yeh YC, Fuh JL, Chen SP, Wang SJ. Clinical features, imaging findings and outcomes of headache associated with sexual activity. *Cephalalgia* 2010;30(11):1329–35.

9. Schwedt TJ, Matharu MS Dodick DW. Thunderclap headache. *Lancet Neurol* 2006;5(7):621–31.

10. Grooters GS, Sluzewski M, Tijssen CC. How often is thunderclap headache caused by the reversible cerebral vasoconstriction syndrome? *Headache* 2014;54(4):732–5.

11. Cuvinciuc V, Viguier A, Calviere L, et al. Isolated acute nontraumatic cortical subarachnoid hemorrhage. *AJNR Am J Neuroradiol* 2010;31(8):1355–62.

12. Fugate JE, Wijdicks EF, Parisi JE, et al. Fulminant postpartum cerebral vasoconstriction syndrome. *Arch Neurol* 2012;69(1):111–17.

13. Lim SY, Evangelou N, Jurgens S. Postpartum headache: diagnostic considerations. *Pract Neurol* 2014;14(2):92–9.

14. Too GT, Hill JB. Hypertensive crisis during pregnancy and postpartum period. *Semin Perinatol* 2013;37(4):280–7.

15. Hart LA, Sibai BM. Seizures in pregnancy: epilepsy, eclampsia, and stroke. *Semin Perinatol* 2013;37(4):207–24.

Moyamoya disease and other non-atherosclerotic cerebral vasculopathies

Dominique Hervé, Manoelle Kossorotoff, and Hugues Chabriat

Introduction

Cerebrovascular disorders are usually responsible for stroke events. However, some of them can be responsible for recurrent episodes of headache, focal manifestations occurring only with physical effort, attacks of migraine with aura, or even diffuse cognitive decline in the total absence of focal deficits. Although infrequent, stroke manifestations are also observed in very young patients during childhood. Moyamoya disease and moyamoya syndromes as well as hereditary small vessel disorders are rare conditions that can be responsible for a large spectrum of clinical manifestations at different life periods. They can be also associated with clinical manifestations related to the involvement of other organs outside the brain. Interestingly, the underlying pathophysiology of these conditions is often complex and related to multiple and distinct mechanisms, but most of them remain of undetermined origin.

During the past two decades, genetic markers in combination with the most classic clinical and radiological tools were used to decipher and better understand these rare vascular conditions with the aim of improving their management.

Today, after the initial work-up, the diagnosis of moyamoya disease is easily performed but determining its exact origin and best clinical management remain challenging tasks in daily practice. This is also the case in the presence of small vessel disease easily diagnosed using MRI when obvious causes are excluded. In this chapter, different cases of moyamoya disease or syndromes and rare small vessel disorders have been selected to illustrate the complex clinical spectrum and multiple potential causes of these conditions.

Case 1. Moyamoya disease in adulthood

Case description

A 40-year-old woman born to parents originating from South Korea and without any vascular risk factor was referred to the neurology department for management of recurrent episodes of transient right-sided hemiparesis. Five years previously, she experienced an episode of left-sided hemiparesis of sudden onset with dysarthria. MRI revealed an acute infarct in the right middle cerebral artery (MCA) territory associated with old ischemic lesions in watershed areas (Figure 14.1). Magnetic resonance angiography (MRA) showed occlusion of both MCAs and severe stenosis of the left anterior cerebral artery (ACA) just after their origin. On digital subtraction angiography (DSA), a typical aspect of "moyamoya" vessels was found in the vicinity of the apex of the carotid arteries with leptomeningeal collaterals arising from distal branches of both posterior cerebral arteries (PCAs) (Figure 14.1). The diagnosis of moyamoya disease was then suspected. Conditions known to be associated with moyamoya syndrome were excluded by a general medical examination and several investigations including cerebrospinal fluid (CSF) analysis, hemoglobin electrophoresis, extensive blood clotting, biochemical, and immunologic work-up, ophthalmologic examination, echocardiography, and imaging of the aorta and its branches. Cerebral blood flow was measured using single photon emission tomography (SPECT) with Tc-99m-HMPAO before and after acetazolamide administration. The results showed that the cerebrovascular reserve was preserved. Surgical revascularization was thus not required. Medical treatment including

Common Pitfalls in Cerebrovascular Disease: Case-Based Learning, ed. José Biller and José M. Ferro. Published by Cambridge University Press. © Cambridge University Press 2015.

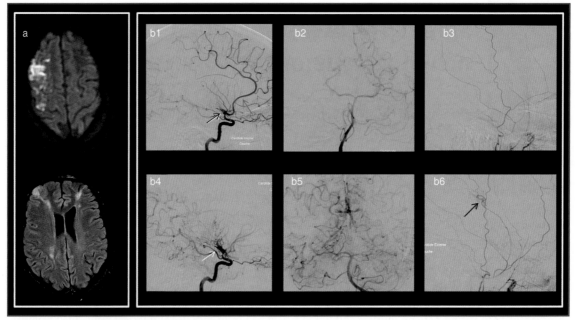

Figure 14.1 (a) Cerebral MRI showing a recent right cortical infarct on diffusion-weighted images (upper image) and old ischemic lesions in watershed areas on FLAIR MRI (bottom image). (b) Initial (b1, b2, b3) and follow-up (b4, b5, b6) digital subtraction angiography showing right ICA on lateral view (b1, b4), cerebral posterior arteries on frontal view (b2, b5), and branches of external arteries (b3, b6). Moyamoya vessels are seen in the vicinity of the carotid artery apex (black arrow, b1 and white arrow, b4). Note the progression of stenosis on the right ACA (blue arrow, b1), the progression of the leptomeningeal anastomosis arising from PCAs, and the appearance of a transdural collateral (red arrow, b6).

aspirin was proposed. During the following 5 years, the patient had no symptoms. Then she presented with several new episodes of transient right hemiparesis always triggered by sustained physical activity such as jogging. No new ischemic or hemorrhagic lesion was detected on MRI but hyperintense vessels were observed on FLAIR images suggestive of low flow in distal branches of MCAs and ACAs. DSA showed stenosis of both terminal ICAs and a significant progression of both ACA stenoses, and an increase of "moyamoya" vessels with several transdural anastomotic vessels in the left hemisphere. A significant decrease of the vascular reserve was detected using Tc-99m-HMPAO and SPECT. A surgical revascularization (encephalo-synangiosis) was then carried out to improve cerebral perfusion. No surgical complication was reported.

Discussion

The medical history of this patient is highly suggestive of moyamoya disease (MMD). All criteria of MMD are present: (a) the location of steno-occlusive lesions that must involve the terminal portions of ICAs or the proximal areas of ACAs or MCAs; (b) the presence of an abnormal vascular network (of so-called "moyamoya" vessels) observed in the vascular territories close to occlusive or stenotic lesions; (c) the intracranial and bilateral aspect of the arteriopathy; and (d) the exclusion of obvious conditions already known to promote appearance of moyamoya vessels and called moyamoya syndromes [1]. The female sex and Asiatic origin of the patient are additional arguments for MMD as the disease is 10 times more frequent in Japan and Korea than in western countries and affects mostly females (sex ratio around 2:1) [2]. Because of its rarity, data concerning the natural history of MMD, particularly in adults, are still limited and were previously reported only from cohorts of small size. The clinical progression of MMD appears variable; development of severe disability can occur rapidly in some cases but the disease can also remain silent over several decades in other cases. The predictive factors of clinical worsening are not well known. In the present case, MMD was revealed by an acute MCA infarct but remained clinically silent during several years after this event. The patient experienced later hemodynamic transient ischemic attacks (TIAs) as often observed during the course of the disease. Transient or permanent ischemic manifestations can be induced by hyperventilation with crying, exertion, or even after induction of anesthesia for a minor surgical procedure. The presumed mechanism is that normal cortical vessels, already maximally dilated with chronic ischemia, may constrict in response to the decrease of carbon dioxide partial pressure resulting in reduced cerebral perfusion [3]. The severity of cerebral hypoperfusion can be evaluated by measuring the cerebrovascular reactivity during CO_2 or acetazolamide administration using SPECT, MR perfusion, or CT perfusion. Decreased perfusion and impaired cerebrovascular reactivity are presumably associated with a higher risk of ischemic manifestations. In the present case, these manifestations were present and led to the decision for revascularization. The efficacy of this type of surgery has not been previously evaluated in a randomized trial. In several reports, the number of ischemic events was found to decrease after revascularization procedures [4–6]. In adults, indications for surgery appear variable between centers and are most often discussed on a case-by-case basis. To evaluate the potential benefit of surgery, the intracranial hemodynamic status has to be evaluated by cerebral perfusion imaging. Detailed analysis of DSA is also needed. In the present case, not only was the vascular reserve impaired despite the development of leptomeningeal and transdural collaterals, but the occurrence of transient ischemic manifestations was also highly suggestive of intracranial hemodynamic failure. In this case, the indirect technique of synangiosis was adopted which consists in using tissues vascularized by the external carotid artery (ECA; spared by the disease) brought into direct contact with hypoperfused cortical areas. Spontaneous development of neovascularization from ECA is supposed to be enhanced by secretion of angiogenic factors from ischemic brain parenchyma. Direct revascularization techniques (such as superficial temporal artery–MCA bypass) are also available for adult patients. When it is successful, the bypass procedure allows a quicker improvement of cerebral hemodynamics. This surgery is, however, associated with a higher risk of hyperperfusion syndrome; the risk can be reduced with specific anesthetic management, which is always needed in MMD to avoid any significant variations in blood pressure and occurrence of hypo- or hypercarbia [7].

Tip

The management of cerebral hemodynamic impairment in moyamoya patients is crucial. In case of ischemic events, the first step is to actively look for triggering factors such as increase of hypotensive drugs, dehydration, or heart failure. The decision of surgery for MMD should follow a multidisciplinary approach for evaluating the spontaneous versus the postoperative risk and be performed by well-trained teams of anesthesiologists and neurosurgeons. For this type of surgery, but also even in the case of minor procedures outside this indication, anesthesia needs particular care to limit the risk of increasing cerebral hypoperfusion.

Case 2. Hereditary moyamoya syndrome

Case description

A 28-year-old man born in Italy with a history of early onset cataract reported repeated episodes of sudden left hemiparesis since the age of 20 years. After the most recent episode, cerebral MRI revealed a recent right-sided cortical MCA infarct and multiple bilateral old subcortical infarcts. DSA showed an occlusion of both ICAs distal to the origin of the ophthalmic artery with a typical aspect of "moyamoya" vessels and leptomeningeal/transdural anastomosis. The posterior cerebral arteries and basilar artery were normal (Figure 14.2). Low dose aspirin was initially recommended. Five years later, the patient had several dyspnea episodes. Echocardiography revealed a severe dilated cardiomyopathy of unknown origin with a significant reduction of the left ventricular ejection fraction (LVEF). Conventional coronary arteriography was normal. From this time, the patient was hospitalized several times for recurrent episodes of heart failure and neurological deficits occurring only when standing and occasionally associated with seizures. Transcranial Doppler suggested hemodynamic impairment on both MCAs. Brain surgical revascularization was declined because of his severe cardiomyopathy. The patient presented with a sudden episode of transient hemiparesis 3 days after his diuretic medication had been increased. Cerebral MRI revealed several new brain infarctions. The patient was 1.50 m tall, had a history of early onset cataract, and had a dysmorphism with bilateral ptosis and long philtrum. Endocrine evaluation revealed partial growth hormone deficiency and hypergonadotropic hypogonadism. Testicular volume was decreased and spermogram showed azoospermia. Information about family history was collected. One

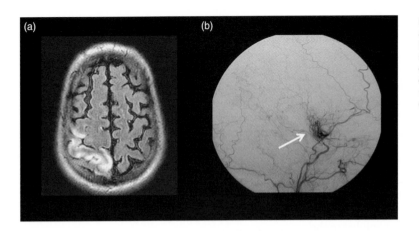

Figure 14.2 (a) Cerebral MRI showing a right cortical infarct on FLAIR MRI. (b) Digital subtraction angiography showing occlusion of the right internal carotid artery distal to the origin of the ophthalmic artery on lateral view with moyamoya vessels in the vicinity of the carotid artery apex.

of his brothers and the son of his sister had a history of stroke during infancy. A Xq28 deletion removing the *BRCC3* and *MTCP1* genes was identified in the patient, his brother, and his nephew.

Discussion

This patient has a moyamoya syndrome related to the loss of *BRCC3* and *MTCP1* genes. Moyamoya syndrome refers to a moyamoya angiopathy associated with other neurological and/or extracranial symptoms, or due to a well-identified acquired or inherited cause. In contrast with MMD, in moyamoya syndrome, the steno-occlusive lesions are not always limited to bifurcations of ICAs. The posterior circulation can be involved and other vascular abnormalities including ectasia, aneurysms, fistula, or mega-dolicho arteries can be observed [8]. In this patient, the characteristics of the intracranial angiopathy are similar to those of MMD. Nevertheless, investigations to identify an acquired condition or an inherited cause of MMS showed several abnormalities. Well-known genetic disorders such as neurofibromatosis type 1, sickle cell disease, or Down syndrome can be easily diagnosed by the presence of café-au-lait macules, sickle cell crisis, or a typical dysmorphism, respectively [9]. But there are several other chromosomal disorders and Mendelian diseases that can lead to a moyamoya syndrome with highly variable penetrance. Questioning about the family history is thus crucial for detecting any abnormality in other affected members and to identify the precise pattern of inheritance. In the present case, all affected individuals were male and related through a maternal lineage which suggested an X-linked pattern of inheritance. Other information may also be crucial such as consanguinity suggestive of an autosomal recessive pattern of inheritance. In this patient, short stature, dysmorphism, dilated cardiomyopathy, azoospermia, and early onset cataract were the main associated features. Investigations must specially include echocardiography, imaging of the aorta and its branches, eye examination, and full body scan. Causative genes have been identified in numerous hereditary moyamoya syndromes. In this family, the disease is caused by an Xq28 deletion that leads to a complete loss of expression of *BRCC3* and *MTCP1* genes [10,11]. *BRCC3* encodes for a member of two protein complexes: a nuclear DNA repair complex and a cytoplasmic complex that might have a role in cardiomyocyte protection. Experimental studies also suggest that *BRCC3* plays an important role in angiogenesis. The exact role of *MTCP1* is undetermined to date. Finally, the pathophysiology of the disease remains unknown. Genetic testing is important to confirm the diagnosis when it is suspected and allows genetic counselling, especially for females at risk of being asymptomatic carriers and transmitters.

Tip

This case points out the importance of obtaining detailed family information in the presence of moyamoya and of assessing all potentially associated clinical manifestations in order to identify a genetic form of moyamoya syndrome. The diagnosis of some moyamoya syndromes can now benefit from genetic testing and allows specific management with multisystemic follow-up and genetic counseling in family members.

Case 3. Pediatric moyamoya disease

Case description

An 11-year-old girl was first investigated after the occurrence of recurrent episodes of severe headache associated with neurological manifestations since the age of 8 years. Each time, she complained of one-sided paresthesia for 1–2 minutes, followed by ipsilateral hemiparesis and facial palsy lasting 3–5 minutes and sometimes associated with speech disturbances. One or two episodes occurred monthly with complete recovery. The patient had normal cognitive development and no school difficulty was reported. The frequency of these episodes progressively increased and repeated episodes of headache also occurred from age of 10 years. Neurological deficits and headache were not associated. The intensity and frequency of headaches dramatically increased within previous few months. Her clinical examination showed only a slight motor deficit of the left hand. The patient had normal cognitive abilities and no difficulty in practicing sports. Brain MRI and angio-MR revealed features suggestive of moyamoya disease with bilateral ICA stenosis associated with MCA occlusion, initial ACA stenosis, and typical "moyamoya" aspects of the basal collateral network. Hyperintensities related to low flow vessels were detected on MRI. In the right watershed posterior region, an old infarction was detected. A single infarction was also observed in the left deep MCA territory (Figure 14.3). The recurrent neurological episodes were considered as possible manifestations of transient ischemia. Bilateral indirect revascularization surgery was proposed based on the frequency of these TIAs, previous occurrence of two cerebral infarctions on MRI, and obvious hypoperfusion on perfusion-weighted MR-sequences. Although the transient neurological manifestations disappeared after surgery, occurrence of headache did not, although their intensity decreased. Cognitive development remained excellent and no further stroke event was observed. Perfusion assessment 3 months after surgery showed a significant improvement compared to the previous examination (Figure 14.4).

Discussion

Moyamoya vasculopathy can present with chronic manifestations in children and is not always responsible for stroke events [12,13]. Recurrent episodes of headache as reported in this case are frequent in children with MMD. Repeated episodes of sensory, motor, and phasic deficits were initially thought to correspond to episodes of migraine with aura although the revised International Headache Society criteria for pediatric migraine with aura were not satisfied in the present case. The patient had transient neurological manifestations without headache. In addition, her neurological examination was abnormal. These findings should have prompted brain imaging much earlier in the present case. In pediatric MMD, stroke can occur without overt clinical manifestations and accurate clinical examination can be particularly helpful for diagnosis. A decision for revascularization surgery should be based on multiparametric aspects [314–16]. The occurrence of (recurrent) ischemic manifestations

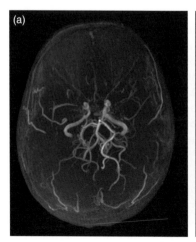
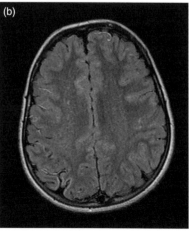

Figure 14.3 (a) 3D time-of-flight angio-MR showing bilateral terminal ICA narrowing, MCA occlusion, proximal ACA stenosis, and typical moyamoya vessels in the collateral network. (b) Fluid attenuation inversion recovery (FLAIR) brain MRI showing a right-hemisphere small old ischemic lesion and multiple bilateral vascular hyperintensities.

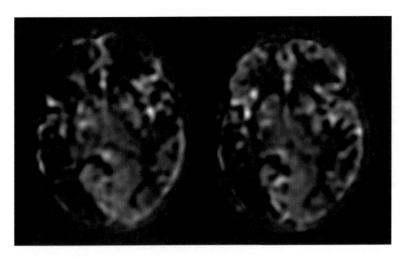

Figure 14.4 Perfusion MRI with arterial spin labeling showing on the right the preoperative assessment with hypoperfused right MCA and ACA and left ACA territories and on the left the postoperative assessment performed 3 months after bilateral multiple burr hole surgery showing perfusion improvement in the right frontal area.

was a strong argument in favor of surgery in the present case as was the presence of old infarcts on MRI. One could object that no actual clinical worsening had been detected over the past 3 years. The recent occurrence of severe episodes of headache was also considered in this case as suggestive of progression of the vasculopathy. Indirect revascularization surgery was considered as the easiest intervention in this patient, who did not present with a rapid progression of the disease that would need an immediate revascularization. Direct artery–artery connection is more difficult with small diameter arteries.

Tip

Pediatric moyamoya may present with recurrent transient ischemic manifestations and headache episodes. Stroke may also occur without obvious clinical manifestations in children. Revascularization surgery may be indicated even in the absence of overt recurrent stroke in the presence of TIAs and silent ischemic lesions on cerebral imaging.

Case 4. Pediatric moyamoya syndrome related to sickle cell disease

Case description

A 5-year-old boy with sickle cell anemia (hemoglobin SS phenotype) presented with abnormal velocities in his annual transcranial Doppler (TCD) evaluation, with time-averaged mean velocity of 221 cm/s for the right MCA, 173 cm/s for the left MCA. His clinical examination and cognitive development were

normal. Brain MRI showed bilateral white matter ischemic lesions in anterior watershed regions and bilateral mild MCA stenosis (Figure 14.5). A monthly transfusion program was started. TCD did not return to normal after repeated transfusions over 6 months (228 cm/s for the right MCA and 234 cm/s for the left MCA) and was not even improved after hydroxycarbamide treatment was added. Four years later, transcranial Doppler velocities dramatically dropped in the right MCA, with no measurable flow. In the left MCA, velocities were still abnormal (208 cm/s). Brain MRI and angio-MR showed right MCA occlusion and a typical moyamoya collateral network (Figure 14.6). No further ischemic lesion was detected. Perfusion assessment showed right hypoperfusion, without major left hypoperfusion. Slight school difficulties were noted and adapted education was needed. The boy had recurrent episodes of headache. Unilateral indirect revascularization surgery was decided on using multicraniostomy. Follow-up showed progressive reperfusion in the right hemisphere. Close follow-up with TCD and angio-MR on the left side showed progressive stenosis of the left ICA and progression towards contralateral moyamoya syndrome. Contralateral surgery is now under consideration.

Discussion

Cerebral vasculopathy associated with sickle cell anemia (SCA) is frequent and occurs mainly during the first decade [17]. Up to 40% of SCA children with hemoglobin SS or Sβ° will have abnormal TCD screening or MRI markers of cerebral vasculopathy,

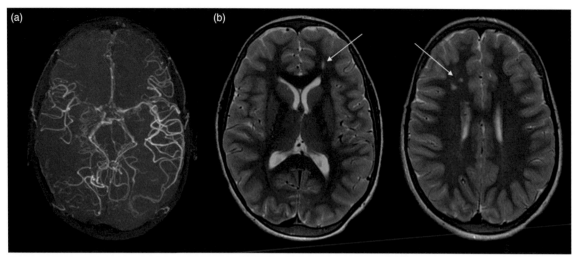

Figure 14.5 Brain MRI and angio-MR at 5 years of age with 3D time-of-flight angio-MR showing bilateral MCA stenosis (a) and T2-weighted images showing bilateral ischemic white matter lesions in the anterior watershed regions (b, arrows).

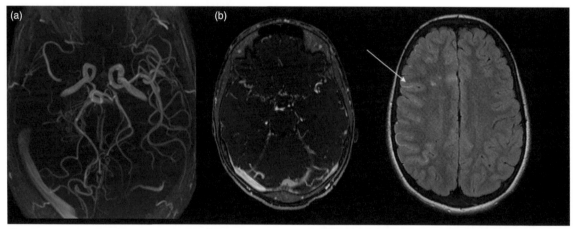

Figure 14.6 Brain MRI and angio-MR at 9 years of age showing (a) right MCA occlusion, moyamoya collateral network and (b) on FLAIR axial images bilateral ischemic white matter lesions in the anterior watershed areas and, as in Figure 14.1, ivy sign or flow hypersignals: arrow.

such as silent infarcts, by the age of 14. Annual TCD screening is recommended from the age of 2 years. Abnormal results (i.e., velocities ≥200 cm/s) lead to chronic transfusion program initiation [18,19]. The chronic reduction of sickle hemoglobin (HbS <30%) dramatically reduces the risk of stroke occurrence. Nevertheless, SCA-associated cerebral vasculopathy is a chronic and progressive condition. In some cases, the transfusion program does not prevent the progression of the cerebral vasculopathy. It is therefore crucial to maintain close clinical and imaging neurological follow-up in children, even under transfusion therapy. This patient had a severe vasculopathy as TCD did not return to normal under transfusion therapy. Hydroxycarbamide, a molecule with promising properties in sickle cell disease and acting by enhancing the fetal protective hemoglobin production, was proposed as it may represent an add-on treatment choice. In this patient, combined transfusion and hydroxycarbamide therapy did not prevent the evolution towards a severe moyamoya syndrome. Although chronic cerebral vasculopathy is frequent in SCA patients, the progression into moyamoya syndrome in well-treated patients is infrequent [20]. Nevertheless, sickle cell disease remains a classical underlying condition that can lead to a moyamoya syndrome. This moyamoya syndrome can initially develop unilaterally and progress later bilaterally. Surgery decision relies on clinical and imaging data used to confirm a typical moyamoya pattern and to assess the clinical, structural, and functional consequences of the vasculopathy (cognitive deterioration, stroke lesions, silent infarcts, and hallmarks of uni- or bilateral hypoperfusion) [18–20]. Even in the absence of overt stroke, revascularization surgery was decided on in this case due to the progression of the vasculopathy, cognitive deterioration, and recurrent headaches despite maximal medical treatment. Usually, indirect revascularization surgery is targeted in territories showing hypoperfusion as hypoperfusion can presumably trigger development of transdural neovascularization through multiple burr holes. A second contralateral surgery may be needed, as in the present case, if contralateral hypoperfusion is further demonstrated.

Tip

The development of a chronic cerebral vasculopathy is frequent in SCA patients. Annual TCD screening is recommended in SCA children from the age of 2 years. Despite maximal medical therapy, including a chronic transfusion program, SCA-associated cerebral vasculopathy may worsen and lead to a severe moyamoya syndrome. Clinical manifestations are identical to those observed in moyamoya disease. Revascularization surgery is considered for SCA children with moyamoya syndrome in the presence of a severe vasculopathy and obvious progression with deleterious consequences at the clinical level.

Case 5. CADASIL in a very old patient

Case description

This 80-year-old man had no vascular risk factors. He had presented at age 60 years with a single episode of scintillating visual scotoma that lasted 30 minutes without headache. Two years later, he had a sudden episode of dysarthria with left-sided numbness of his face lasting 3 days. At age 75 years, he complained of a few memory and attention problems and difficulties with reading or following long movies on television. Although still independent, he was also more apathetic and much less active in daily life according to his wife. His neuropsychological evaluation confirmed the presence of executive dysfunction, decreased performances in attention with increased time at different tests such

as the Trail Making or Wisconsin tests. MRI showed diffuse white matter hyperintensities with symmetrical distribution and large hyperintensities in the centrum semi-ovale predominating in frontal areas as well as in anterior parts of the temporal lobes in contact with the cortex. Thin slices of FLAIR images showed multiple dilated perivascular spaces between the cortex and the white matter in the same areas (Figure 14.7). Complete work-up for ischemic stroke was negative. Electrocardiogram was normal. Magnetic resonance angiography was normal as well as cardiac echography. CSF examination was normal. Genetic testing showed a typical mutation leading to an odd number of cysteine residues in the NOTCH3 gene on chromosome 19 responsible for CADASIL.

Discussion

Cerebral autosomal dominant arteriopathy with subcortical infarcts and leukoencephalopathy (CADASIL), is the most frequent hereditary ischemic small vessel disease of the brain responsible for attacks of migraine with aura, and ischemic stroke and can lead progressively to severe cognitive decline associated with gait and balance difficulties. The disease occurs during mid-adulthood. Disability progresses with aging and most patients present before death with severe neurological deficits and become bedridden. The clinical presentation is, however, extremely variable among affected subjects. In the present case, focal neurological symptoms occurred only after 60 years of age and were transient and benign. At age 80 years, the patient was still independent and presented with typical features of the disease usually observed earlier at age 50–60 years. The cognitive deficit is as reported in subcortical ischemic vascular disorders with prominent executive dysfunction, attention difficulties, and relatively preserved memory. Memory performances, when altered, usually improved with cues as in other subcortical disorders contrasting with memory deficit of hippocampic type detected at the onset of Alzheimer's disease. The lack of any typical infarction on MRI is also of interest in this case and illustrates that focal ischemic lesions can be totally absent in some individuals with CADASIL. Diagnostic confirmation is now easy with genetic testing that should reveal a typical mutation leading to an odd number of cysteine residues in epidermal growth factor (EGF) domains of the NOTCH3 receptor. In difficult cases, skin biopsy with electron microscopy can be used to search for typical accumulation of granular

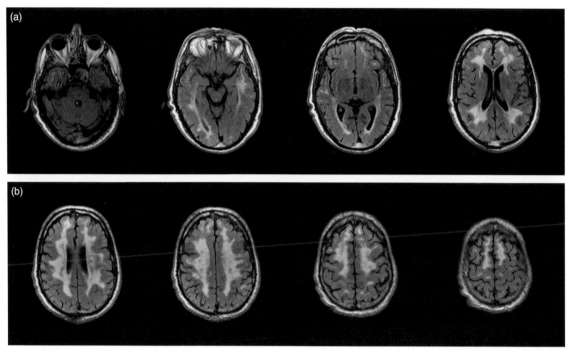

Figure 14.7 FLAIR MRI showing diffuse white matter hyperintensities with characteristic multiple punctiform hypointensities corresponding to dilated perivascular spaces between the cortex and the underlying white matter in the temporal lobes (first image of the upper panel). Note in this 80-year-old patient with preserved cognitive abilities and who was still independent, the lack of any CSF-like infarction and absence of cerebral atrophy in a diffuse small vessel disease.

osmiophilic material (so-called GOM) within the wall of small arteries and capillaries.

Tip

The diagnosis of CADASIL should not be ruled out in old patients in the absence of a typical history of stroke events and with mild neurological symptoms when diffuse white matter hyperintensities are detected on MRI, even in the total absence of lacunar infarction [21,22]. The occurrence of typical migraine with aura is only observed in one-third of patients; aura without headache as reported in this patient is a possible clinical manifestation of the disease [21]. The involvement of temporal lobes at MRI examination with widespread white matter hyperintensities associated with multiple dilated perivascular spaces between the cortex and white matter in the same area is highly suggestive of the disease although inconstant. A positive family history is particularly suggestive, and the diagnosis can be easily confirmed today by genetic testing [23,24]. Skin biopsy with electron microscopy should be used only in difficult or doubtful cases.

Case 6. CADASIL with isolated cognitive complaints

Case description

This 64-year-old patient was initially evaluated because of cognitive complaints. He had been treated for hypertension for the previous 2 years and did not have any other vascular risk factors. He had no history of stroke. This highly educated patient mainly complained of rapid tiring after prolonged cognitive efforts. He had difficulties with reading long texts, which made him fall asleep. The patient complained also about difficulties finding the right word at the appropriate time. However, he was fully autonomous, had paperwork, followed very well his medication, his expenses and fees, prepared meals, and daily used transportation for many activities. The patient was not depressed or anxious but described a loss of desire and that all activities were still possible but with more effort than previously. The cognitive evaluation showed that his global efficiency was preserved, and memory performances were correct with both encoding and storage

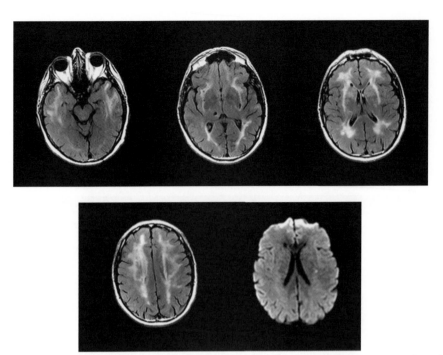

Figure 14.8 MRI in the presence of isolated cognitive complaints in CADASIL. FLAIR MRI showing diffuse white matter hyperintensities with typical involvement of both temporal lobes. Note the presence of an old infarction in the right thalamus and a recent ischemic lesion on diffusion-weighted images in the right white matter.

processes in the normal range. A slowing of speed processing was, however, detected with slight alterations in mental flexibility, ability to concentrate and maintaining selective attention. His capacity for manipulating information in working memory was correct, and recall of teaching and cultural knowledge was perfect. Since he belonged to a large CADASIL family, an MRI was performed showing widespread white matter hyperintensities involving the anterior parts of temporal lobes (Figure 14.8). The diagnosis was confirmed by genetic testing.

Discussion

The presence of hypertension in the presence of diffuse white matter lesions should not be considered as only responsible for ischemic small vessel disease. Hypertension is frequent after 60 years of age and can be associated with other types of small vessel disease. It is present in one-fifth of CADASIL patients. Cognitive complaints can remain totally isolated in ischemic small vessel disease as in the present case [25,26]. They can occur without any stroke event. Cognitive manifestations can vary widely in CADASIL. At onset, cognitive manifestations are moderate, and extensive cognitive testing reveals symptoms related to executive dysfunction [25]. At the early onset, only slowing of cognitive processes is detected, therefore tests involving speed processing are the most sensitive to the earliest subtle cognitive changes. With progression of the disorder, all cognitive domains can be affected, even memory that is preserved initially [25]. Hippocampic memory impairment as detected in Alzheimer's disease with major alterations in encoding, although unusual, can be detected in 20% of CADASIL patients with memory impairment [27]. This is, however, most often observed at the late stage of the disorder after stroke events or in the presence of dementia. Cognitive manifestations are related both to white matter lesions that may be responsible for the earliest neuropsychological symptoms of the disease and to the accumulation of lacunar infarcts and progression of cerebral atrophy over the course of the disease [28,29]. The accumulation of lacunar infarcts and development of atrophy are associated with apathy and dementia in CADASIL, not the extent of white matter hyperintensities [30,31].

Tip

In CADASIL, cognitive manifestations can be totally isolated and can occur quite late in the absence of stroke events. The family history and MRI features should help in the diagnosis of small vessel disease. The degree of cognitive impairment is mostly related to the number of lacunar infarcts and degree of cerebral atrophy. It is not related to the extent of white matter hyperintensities.

Case 7. COL4A1 microangiopathy

Case description

This 37-year-old woman had no cardiovascular risk factors. A detailed familial history indicated no remarkable cerebrovascular or ocular event in her parents and four siblings. She had a long history of bilateral Raynaud's phenomenon since childhood. At the age of 13, she was hospitalized after a traumatic vitreous hemorrhage in the right eye followed by postsurgical retinal detachment and cataract. At the age of 28, an episode of sudden deafness occurred that completely recovered in a few months. The patient had neither cramp nor hematuria. At the age of 35 she had an acute left hemiplegia with headache and vomiting. MRI showed several intracerebral hemorrhages including two large hemorrhagic lesions in the right and left caudate nucleus. On FLAIR and T2-weighted images, there were widespread and symmetrical hyperintensities located predominantly in the periventricular white matter and to a lesser extent in the deep gray nucleus and within the pons. Multiple small hypointense foci suggestive of microbleeds were present on T2*-weighted images. Cerebral angiography revealed two types of abnormalities. First, there were several occlusions of distal branches of the right MCA. Second, there were areas with numerous tortuous abnormal small vessels suggestive of neovascularization (Figure 14.9). When

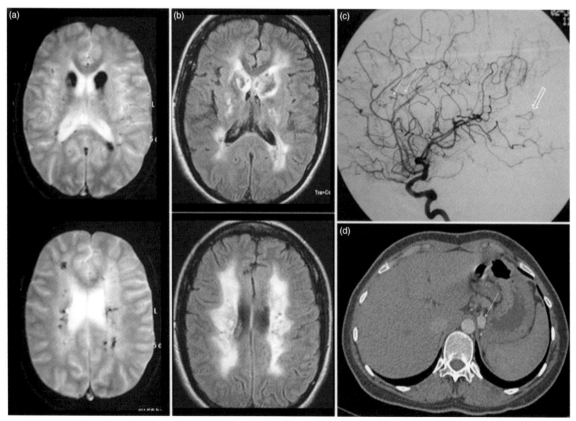

Figure 14.9 Gradient echo MRI showing multiple hypointensities corresponding to macro- and microbleeds in deep brain areas (a) associated with periventricular white matter hyperintensities (b), abnormal vessels on cerebral angiography (c), and an aneurysm of the splenic artery (d) in the presence of a mutation of *COL4A1* gene.

examined at the age of 37, she had a left hemiparesis and a slight impairment in attention and executive functions without other neurological signs. Blood pressure was 104/62 mmHg. Visual acuity was decreased in the left eye. Fundus examination showed a left optic atrophy. Retinal arteries were normal in both eyes. Conventional capillaroscopy revealed a nonspecific microangiopathy with enlarged capillaries, hemorrhages, sludge phenomenon, dystrophy, and microaneurysms. Computed tomographic angiography of the aorta and its branches showed a splenic artery aneurysm (14 mm diameter). There was neither renal failure nor hematuria or proteinuria. Other investigations, including computed tomographic scan of kidneys, cervical and transcranial ultrasound examination, transthoracic echocardiography, ECG, anticardiolipin antibodies, lupus anticoagulant, antinuclear factor, creatine kinase, glucose, and cholesterol blood level, were normal.

Discussion

Multiple manifestations have been associated with mutations in the COL4A1 gene and more recently with those in the COL4A2 gene. Type IV collagens are structural components of the extracellular matrix and play a key role in basement membranes. Half of the heterozygous mutant mice with mutations in the COL4A1 gene developed porencephaly or perinatal intracerebral hemorrhages [32]. Multiple clinical phenotypes have been associated with such mutations in humans: pediatric phenotypes include intracerebral hemorrhage, infantile hemiparesis, and porencephaly. In children as well as in adults, other phenotypes include deep intracerebral hemorrhages, microbleeds, and white matter hyperintensities or more rarely small infarcts with leukoencephalopathy. At the ocular level, multiple abnormalities have been previously reported as associated manifestations such as juvenile or congenital cataract, increased intraocular pressure, optic nerve abnormalities, and/or more severe defects such as the Axenfeld–Rieger anomaly. The disease can also promote the development of intracranial aneurysms at sometimes peculiar locations (carotid siphon), hepatic cysts, muscle cramps, elevated serum creatine kinase, or proteinuria (as observed in the HANAC syndrome). In the present case, large and unexplained hemorrhagic lesions occurred in the brain associated with periventricular white matter hyperintensities and deep microbleeds. Abnormalities were detected

in intracranial medium-sized arteries and in large abdominal arteries. The ocular manifestations are suggestive of the diagnosis with their post-traumatic onset, the early occurrence of cataracts, and postsurgical complications possibly related to the fragility of basement membranes.

Tip

Manifestations related to COL4A1 or COL4A2 gene mutations have not been definitely described [33–37]. Complex features can be observed with one or multiple clinical manifestations; silent or symptomatic lesions, post-traumatic or spontaneous clinical events, and the possible involvement of multiple organs. Not only small vessels (leukoencephalopathy, small or large hemorrhages, small infarcts), large vessels (intracranial or extracranial as in the present case), and the eyes (with multiple types of abnormalities) can be affected but also kidney, muscle, and liver. Sometimes vascular abnormalities can be detected by detailed eye fundus examination (tortuosities, microaneurysms) or with cerebral or aorta angiography. This difficult diagnosis should be raised in the presence of unexplained hemorrhagic cerebral lesions [38]), periventricular white matter lesions after detailed examination of the eyes, and family investigation searching for any history of ocular cataracts, porencephaly [39], infantile hemiparesis, renal or hepatic cysts, and artery aneurysms. Genetic diagnosis is particularly helpful for avoiding high-risk situations and for genetic counseling in parents before pregnancy.

References

1. Guidelines for diagnosis and treatment of moyamoya disease (Spontaneous Occlusion of the Circle of Willis). Neurol Med Chir 2012;52(5):245–66.

2. Ahn IM, Park DH, Hann HJ, Kim KH, Kim HJ, Ahn HS. Incidence, prevalence, and survival of moyamoya disease in Korea: a nationwide, population-based study. Stroke 2014;45(4):1090–5.

3. Scott RM, Smith ER. Moyamoya disease and moyamoya syndrome. N Engl J Med 2009;360(12):1226–37.

4. Kim SK, Cho BK, Phi JH, et al. Pediatric moyamoya disease: an analysis of 410 consecutive cases. Ann Neurol 2010;68(1):92–101.

5. Guzman R., Lee M, Achrol A, et al. Clinical outcome after 450 revascularization procedures for moyamoya disease. Clinical article. J Neurosurg 2009;111(5):927–35.

6. Scott RM, Smith JL, Robertson RL, Madsen JR, Soriano SG, Rockoff MA. Long-term outcome in children with moyamoya syndrome after cranial revascularization by pial synangiosis. *J Neurosurg* 2004;100(2 Suppl Pediatrics):142–9.

7. Pandey P, Steinberg GK. Neurosurgical advances in the treatment of moyamoya disease. *Stroke* 2011;42(11):3304–10.

8. Rosser TL, Vezina G, Packer RJ. Cerebrovascular abnormalities in a population of children with neurofibromatosis type 1. *Neurology* 2005;64(3):553–5.

9. Kuroda S, Houkin K. Moyamoya disease: current concepts and future perspectives. *Lancet Neurol* 2008;7(11):1056–66.

10. Herve D, Touraine P, Verloes A, et al. A hereditary moyamoya syndrome with multisystemic manifestations. *Neurology* 2010;75(3):259–64.

11. Miskinyte S, Butler MG, Hervé D, et al. Loss of BRCC3 deubiquitinating enzyme leads to abnormal angiogenesis and is associated with syndromic moyamoya. *Am J Hum Genet* 2011;88(6):718–28.

12. Smith ER, Scott RM. Spontaneous occlusion of the circle of Willis in children: pediatric moyamoya summary with proposed evidence-based practice guidelines. A review. *J Neurosurg Pediatr* 2012;9(4):353–60.

13. Ezura M, Yoshimoto T, Fujiwara S, Takahashi A, Shirane R, Mizoi K. Clinical and angiographic follow-up of childhood-onset moyamoya disease. *Childs Nerv Syst* 1995;11(10):591–4.

14. Scott RM, Smith JL, Robertson RL, Madsen JR, Soriano SG, Rockoff MA. Long-term outcome in children with moyamoya syndrome after cranial revascularization by pial synangiosis. *J Neurosurg* 2004;100(2 Suppl Pediatrics):S142-9.

15. Fung L-WE, Thompson D, Ganesan V. Revascularisation surgery for paediatric moyamoya: a review of the literature. *Childs Nerv Syst* 2005;21(5):358–64.

16. Ng J, Thompson D, Lumley JPS, Saunders DE, Ganesan V. Surgical revascularisation for childhood moyamoya. *Childs Nerv Syst* 2012;28(7):1041–8.

17. Park EK, Lee Y-H, Shim K-W, Choi J-U, Kim D-S. Natural history and progression factors of unilateral moyamoya disease in pediatric patients. *Childs Nerv Syst* 2011;27(8):1281–7.

18. Roach ES, Golomb MR, Adams R, et al. Management of stroke in infants and children: a scientific statement from a Special Writing Group of the American Heart Association Stroke Council and the Council on Cardiovascular Disease in the Young. *Stroke* 2008;39(9):2644–91.

19. Switzer JA, Hess DC, Nichols FT, Adams RJ. Pathophysiology and treatment of stroke in sickle-cell disease: present and future. *Lancet Neurol* 2006;5(6):501–12.

20. Dobson SR, Holden KR, Nietert PJ, et al. Moyamoya syndrome in childhood sickle cell disease: a predictive factor for recurrent cerebrovascular events. *Blood* 2002;99(9):3144–50.

21. Chabriat H, Joutel A, Dichgans M, Tournier-Lasserve E, Bousser MG. CADASIL. *Lancet Neurol* 2009;8(7):643–53.

22. Chabriat H, Levy C, Taillia H, et al. Patterns of MRI lesions in CADASIL. *Neurology* 1998;51(2):452–7.

23. Joutel A, Bousser MG, Biousse V, et al. A gene for familial hemiplegic migraine maps to chromosome 19. *Nat Genet* 1993;5(1):40–5.

24. Joutel A, Vahedi K, Corpechot C, et al. Strong clustering and stereotyped nature of Notch3 mutations in CADASIL patients. *Lancet* 1997;350(9090):1511–15.

25. Buffon F, Porcher R, Hernandez K, et al. Cognitive profile in CADASIL. *J Neurol Neurosurg Psychiatry* 2006;77(2):175–80.

26. Chabriat H, Bousser MG. Neuropsychiatric manifestations in CADASIL. *Dialogues Clin Neurosci* 2007;9(2):199–208.

27. Epelbaum S, Benisty S, Reyes S, et al. Verbal memory impairment in subcortical ischemic vascular disease: a descriptive analysis in CADASIL. *Neurobiol Aging* 2011;32(12):2172–82.

28. Jouvent E, Reyes S, Mangin JF, et al. Apathy is related to cortex morphology in CADASIL. A sulcal-based morphometry study. *Neurology* 2011;76(17):1472–7.

29. Jouvent E, Viswanathan A, Mangin JF, et al. Brain atrophy is related to lacunar lesions and tissue microstructural changes in CADASIL. *Stroke* 2007;38(6):1786–90.

30. Reyes S, Viswanathan A, Godin O, et al. Apathy: a major symptom in CADASIL. *Neurology* 2009;72(10):905–10.

31. Viswanathan A, Godin O, Jouvent E, et al. Impact of MRI markers in subcortical vascular dementia: a multi-modal analysis in CADASIL. *Neurobiol Aging* 2010;31(9):1629–36.

32. Yoneda Y, Haginoya K, Kato M, et al., Phenotypic spectrum of COL4A1 mutations: porencephaly to schizencephaly. *Ann Neurol*, 2013;. 73(1): p. 48–57.

33. Mine M, Tournier-Lasserve E. Intracerebral hemorrhage and COL4A1 mutations, from preterm infants to adult patients. *Ann Neurol* 2009;65(1):1–2.

34. Plaisier E, Chen Z, Gekeler F, et al. Novel COL4A1 mutations associated with HANAC syndrome: a role for

the triple helical CB3[IV] domain. *Am J Med Genet A* 2010;152A(10):2550–5.

35. Plaisier E, Gribouval O, Alamowitch S, et al. COL4A1 mutations and hereditary angiopathy, nephropathy, aneurysms, and muscle cramps. *N Engl J Med* 2007;357(26):2687–95.

36. Sibon I, Coupry I, Menegon P, et al. COL4A1 mutation in Axenfeld-Rieger anomaly with leukoencephalopathy and stroke. *Ann Neurol* 2007;62(2):177–84.

37. Vahedi K, Alamowitch S. Clinical spectrum of type IV collagen (COL4A1) mutations: a novel genetic multisystem disease. *Curr Opin Neurol* 2011;24(1):63–8.

38. Vahedi K, Kubis N, Boukobza M, et al. COL4A1 mutation in a patient with sporadic, recurrent intracerebral hemorrhage. *Stroke* 2007;38(5):1461–4.

39. Weng YC, Sonni A, Labelle-Dumais C, et al. COL4A1 mutations in patients with sporadic late-onset intracerebral hemorrhage. *Ann Neurol* 2012;71(4):470–7.

Chapter 15

Vascular dementia and vascular cognitive impairment

Ana Verdelho

This chapter focuses on the presentation and management of vascular cognitive impairment and dementia. With the aging of the population and improved stroke care, we are facing a growing number of stroke survivors, many of them with cognitive impairment due to vascular disease. Vascular cognitive impairment is a concept that has evolved over the last decades, ranging in severity from mild to major disability. Six cases are presented and discussed, focusing on the different types of presentations of vascular cognitive impairment, including behavioral changes. Unlike other areas in the cerebrovascular field, there is a lack of evidence-based data to guide treatment, so many of the proposals for management are often based on the empirical experience of daily practice.

Case 1. Cognitive impairment after recurrent stroke

Case description

A 78-year-old woman had her first stroke 6 years earlier when she experienced sudden onset of aphasia and right hemiparesis. She was a retired primary school teacher, widowed and living alone. She had a history of hypertension. She was admitted to hospital due to her stroke, was diagnosed with atrial fibrillation, and started on warfarin. She had a fine recovery except for a very mild anomia. She returned home and restarted all her usual activities, and remained very active, participating at a Senior University and fully independent in all activities of daily-living. Three years later she had her second stroke, despite adequate anticoagulation, with sudden onset of walking difficulties, and dysesthesias of her left arm and leg. She was readmitted, and again had a good recovery. At that time, she was switched

from warfarin to a new oral anticoagulant, although she was compliant and the International Normalized Ratio (INR) had been quite stable. After her second stroke she again become fully independent and returned home. Although she needed more time to complete usual tasks, she had no memory complaints and her daughters did not notice any memory difficulties. Until one year ago she was able to organize Christmas at her home, although the house was less ornamented than usual. She continued to cook for all her family but the meals were simpler. She was able to buy presents for her grandchildren without assistance. Then she had influenza and after that her daughters decided to organize Christmas at one of their homes. Since then, the patient seemed unmotivated, had less initiative for usual duties, and requested assistance with shopping. The daughters found out that she had given up Senior University, without an obvious explanation, and they assumed she was depressed. She was brought to hospital because a week earlier she was unable to recall which of the daughters had visited her. Until then, no memory complaints were noted by the daughters. However, she kept her house clean and tidy, she had no apparent difficulties in basic activities, and her grooming and hygiene were unremarkable. She had a Mini-Mental State Examination (MMSE) score of 28 (lost 2 points on temporal orientation). The brain CT (Figure 15.1) showed two cortical strokes (one involving the left frontal lobe, and the other involving the right fronto-parietal region), white matter changes, and several subcortical lesions. This scan was similar to another performed 2 years earlier. A brain MRI was conducted, and did not show any recent lesion on diffusion or different lesions other than those identified in the brain CT. Laboratory evaluation and electroencephalogram (EEG) showed no relevant abnormalities. Neuropsychological evaluation showed

Common Pitfalls in Cerebrovascular Disease: Case-Based Learning, ed. José Biller and José M. Ferro. Published by Cambridge University Press. © Cambridge University Press 2015.

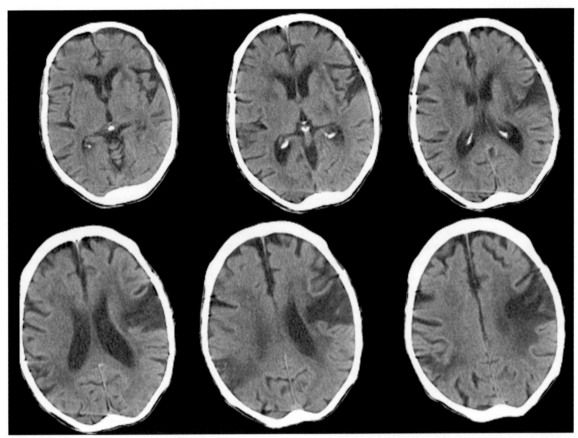

Figure 15.1 Brain CT showing two cortical strokes (left frontal lobe and right parieto-frontal lobe) and several subcortical vascular lesions.

temporal disorientation, deficit of sustained attention, dysexecutive syndrome with relevant slowness, and diminished verbal and motor initiative. She had very mild anomia. Visual and even verbal memory was quite preserved. She had no criteria for depressive episode. During hospitalization she remained quite stable, with no further deterioration. No other misidentification of daughters happened again.

Discussion

This patient had recurrent strokes and imaging evidence of severe vascular brain involvement beyond two clinically evident stroke episodes. She could represent the old concept of "multi-infarct dementia." She had some minor cognitive sequel from each clinical stroke, but progressive cognitive deterioration started a few years after the last clinical stroke. The first question posed by the daughters was "did she have a new stroke?" The clinical picture was not suggestive of a new stroke and brain imaging did not

show new lesions. Laboratory evaluation did not show concomitant metabolic comorbidity that could explain her clinical deterioration observed over the previous months. Slow progression of the picture before hospitalization, stability of the clinical status after admission, and absence of other changes in brain imaging and EEG did not become suspicious of other etiologies (as for instance encephalitis). She did not have a depressive episode to explain the neuropsychological deficits. Furthermore, the neuropsychological deficits were not suggestive of a concomitant degenerative disorder as Alzheimer's disease; instead, they were more compatible with vascular cognitive impairment. Traditional criteria for vascular dementia implicate the following key elements: (1) cognitive impairment enough to implicate functional impairment and loss of autonomy; (2) evidence of cerebrovascular disease; and (3) a relationship between the cognitive deficit and the cerebrovascular disorder [1]. The relationship between cerebrovascular disease and cognitive impairment is usually defined in classical clinical criteria by a temporal relationship, and evolution should be sudden, with stepwise progression. However, vascular cognitive impairment can start slowly and frequently subtle difficulties are not identified in early stages and can be misdiagnosed. After a certain vascular lesion load, the disease becomes progressive (as was the case with our patient), and even without any further vascular lesions, the clinical picture continues to deteriorate. In the past two decades, the concept has progressively evolved and new concepts such as "vascular cognitive impairment" [2–4] and "vascular cognitive disorder" [5,6] have been proposed to include the spectrum of cognitive and behavioral manifestations between mild and severe forms of cognitive involvement. The key aspect is, as in this case, that prevention of further strokes can prevent future damage and delay functional loss. Appropriate management of vascular risk factors, including antiplatelets and anticoagulants, was recently associated with improved protective effect on long-term cognitive outcome among stroke patients [7] in a population-based study. Considering isolated treatment, the best effect was noted after 10 years, using anticoagulants. However, the most impressive effect was from the use of optimal treatment, defined as concomitant treatment: antihypertensive, antiplatelets or anticoagulants, and lipid-lowering agents for ischemic strokes, and antihypertensive agents for hemorrhagic strokes [7].

There is no approved symptomatic treatment for vascular cognitive impairment [8] but there is some evidence of a small benefit using cholinesterase inhibitors and memantine, probably related to the coexistence of Alzheimer's disease pathology [9]. Use of these drugs must be cautious, as relevant side effects have been reported with cholinesterase inhibitors [9,10]. Moreover, in most countries, these drugs are not approved for this indication, thus, limiting their use.

Tip

Recurrent stroke is one of the most important risk factors for cognitive impairment after initial stroke. Even without clear memory complaints, professionals who manage stroke patients should be attentive to identify subtle cognitive difficulties (mainly in recurrent stroke patients) that frequently are mistakenly ascribed to

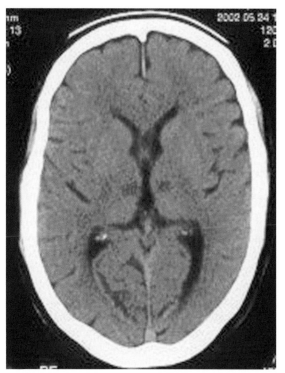

Figure 15.2 Brain CT showing bilateral median thalamic infarcts.

depression. Prevention of further strokes is essential to prevent cognitive impairment.

Case 2. Cognitive impairment after strategic infarct

Case description

A 60-year-old civil engineer, running his own company at the time of admission, and a current smoker, was admitted to hospital with acute onset of somnolence and impaired vertical gaze. CT scan showed acute bilateral median thalamic infarcts (Figure 15.2).

He was hypertensive (unknown until then) and further ancillary evaluation was unremarkable. Initially, disturbed sleep–wake cycles and severe loss of initiative made neuropsychological testing quite difficult. In the following days, the somnolence and vertical gaze palsy improved. Neuropsychological evaluation showed a deficit in sustained attention, slowness, diminished verbal and motor initiative, and disturbed motor control. He also had a severe learning deficit for new facts, and episodic memory was severely impaired. Over the following months his attention and executive deficits improved, but memory was severely impaired with deficit in learning new information, even after repeated presentations of stimuli. Over the following years he continued to show improvement in his executive functions, but learning new facts did not return to normal levels and he was unable to return to work. The picture became stable, and no further deterioration was observed after 5 years of being followed as outpatient.

Discussion

This patient had an acute cognitive deficit, temporally related with the thalamic vascular lesions. The cognitive deficit was not related to the volume of tissue that was damaged, but instead was associated with the strategic location of the lesion [1]. Infarcts involving the paramedian territory of the thalamus can be bilateral due to involvement of the paramedian arteries, as these may arise from a single pedicle with a common origin, the Percheron artery, a single arterial trunk arising from the P1 segment of one of the posterior cerebral arteries. Paramedian thalamic arterial lesions cause the symptoms observed: decreased level of consciousness, vertical gaze palsy, and characteristic cognitive deficits. In the acute stage, loss of self-activation, abulia, and apathy are frequent. Difficulty in learning due to the lack of encoding of new information can be quite severe and persistent without improvement. Frequently, the infarct is due to a cardioembolic source, although no embolic source was identified in our patient. Cognitive rehabilitation can be useful in these patients; although it is usually described that the deficit in learning new facts remains without change, this patient learned how to adapt to daily-life routine. The patient continued to be stable after 5 years of evolution. There are no data to support the use of cholinesterase inhibitors in strategic infarct dementia. Although data from animal studies suggest that memantine could improve motor control [11,12], further studies with better cognitive outcomes are needed.

Tip

Strategic infarct dementia is one of the causes of rapidly progressive dementia and is quite disabling in younger ages, when subjects are usually active. Cognitive rehabilitation may be effective, when done by experienced technicians.

Case 3. Challenging diagnosis of comorbidities in vascular cognitive impairment

Case description

A 76-year-old retired university teacher was admitted to hospital due to severe anorexia with weight loss of >10 kg over 3 months. He had hypertension, diabetes, hypercholesterolemia, and chronic obstructive pulmonary disease. He also had previous recurrent depressive episodes for more than 30 years, and was diagnosed with vascular cognitive impairment 2 years earlier. On admission, he was emaciated and dehydrated, with depressive mood. Whenever he tried to eat, he quickly gave up after attempting to ingest two or three spoonfuls, and refused to continue eating. Prior to his admission to the Dementia Unit, an ear, nose, and throat evaluation excluded structural changes. Electrodiagnostic studies excluded motor neuron involvement. Ancillary laboratory data demonstrated mild anemia and moderate renal insufficiency. No infectious or inflammatory changes were noted.

Discussion

Immediate approach and evolution

On admission we had three major hypotheses: (1) the dysphagia could be accounted for on the basis of cerebrovascular disease, or (2) his anorexia was due to worsening of depression, or (3) he could have a concomitant underlying disease accounting for his anorexia and weight loss. Unlike Alzheimer's disease, several changes in the neurologic examination can be found in patients with vascular cognitive impairment even in the initial stages, such as balance and gait abnormalities, dysphonia and dysphagia, paratonia, urinary incontinence, emotionalism with inappropriate crying and laughing, and presence of primitive reflexes. To further explore the hypothesis that our patient had one of the possible neurologic symptoms in the context of vascular dementia, a multidisciplinary approach was undertaken. Speech therapy and specialist nurse in swallowing evaluation excluded dysphagia as a cause of his inability to be fed, although the patient continued to refuse to eat. A psychiatrist adjusted the pharmacological treatment of his depression. His depression improved and was not considered severe enough to interfere with his

(a) (b) (c)

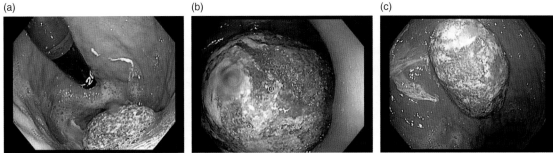

Figure 15.3 Upper gastrointestinal endoscopy showing massive gastric bezoar.

ability to be fed. Investigations for associated comorbidities were conducted simultaneously, and upper gastrointestinal endoscopy showed a massive gastric bezoar (Figure 15.3). Attempts at endoscopic bezoar removal were not successful and open surgery was undertaken.

Discussion of the approach

This patient illustrates several important aspects in the setting of vascular cognitive impairment.

First of all, vascular cognitive impairment is a challenging disorder, as patients often have several comorbidities that potentially influence their health status. Unlike other degenerative dementias, patients with cardiovascular and cerebrovascular diseases may have complex medical disorders and are often receiving several medications that could negatively impact on cognition. Adequate vascular risk factor control is of major importance, but frequently other comorbidities can also influence outcome.

Second, notwithstanding some symptoms can be part of the disease, cognitively impaired subjects deserve systematic investigations searching for treatable causes of deterioration, even if demented. A thorough assessment of comorbidities is recommended in cognitively impaired subjects, either during the initial encounter or throughout the course of the disease [13]. In our patient, a gastrointestinal pathology was the cause, but other diseases should be looked for and adequately approached.

Third, the best approach to a cognitively impaired patient should involve a multidisciplinary team. Although the effectiveness of multidisciplinary teams has not been studied in detail in vascular cognitive impairment, other examples already exist in the dementia field [14]. The objectives of a multidisciplinary team from a Dementia Unit include making an accurate diagnosis, staging the disease, and anticipating possible complications. The Dementia Unit team also

aims to identify medical comorbidities and coordinate and monitor a plan of intervention. The team should include primary care/general physicians, nurses, and specialists in psychiatry, neurology, internal medicine, and rehabilitation medicine. The team should also count on nurses and nurse assistants, neuropsychologists and clinical psychologists, physical, occupational, and speech therapists and social workers.

Tip

Cognitive impairment and dementia should not preclude a thorough investigation and treatment of complications, unless a plan for palliative care has been predetermined. Decisions should be individualized, and optimal control of other complications should be the goal in cognitively impaired subjects.

Case 4. Challenging management in subcortical vascular cognitive impairment

Case description

A 75-year-old retired computer technician, married, living with his spouse was brought for neurology consultation due to multiple falls.

The patient had a previous history of a myocardial infarction 6 years earlier. He also had peripheral arterial disease (PAD), asymptomatic bilateral internal carotid stenosis (<50%), and an unruptured abdominal aortic aneurysm. His father and older brother had died from myocardial infarction. He had been diagnosed with vascular parkinsonism and was on selegiline 5 mg/day.

Of note, in recent years he had abandoned his usual hobbies and his interest in reading had decreased considerably. He had difficulties using the television remote control and video recording. His loss of initiative was disturbing to the family and he was also concerned about his own difficulties.

Neuropsychological evaluation showed a mild executive function deficit (namely in planning and organization), but no memory deficits. He was started on fluvoxamine 50 mg/day, 3 weeks before his first observation at the memory clinic. Since then, the patient had had several falls. In one of these falls he fractured his right hand. At the outpatient clinic, the patient appeared calm, with coherent speech, but was concerned about his multiple falls. On examination he had very mild bilateral hypertonia. He had no cogwheel rigidity. Muscle stretch reflexes were symmetrical. He had no tremor at rest. Cranial nerve function was unremarkable, including vertical gaze movements.

MMSE was 28 (two items lost due to orientation error: day of the month and day of the week). A previous brain CT showed moderate periventricular white matter changes and ventricular enlargement with widening of cortical sulci suggestive of cortical-subcortical atrophy. Electrocardiogram (ECG) showed mild bradycardia (56/min). Carotid ultrasound and transcranial Doppler (TCD) were similar to previously obtained studies. A prolonged 12-lead ECG showed periods of severe bradyarrhythmia that were symptomatic (feeling dizzy), even in the lying position. He was admitted to the coronary care unit with continuous ECG monitoring, and selegiline and fluvoxamine were discontinued. The bradycardia slowly improved and no severe bradyarrhythmia episode was further identified. The patient had no recurrent syncope. However, he became confused and progressively agitated. Haloperidol was initiated, as he insisted on walking around the coronary care unit.

He returned home after 3 days in the coronary unit, and his confusional syndrome continued to worsen, with agitation and severe circadian sleep disruption despite the administration of neuroleptics in high dosages. He was then admitted to the Dementia Unit, with severe agitation and dehydration. On admission, he was agitated and had visual hallucinations and delusions. He drew his visual hallucinations while he was making the drawing of the MMSE (see first and second attempts – Figure 15.4a and b).

Management and discussion

All pharmacological treatments were discontinued except for platelet antiaggregants. Over the first weeks he continued to deteriorate, and he became bedridden. The visual hallucinations increased and his circadian-sleep disruption became worse. Feeding the patient was challenging as he did not cooperate. At this point, we thought he had a different pathology, and proceeded with further investigations, trying to exclude: (1) rapidly progressive dementia due to the continuous and rapid deterioration and (2) Lewy body dementia due to the persistence of hallucinations and cognitive fluctuation. EEG showed diffuse slowing without other relevant changes, namely no periodic sharp-wave complexes or epileptic discharges. MRI (Figure 15.5) showed mild cortical and subcortical atrophy and hyperintensities compatible with small vessel disease on FLAIR imaging. No acute vascular lesions were noted on diffusion-weighted imaging. Due to the ventricular enlargement noticed on MRI (although there was no widening of the cortical sulci), a lumbar puncture was done with withdrawal of a large amount of cerebrospinal fluid (CSF). Opening pressure was normal and CSF biochemical, serological, and cultural tests were negative. The CSF protein 14-3-3 was negative. The dopamine transporter (DAT) SPECT scan showed no reduced tracer uptake (Figure 15.6).

(a)

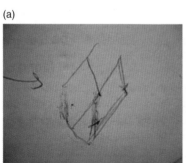

(b)

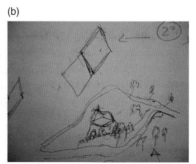

Figure 15.4 The patient's drawing of MMSE figure at admission. The patient tried to copy twice. (a) First attempt; (b) second attempt, when he drew the visual hallucination.

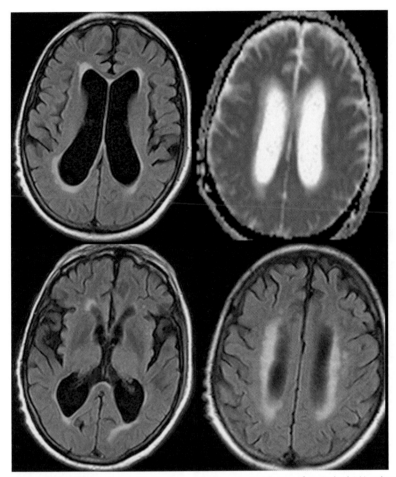

Figure 15.5 MRI showing ventricular enlargement without widening of cortical sulci. No relevant changes in diffusion.

At this point, we admitted that he could have a systemic process, as he had mild hypotension. A follow-up thoracic and aortic CT showed a stable unruptured aneurysm, similar to previous exam 2 years before, and no other relevant changes.

Meanwhile, the multidisciplinary team conducted daily interventions; the speech therapist and specialist nurse in swallowing worked together training swallowing; the physical and occupational therapists stimulated the patient. He also received subcutaneous hydration overnight, and 24-hour nursing care. Mild rigidity was present and levodopa was added in low dosage, after exclusion of other etiologies. No dopaminergic agonists were added. Slowly, after a month he became more cooperative, and feeding became possible. He started to cooperate with physical therapy and he was released after 2 months. A few months later, he had full independent gait but required help with some

complex activities, but overall, he was independent in basic activities. He returned home with his wife, and follow-up re-evaluation 6 months later showed moderate deficits in executive functions (mental flexibility, motor and verbal initiative), and very mild memory deficit (immediate logical memory, recovering to normal level with cueing, no learning deficit). He remained stable in neuropsychological status 2 years and 4 years after and during his last evaluation in 2011 he had an MMSE of 25 (lost 4 points in temporal orientation, 1 in recall). He died in 2012 at the age of 80 years, due to sudden cardiac arrest.

This patient illustrates a prolonged delirium, which was probably caused by the association of drugs (selegiline – a selective MAO-B inhibitor – and fluvoxamine – a selective serotonin reuptake inhibitor) with consequent cardiac bradyarrhythmia in a patient with previous mild cognitive impairment of vascular

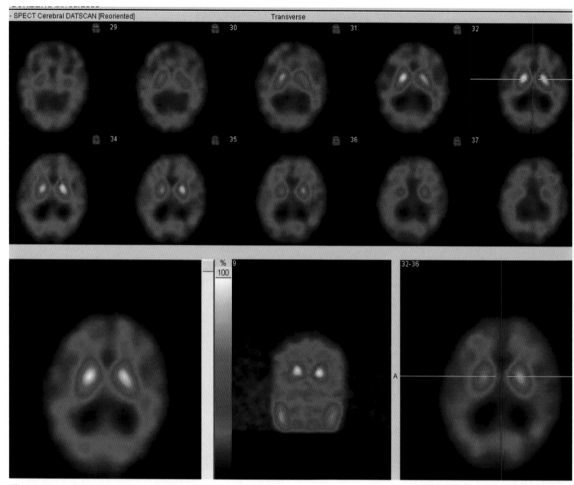

Figure 15.6 DAT-SPECT with normal tracer uptake.

etiology. Delirium is a frequent complication in patients with cognitive impairment, even among those who are slightly impaired. Delirium can reach a prevalence of 89% among hospitalized demented patients [15]. Persistence of delirium over weeks and months after an acute insult has been described, and some evidence suggests that patients with dementia and an increasing number of medical conditions have an increased risk of prolonged delirium [16]. There is suggestive evidence that delirium can partly represent a cholinergic deficit but there is no evidence that cholinesterase inhibitors can reduce the duration of delirium [17].

This patient also illustrates the subcortical type of vascular cognitive impairment [18,19]. Typically, subcortical vascular cognitive impairment is the expression of small vessel disease that is visible in brain imaging through white matter changes, lacunar infarcts, and microbleeds. The clinical picture is characterized by executive dysfunction, slowness and reduced processing speed, usually with some attention deficit, but memory can be preserved until later stages of the disease, so it can be underdiagnosed for years. There is some evidence that the cholinesterase inhibitor donepezil can improve executive function in a form of subcortical vascular dementia (CADASIL), but results must still be replicated [20]. The patient described also had signs that usually appear in cognitive vascular disorder, such as balance and gait abnormalities, usually more symmetrical with pyramidal signs, and less responsive to levodopa. Although vascular parkinsonism has been increasingly recognized, as yet, there are no accepted international criteria for its diagnosis [21].

Tip

A confusional state can be prolonged. Investigation of precipitants must be conducted and prolonged adequate medical support is mandatory. Discontinuation of all medications that can potentially interfere with the central nervous system, mainly those with cholinergic interference, is recommended.

Case 5. Behavioral changes in vascular cognitive impairment

Case description

In March 2010, a 58-year-old married man, a university teacher and previously healthy, was admitted due to a ruptured anterior communicating artery aneurysm. In the acute stage of his subarachnoid hemorrhage (SAH), he developed cerebral ischemia secondary to vasospasm as well as acute hydrocephalus requiring ventricular drainage. A favorable outcome was noticeable after one month in the intensive care unit, with recovery of the level of alertness. At that time he was paretic on the left side, and a severe delirium then emerged. He was admitted to a rehabilitation unit 2 months later, and imaging studies demonstrated asymmetric bifrontal damage, more extensive on the right frontal lobe (Figure 15.7).

On admission, he was disorientated in time and space and appeared disinhibited. Within a few days, he was delirious, and was convinced that the Pope would arrive at the hospital to visit him. He explained to everyone that he came to the hospital by helicopter and that the Pope would come in the same way. At the same time he had sexual disinhibition with the caregivers.

Management and discussion

This case exemplifies how vascular lesions can be associated with severe behavioral changes [22]. Inappropriate sexual behaviors can be very difficult to manage, and pharmacological treatments (including several psychoactive medications even in high dosages) are frequently quite ineffective [23,24]. The patient received paroxetine, with good response. At the same time, the patient was evaluated by the neuropsychologist and a program of rehabilitation was delineated. Cognitive rehabilitation involves individually designed interventions designed according to the recognition of specific deficits and also the behavioral symptoms. Several studies support cognitive rehabilitation [25], but evidence of benefit is still weak and limited to patients following an acute event, due to several methodological limitations [26,27]. Goals must be established in a realistic way, according to available resources for each center and possible interventions. Discussion over time with patients and caregivers is essential to success. Training repetitively under supervision increases the automaticity of strategies, and facilitates independence and efficacy of tasks. Over time, our patient learned how to apply newly acquired skills and he learned strategies in order to replicate daily-life activities. After one year, he fully recovered his autonomy and was able to go out of the house without getting lost. He never repeated his inappropriate sexual behaviors.

However, after 2 years of training, his executive deficits and difficulty in encoding new memories precluded him returning to work and he was forced to quit his job in the university. Then he decided to retire, but became depressed requiring additional psychological and psychiatric support. Antidepressant treatment was adjusted for a few months. After 4 years from the index SAH, he was capable of restructuring his life, and is currently in the second year of a history of art course.

Tip

Cognitive rehabilitation is effective following acute vascular lesions, not only in regard to cognitive recovery, but also for improved behavioral control. Results can be only observed after months or even years of continued training. Similarly to physical rehabilitation, an individualized program has to be drawn up. Adequate strategies can dramatically change outcomes.

Case 6. When Alzheimer and vascular pathology mix

Case description

An 82 -year-old housewife, widowed and living alone for the last 40 years, was evaluated in the outpatient clinic due to memory problems of 5 years duration. The memory complaints were reported by her sons, and were described as slowly progressive, with deficits recalling recent events as well as multiple errors with activities of daily living. She was quite apathetic unless she was contradicted. The patient refused to be assisted at home or to move to an assisted-home facility. The MMSE was 21 on first visit (lost points in orientation, recall, and attention/calculation). Memory deficits did not improve with cueing and the patient did not

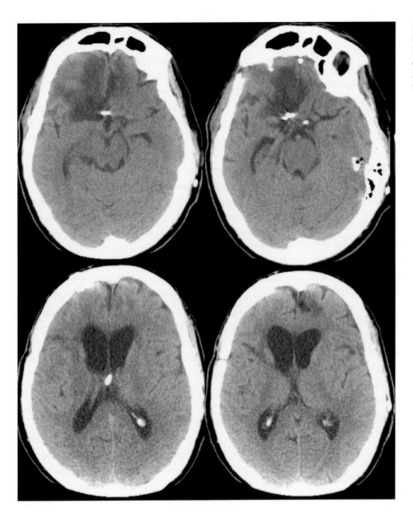

Figure 15.7 Asymmetric frontal lobe lesions 2 months after subarachnoid hemorrhage due to ruptured anterior communicating artery aneurysm. Artifacts after aneurysm clipping and shunting surgery can also be seen.

recognize the deficits. Brain CT showed bitemporal atrophy, white matter changes, and two old small vascular lesions. A diagnosis of Alzheimer's disease with vascular component was made. The patient was stabilized with donepezil, and after that became more attentive to usual duties. However, she continued to refuse help. After a few months, the patient deteriorated suddenly, with increased agitation and sleep problems. A urinary infection was diagnosed and she improved following antibiotic therapy. After a few months, she again deteriorated with severe agitation and she ran away from own home one night, and was returned home by the police as she was found wandering at a metro station. A recurrent urinary tract infection was diagnosed and appropriate antimicrobial treatment was made with subsequent improvement. After this episode, she was admitted to a nursing home and was supervised in all activities. Her behavior and cognition progressively stabilized for 6 months. After that, she refused to leave the nursing home and was agitated whenever requested to participate in any outdoor activity. Otherwise, she was very stable if her routines were kept unchanged. In October 2013 she had sudden language disturbances, with anomia and a few paraphasias. She recovered partially after a few days, although she did not recover full normal speech. The sons thought she had another urinary tract infection and did not take her to the emergency room. Urine cultures showed a *Klebsiella* infection, which was again treated with appropriate antimicrobials. An ischemic stroke was suspected, but a CT scan obtained one month after the episode did not show any new lesion compared to previous scans.

Carotid ultrasound showed no relevant changes. ECG showed normal sinus rhythm. She was started

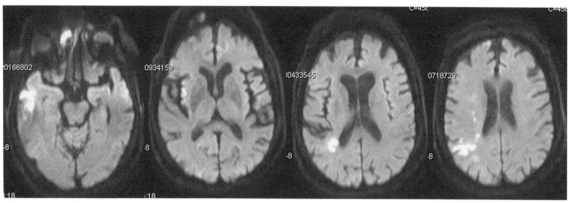

Figure 15.8 Diffusion changes in right frontal, parietal and temporal lobes, both cortical and subcortical, (MCA but also ACA/MCA and PCA/MCA watershed territory involvement).

on clopidogrel and speech therapy and recovered quite well.

Then, 5 months later, she had a sudden episode of left hemiparesis and dysarthria. MRI showed recent ischemic changes (Figure 15.8).

Paroxysmal atrial fibrillation was suspected. A 24-hour electrocardiogram (ECG) monitor was planned, but the patient was agitated and her sons decided she should return home. She left the hospital before completion of the 24-hour ECG. At that time, she received dual antiplatelet treatment, with clopidogrel and aspirin. She started physiotherapy, continued with speech therapy, and again she recovered quite well. However, her apathy was more prominent as compared to the previous evaluation. She was independent with daily-living basic activities.

Two months later, she was admitted with sudden onset of global aphasia, gaze deviation to the left, and right hemiplegia.

CT scan showed an acute infarct of the left middle cerebral artery (MCA) territory (Figure 15.9).

ECG showed atrial fibrillation with rapid ventricular response, with prompt control with amiodarone. She also had aspiration pneumonia, which evolved well and one month later the patient was alert, spontaneously opening her eyes, but unable to communicate, even with non-verbal means. She was transferred to a rehabilitation care home, but no improvement in speech was noticed after 3 months and no spontaneous movement was achieved in the paretic limbs. She was finally transferred to a palliative care home.

Discussion

This case illustrates the fact that Alzheimer's and vascular disease frequently coexist, mainly among older patients. Vascular events usually accelerate the course of a degenerative disease, and the treatment of vascular events and decision about how aggressive treatments should be in demented subjects is never easy. The first principle is that dementia should not preclude investigation of a vascular event, and accurate diagnosis is desirable. The second principle is that secondary prevention should always be considered, and the adequacy of the type of prevention must take into account the environment, condition of the patient, and benefit–risks ratio. In our patient we were unable to prove that she had atrial fibrillation although it was highly suspected. Even though dual antiplatelet therapy was started, a new stroke occurred, with a bad outcome, rendering the patient fully dependent.

Because patients with severe leukoaraiosis are at higher risk of parenchymal hemorrhage, decisions regarding anticoagulation are never easy in older patients, mainly when demented and with risk of falls increased.

Tip

Cerebrovascular and Alzheimer pathology coexist and vascular events must be suspected in the presence of sudden focal signs. Treatment decisions must always be individualized.

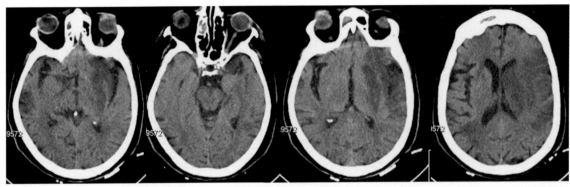

Figure 15.9 Left MCA acute stroke; old right parietal and temporal ischemic lesions can be seen.

Final considerations

Vascular cognitive impairment is a complex disease, highly heterogeneous in etiology and in the spectrum of manifestations. Identification and management requires expertise and training, and although evidence for pharmacological treatments is as yet weak, other non-pharmacological measures and a multidisciplinary approach can be quite effective.

References

1. Román GC, Tatemichi TK, Erkinjuntti T, Cummings JL, Masdeu JC, Garcia JH, Amaducci L, Orgogozo JM, Brun A, Hofman A, et al. Vascular dementia: diagnostic criteria for research studies. Report of the NINDS-AIREN International Workshop. *Neurology* 1993;43:250–60.

2. Bowler JV, Hachinski V. The concept of vascular cognitive impairment. In: Erkinjuntti T, Gauthier S, eds. *Vascular Cognitive Impairment*. London: Dunitz; 2002:9–25.

3. Bowler JV, Hachinski V. Vascular cognitive impairment – a new concept. In: Bowler JV, Hachinski V, eds. *Vascular Cognitive Impairment. Preventable Dementia*. Oxford: Oxford University Press; 2002:321–37.

4. Hachinski V, Iadecola C, Petersen RC, Breteler MM, Nyenhuis DL, Black SE, Powers WJ, DeCarli C, Merino JG, Kalaria RN, Vinters HV, Holtzman DM, Rosenberg GA, Wallin A, Dichgans M, Marler JR, Leblanc GG. National Institute of Neurological Disorders and Stroke-Canadian Stroke Network vascular cognitive impairment harmonization standards. *Stroke* 2006;37:2220–41.

5. Sachdev P. Is it time to retire the term "dementia"? *J Neuropsychiatry Clin Neurosci* 2000;12:276–9.

6. Sachdev P, Kalaria R, O'Brien J, Skoog I, Alladi S, Black SE, Blacker D, Blazer DG, Chen C, Chui H, Ganguli M, Jellinger K, Jeste DV, Pasquier F, Paulsen J, Prins N, Rockwood K, Roman G, Scheltens P. Alzheimer Diagnostic Criteria for Vascular Cognitive Disorders: a VASCOG statement. *Alzheimer Dis Assoc Disord* 2014;28(3):206–18.

7. Douiri A, McKevitt C, Emmett ES, Rudd AG, Wolfe CD. Long-term effects of secondary prevention on cognitive function in stroke patients. *Circulation* 2013;128:1341–8.

8. Dichgans M, Zietemann V. Prevention of vascular cognitive impairment. *Stroke* 2012;43:3137–46.

9. Kavirajan H, Schneider LS. Efficacy and adverse effects of cholinesterase inhibitors and memantine in vascular dementia: a meta-analysis of randomised controlled trials. *Lancet Neurol* 2007;6:782–92.

10. Birks J, McGuinness B, Craig D. Rivastigmine for vascular cognitive impairment. *Cochrane Database Syst Rev* 2013;5:CD004744.

11. Shih AY, Blinder P, Tsai PS, Friedman B, Stanley G, Lyden PD, Kleinfeld D. The smallest stroke: occlusion of one penetrating vessel leads to infarction and a cognitive deficit. *Nat Neurosci* 2013;16:55–63.

12. López-Valdés HE, Clarkson AN, Ao Y, Charles AC, Carmichael ST, Sofroniew MV, Brennan KC. Memantine enhances recovery from stroke. *Stroke* 2014;45:2093–100.

13. Sorbi S, Hort J, Erkinjuntti T, Fladby T, Gainotti G, Gurvit H, Nacmias B, Pasquier F, Popescu BO, Rektorova I, Religa D, Rusina R, Rossor M, Schmidt R, Stefanova E, Warren JD, Scheltens P; EFNS Scientist Panel on Dementia and Cognitive Neurology. EFNS-ENS Guidelines on the diagnosis and management of disorders associated with dementia. *Eur J Neurol* 2012;19:1159–79.

14. Gould N. Guidelines across the health and social care divides: the example of the NICE-SCIE dementia guideline. *Int Rev Psychiatry* 2011;23:365–70.

15. Fick DM, Agostini JV, Inouye SK. Delirium superimposed on dementia: a systematic review. *J Am Geriatr Soc* 2002;50:1723–32.

16. Dasgupta M, Hillier LM. Factors associated with prolonged delirium: a systematic review. *Int Psychogeriatr* 2010;22:373–94.

17. van Eijk MJ, Roes KCB, Honing MLH, et al. Effect of rivastigmine as an adjunct to usual care with haloperidol on duration of delirium and mortality in critically ill patients: a multicentre, double-blind, placebo-controlled randomised trial. *Lancet* 2010; 376:1829–37.

18. Erkinjuntti T, Inzitari D, Pantoni L, Wallin A, Scheltens P, Rockwood K, Roman GC, Chui H, Desmond DW. Research criteria for subcortical vascular dementia in clinical trials. *J Neural Transm Suppl* 2000;59:23–30.

19. Román GC, Erkinjuntti T, Wallin A, et al. Subcortical ischaemic vascular dementia. *Lancet Neurol* 2002;1:426–36.

20. Dichgans M, Markus HS, Salloway S, Verkkoniemi A, Moline M, Wang Q, Posner H, Chabriat HS. Donepezil in patients with subcortical vascular cognitive impairment: a randomised double-blind trial in CADASIL. *Lancet Neurol* 2008;7:310–18.

21. Kalra S, Grosset DG, Benamer HT. Differentiating vascular parkinsonism from idiopathic Parkinson's disease: a systematic review. *Mov Disord* 2010;25:149–56.

22. McKeith I, Cummings J. Behavioural changes and psychological symptoms in dementia disorders. *Lancet Neurol* 2005;4:735–42.

23. Tucker I. Management of inappropriate sexual behaviors in dementia: a literature review. *Int Psychogeriatr* 2010;22:683–92.

24. Ozkan B, Wilkins K, Muralee S, Tampi RR. Pharmacotherapy for inappropriate sexual behaviors in dementia: a systematic review of literature. *Am J Alzheimers Dis Other Demen* 2008;23:344–54.

25. Cicerone KD, Langenbahn DM, Braden C, Malec JF, Kalmar K, Fraas M, Felicetti T, Laatsch L, Harley JP, Bergquist T, Azulay J, Cantor J, Ashman T. Evidence-based cognitive rehabilitation: updated review of the literature from 2003 through 2008. *Arch Phys Med Rehabil* 2011;92:519–30.

26. van Heugten C, Gregório GW, Wade D. Evidence-based cognitive rehabilitation after acquired brain injury: a systematic review of content of treatment. *Neuropsychol Rehabil* 2012;22:653–73.

27. Chung CS, Pollock A, Campbell T, Durward BR, Hagen S. Cognitive rehabilitation for executive dysfunction in adults with stroke or other adult non-progressive acquired brain damage. *Cochrane Database Syst Rev* 2013;4:CD008391.

Chapter 16

Pitfalls in the diagnosis of subarachnoid hemorrhage

Christopher P. Robinson and Sean Ruland

Introduction

Subarachnoid hemorrhage is the most catastrophic form of stroke. Its early recognition and diagnosis are vital. The aim of this chapter is to focus on the many diagnostic dilemmas a physician may encounter in the acute setting of this disease.

Case 1

A 65-year-old man was at home with his wife when he experienced nausea and lightheadedness. En route to the emergency department (ED), the patient screamed "Oh, my head" and acutely became unresponsive. On ED arrival, blood pressure was 198/97 mmHg and heart rate 112 beats per minute. His wife reported a family history of multiple ruptured intracranial aneurysms in first degree family members. He was comatose with Cheyne–Stokes respirations, pinpoint pupils, and a Glasgow Coma Scale (GCS) of 4 (eye = 1, verbal = 1, motor = 2). He was emergently intubated and was subsequently sent for cranial computed tomography (CCT). CCT showed a diffuse, high density collection in the suprasellar cistern extending bilaterally into the Sylvian fissures (Figure 16.1).

Discussion

Subarachnoid hemorrhage (SAH) accounts for only 3% of all strokes and affects nearly 24 000 individuals annually throughout the United States [1]. However, it is the most catastrophic stroke type with a case-fatality rate of 50%. Up to a third of survivors are physically disabled and many more are left with cognitive impairment. The overall incidence reported in most populations is 6–7 per 100 000 person-years and increases with age. The incidence in Japan and

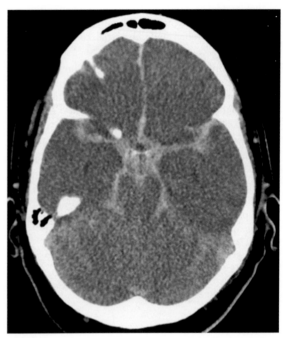

Figure 16.1 Axial cranial computed tomography showing diffuse high density collection in the suprasellar cistern extending bilaterally into the Sylvian fissures consistent with subarachnoid hemorrhage.

Finland is up to 20 per 100 000 person-years [2]. The most common symptom is a sudden and severe (i.e., thunderclap) headache. When a patient presents with a thunderclap headache and impaired consciousness as in the case above, the diagnosis is typically straightforward. However, this is not invariably the case and the headache need not be severe. Other symptoms may predominate (see below). SAH can be traumatic or non-traumatic. Non-traumatic etiologies are subclassified into

Common Pitfalls in Cerebrovascular Disease: Case-Based Learning, ed. José Biller and José M. Ferro. Published by Cambridge University Press. © Cambridge University Press 2015.

Table 16.1 Rare causes of SAH

Inflammatory arteriopathies:

- Primary angiitis of the CNS
- Infectious aneurysm
- Granulomatosis with polyangiitis
- Polyarteritis nodosa
- Churg–Strauss syndrome
- Behçet's disease

Noninflammatory arteriopathies:

- Moyamoya disease
- Intracranial arterial dissection
- Intracranial vascular malformations
- Cerebral amyloid angiopathy
- Reversible cerebral vasoconstriction syndrome

Cerebral venous sinus thrombosis

Spinal cord vascular malformations

Sickle cell disease

CNS tumors

Bleeding diatheses

Drugs:

- Cocaine
- Antiplatelets, anticoagulants, and fibrinolytics

aneurysmal or non-aneurysmal. Approximately 85% of non-traumatic SAHs occur due to ruptured saccular intracranial aneurysms (aSAH). Of the remaining 15%, non-aneurysmal perimesencephalic hemorrhages account for half, with rarer causes in only 5% [3] (Table 16.1, Figures 16.2–16.4).

Intracranial aneurysms develop over time. They are not congenital contrary to previous belief. The best estimate of aneurysm frequency for an average adult without risk factors is 3.2% [4]. Modifiable risk factors such as hypertension, smoking, and excessive alcohol intake more than double the lifetime risk of aneurysm formation. Patients with autosomal dominant polycystic kidney disease (ADPKD) or aortic coarctation are also at increased risk for intracranial aneurysms. The chance of harboring an aneurysm in patients with ADPKD is increased nearly sevenfold [4]. The annual risk of aneurysmal rupture varies, and depends on multiple factors including age, aneurysm size and location, sex, race, and ethnicity [5] (Table 16.2). Individuals with a first degree relative in whom an aneurysm rupture occurred carry a lifetime risk of 2–5% for aSAH [6].

Early recognition and diagnosis of aSAH is imperative to reduce overall mortality and improve functional outcomes. Nearly half of patients die from the initial rupture regardless of intervention and the mortality rate

for those whose aneurysms rebleed prior to obliteration is even higher. Of surviving patients, 25% incur moderate to severe disability and require long term supportive care. Early diagnosis leading to early intervention reduces short term complications including recurrent bleeding and delayed ischemic neurological deficit (Figure 16.5), improving long term outcomes [7].

Despite the current widespread availability of neurodiagnostic technology, initial missed diagnosis is common [8]. The impact of missing an early diagnosis of aSAH can be devastating. In a review of patients with aSAH who initially presented to the ED with a headache and normal neurologic exam (Hunt–Hess grade 1 or 2, Table 16.4), misdiagnosis resulted in a fourfold increase in 12-month mortality and worse functional outcomes amongst survivors [8]. The higher mortality and morbidity associated with delayed diagnosis is primarily due to early aneurysmal rebleeding. The recurrent bleeding frequency amongst patients with aSAH is 6.9–17.3% and is highest within the first few hours. Without treatment, 15% of ruptured intracranial aneurysms rupture again within the first 24 hours; 4% on the first day after initial hemorrhage, and 1–2% over the following 2 weeks [9].

Misdiagnosis of SAH may stem from three recurring and correctable factors: (1) lack of appreciation for the clinical spectrum of presenting signs and symptoms, (2) insufficient knowledge of the limitations of imaging, and (3) difficulty interpreting the results of cerebrospinal fluid (CSF) analysis [10]. Knowledge of these factors will assist the physician in correctly identifying patients with SAH and delivering timely treatment.

Tip

This case is a straightforward presentation of aSAH. Following emergent stabilization of airway, breathing, and circulation, immediate attention should be given to management of elevated intracranial pressure (ICP) and rapid identification and treatment of an intracranial aneurysm if present. Hyperventilation, mannitol, and hypertonic saline can be employed. CSF diversion via an external ventricular drain (EVD) may be necessary as acute obstructive hydrocephalus commonly develops. The patient should receive CT angiography (CTA) or conventional catheter-based cerebral digital subtraction angiography (DSA) to assess for an intracranial aneurysm. The latter may also permit therapeutic aneurysm obliteration with endovascular techniques such as detachable platinum coils when feasible based on aneurysm location and configuration.

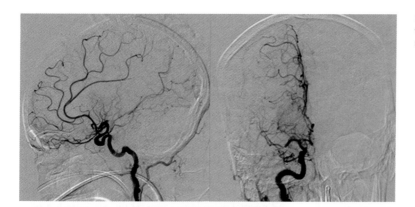

Figure 16.2 Reversible cerebral vasoconstriction syndrome with severe right MCA vasospasm.

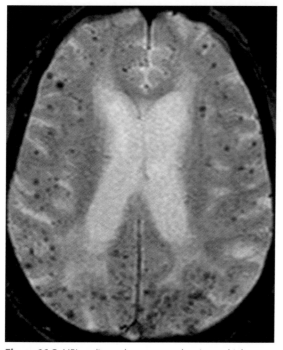

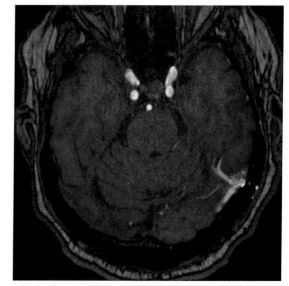

Figure 16.4 MRA of the head following SAH showing a left dural AV fistula. Image courtesy of Michael Star, MD.

Figure 16.3 MRI gradient echo sequence showing multiple microbleeds indicative of cerebral amyloid angiopathy. Image courtesy of Amre Nouh, MD.

Table 16.2 Annual risk of aneurysmal rupture in relation to size and anatomic location [5]

Territory	<7 mm	7–12 mm	13–24 mm	≥25 mm
Anterior circulation (ICA, ACOM, ACA, MCA)	0%	2.6%	14.5%	40%
Posterior circulation (PCOM, basilar, PICA)	2.5%	14.5%	18.4%	50%

ACOM, anterior communicating artery; PCOM, posterior communicating artery; PICA, posterior inferior cerebellar artery.

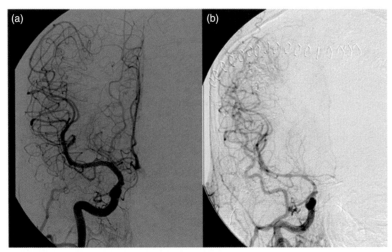

Figure 16.5 (a) Digital subtraction angiography (DSA) post-SAH day 1 following SAH, showing widely patent anterior circulation. (b) DSA post-SAH day 5 showing severe vasospasm of the anterior cerebral artery.

Pitfalls in the diagnosis of SAH in patients with thunderclap headache, negative CCT scans, and atypical presentations

Case 2

A 38-year-old woman presented to the ED with a sudden onset of the "worst headache of my life" that had been unremitting for the past week. She reported mild neck stiffness but no photophobia, nausea, vomiting, recent illness, or history of previous headaches. She had no known family history of intracranial aneurysms. Her neck was supple and funduscopy was unremarkable. She was alert and oriented with no abnormal sensorimotor signs on neurologic examination. CCT was unremarkable.

Discussion

The estimated yearly frequency of ED visits for headache is 3 million, comprising 2.4% of all visits [11]. The majority of patients with headache seen in the ED have primary headache disorders such as migraine or secondary tension-type headaches [12]. The most characteristic symptom of SAH is thunderclap headache, which occurs in nearly 60% of cases. Thunderclap headaches reach their peak within seconds to minutes, are generally diffuse, and may last up to 2 weeks. In addition to aSAH, thunderclap headaches may also stem from other life-threatening neurologic conditions

including meningitis, cerebral venous thrombosis, cervicocerebral artery dissection, pituitary apoplexy, ischemic stroke, colloid cyst of the third ventricle, spontaneous intracranial hypotension, central nervous system vasculitis, and reversible cerebral vasoconstriction syndrome (RCVS). Primary idiopathic thunderclap headache is also possible but requires exclusion of known etiologies. Misdiagnosis of patients that present with thunderclap headache is common and may be due to misinterpretation or misrepresentation of the temporal onset of a primary or secondary headache disorder. In a prospective review, only 10% of patients that presented with sudden headache in general practice were diagnosed with SAH [13]. Clinicians must identify associated red flags so that a prompt clinical diagnosis of a life-threatening etiology can be made. These include sudden onset, age older than 50 years, meningeal signs, altered sensorium, and focal neurologic deficits lasting greater than one hour [14]. Notably, the most important feature of a headache due to SAH is not its presenting severity but rather the suddenness of onset, which is a common misunderstanding.

A sentinel headache in the days to weeks preceding presentation of patients with confirmed SAH has been reported in 1–19% of cases [13,15]. Sentinel headaches are thought to be due to a small rupture and blood leakage, or acute aneurysm expansion. They also have an abrupt onset, although less severe, and should be another red flag for clinicians. The occurrence of a sentinel headache in patients subsequently presenting with aSAH predicts a higher incidence of

Table 16.3 Presenting signs and symptoms of SAH

Thunderclap headache

Sentinel headache

Decreased level of consciousness

Nausea and vomiting

Neck stiffness

Nuchal rigidity

Papilledema

Cranial nerve III palsy

Cranial nerve VI palsy

Anisocoria

Seizure

Terson's syndrome

    Subretinal hemorrhage

    Retinal hemorrhage

    Pre-retinal hemorrhage

    Subhyaloid hemorrhage

Low back or leg pain

Cardiac arrest

early recurrent bleeding, overall mortality, and delayed ischemic neurologic deficit [9].

Although up to two-thirds of all patients with SAH have depressed consciousness on admission, there are a number of other clinical manifestations that have been shown to be associated with SAH that can confound diagnosis [16] (Table 16.3). Acute confusion can be misinterpreted as a psychiatric disorder. Neck stiffness due to meningeal inflammation by blood products is common but not invariable. Patients with SAH can present with seizures, and seizure on presentation concomitant with sudden severe headache is a strong indicator of aneurysmal rupture [17]. Focal neurologic deficits such as cranial nerve palsies and hemiparesis can also occur based on anatomic location and volume of hemorrhage. Terson's syndrome, the presence of associated vitreous hemorrhage, occurs in 13% of patients with SAH [18] (Figure 16.6). Intraocular hemorrhage may also involve the subretinal, retinal, preretinal, or subhyaloid space. Any intraocular hemorrhage in the setting of altered consciousness strongly suggests intracranial hemorrhage with acutely elevated ICP as the cause [19]. Up to 10% of patients with SAH present without headache or focal neurologic deficits. Several aSAH grading systems based on the clinical presentation and CCT findings have been established

to estimate surgical mortality, functional outcome, and vasospasm risk (Table 16.4).

Neuroimaging

Determining a subsequent diagnostic plan for patients with possible SAH and negative CCT scans requires familiarity with the sensitivity and limitations of CCT for detecting SAH. Many tertiary care centers employ third or fourth generation scanners for CCT. With each subsequent generation in development, sensitivity and specificity of CCT for detecting SAH has increased. In the International Cooperative Study of the Timing of Aneurysm Surgery study, the sensitivity of CCT using first and second generation scanners was 92% on the day of aneurysm rupture. It dropped to 86% after only 24 hours and approached 0% at 3 weeks [20]. With more recent technology, sensitivity of CCT for SAH reportedly ranges between 90% and 100%, initially. However, it also diminishes over time [21,22]. The decrease is due to rapid lysis and clearance of red blood cells (RBCs) within the CSF compartment. Thin (3–5 mm) slices are recommended to maximize detection. In alert patients who present within 6 hours of symptom onset, the sensitivity of CCT is as high as 98.5% and decreases thereafter [23]. Therefore, interpretation should be considered based on acquisition time from the ictus. Small volume low-lying SAH in the posterior fossa or above the orbits may also elude detection due to bony artifact from surrounding structures. Magnetic resonance imaging (MRI) has an emerging role in the evaluation of patients with SAH. In the 6 days following SAH, CT and MRI have proven similarly sensitive in the detection of SAH. During the subacute phase (6–30 days) the sensitivity of susceptibility-weighted gradient-recalled echo (GRE) imaging and fluid-attenuated inversion recovery (FLAIR) sequences has been reported to be superior to CT (100% vs. 45%) [24]. Furthermore, MRI may detect other potential etiologies of thunderclap headache that are beyond the resolution capability of CT.

Cerebrospinal fluid analysis

A lumbar puncture (LP) and CSF analysis can be an important diagnostic tool in the evaluation of CT negative patients or those with atypical presentations. Normal CSF is clear and colorless. It has less protein than serum (350 mg/L) and contains no RBCs. Pigment changes that occur within CSF are due to the presence of additional substances, including hemoglobin (red) and

Table 16.4 SAH grading scales

Grade	Hunt and Hess[a]	WFNS scale[b]	Fisher scale[c]
0	Unruptured aneurysm	Unruptured aneurysm	n/a
1	Asymptomatic or mild HA	GCS 15 and no motor deficit	No SAH on CCT
2	Moderate to severe HA, nuchal rigidity, cranial nerve deficit	GCS 13–14 and no motor deficits	Diffuse SAH <1 mm thick, no clot
3	Confusion, lethargy, or mild focal neurologic deficit	GCS 13–14 and motor deficit	Localized clot or layers of blood >1 mm thick
4	Stupor and/or hemiparesis	GCS 7–12 ± motor deficit	IVH and ICH without significant SAH
5	Coma and/or extensor posturing	GCS 3–6 ± motor deficit	n/a

WFNS· World Federation of Neurological Surgeons; IVH, intraventricular hemorrhage; ICH, intracerebral hemorrhage; HA, headache; GCS, Glasgow Coma Scale.

[a] Surgical mortality by Hunt and Hess grade: grade 0–1 = 0–5%, grade 2 = 10%, grade 3 = 10–15%, grade 4 = 60–70%, grade 5 = 70–100%.

[b] Hospital mortality and WFNS grade: grade 0 = 1%, grade 1 = 5%, grade 2 = 9%, grade 3 = 20%, grade 4 = 33%, grade 5 = 76%.

[c] Fisher scale grade 3 carries the highest risk of symptomatic vasospasm of the Fisher grades.

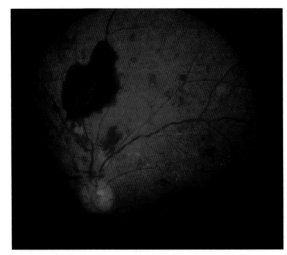

Figure 16.6 Terson's syndrome with subhyaloid and retinal hemorrhages. Image courtesy of Loyola Medical Center Ophthalmology.

bilirubin (yellow). Xanthochromia is a yellow discoloration of the CSF and, when present, is most commonly due to the enzymatic breakdown of hemoglobin. The breakdown process results in the formation of oxyhemoglobin, methemoglobin, and bilirubin. Oxyhemoglobin is released both in vitro and in vivo. However, bilirubin formation requires in-vivo transformation via hemoxygenase (heme to biliverdin) and biliverdin reductase (biliverdin to bilirubin) produced by ependymal cells [25]. Using spectrophotometry, the presence of oxyhemoglobin in CSF is detected rapidly but the formation of bilirubin takes 6–12 hours. This raises the question of whether LP should be delayed when SAH is suspected [25]. There is currently no US guideline addressing this issue. The UK guideline advises waiting 12 hours from symptom onset before performing LP to allow sufficient in-vivo conversion of heme into bilirubin [(26].

Longstanding debate exists as to whether visual inspection or spectrophotometry for CSF fluid pigment analysis is superior. Most hospital laboratories in the US use visual inspection and few possess spectrophotometry. In contrast, spectrophotometry is utilized in nearly all hospitals in the UK [27]. Both techniques involve centrifugation of CSF from the fourth tube collected, followed by examination of the supernatant. Visual inspection compares the CSF supernatant to a tube of water against a white background to assess for xanthochromia (Figure 16.7). Spectrophotometry measures specific amounts of light transmitted at different wavelengths through the CSF and is superior to the photoreceptor cone cells of the human retina for threshold detection and discrimination of pigment wavelengths within the spectral ranges of bilirubin and oxyhemoglobin, particularly at low concentrations.

Several studies comparing spectrophotometry to visual inspection for detection of xanthochromia in the

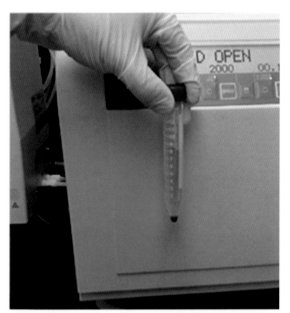

Figure 16.7 Visual inspection of CSF supernatant for detection of xanthochromia. Courtesy of William Ashley Jr., MD, PhD.

Table 16.5 Conditions that may give rise to CSF xanthochromia

Small spinal needles
- Pneumatic tube delivery systems
- Delayed analysis or centrifugation
- Carotenoids
- Compounds containing bromide
- Elevated CSF protein >150 mg/dL
- Hyperbilirubinemia
- Other sources of a bleed in the neuraxis (i.e., hemosiderosis)
- Rifampin
- Tissue necrosis within the CSF
- Meningeal melanomatosis

CSF of patients diagnosed with SAH have been reported. A review of CSF samples obtained at a neurological hospital in London from 1996 to 2004 revealed that nearly 80% of samples containing substantial amounts of bilirubin detected by spectrophotometry were not perceived visually to have xanthochromia [28]. A study using spectrophotometry as a gold standard showed that visual inspection of purposefully lysed RBCs in samples of CSF had a sensitivity of 27% and specificity of 98% [29]. Another study of 111 patients with CT proven SAH concluded that spectrophotometry performed on CSF specimens collected between 12 hours and 2 weeks of SAH is 100% sensitive for xanthochromia [30]. Despite its high sensitivity, the specificity of spectrophotometry has been questioned by some investigators [30,31]. These authors have raised concerns that the false positive results from universal spectrophotometric analysis could unnecessarily increase DSA utilization leading to the discovery of incidental aneurysms and exposure to unnecessary interventions with periprocedural risks [31]. Moreover, there are other causes of CSF xanthochromia, including ex-vivo lysis of CSF RBCs, that may confound CSF interpretation (Table 16.5).

Another common issue is distinguishing a traumatic LP from true SAH when CSF RBCs are present and xanthochromia is absent. This may be particularly problematic when the LP is performed early after symptom onset. The frequency of traumatic taps in standard bedside LPs ranges from 14% to 20%. Some authors have advocated 400×10^6 erythrocytes/L as a cutoff to distinguish a traumatic tap from SAH [21,32]. Others have considered a decrease in RBCs from the first to fourth tube during CSF collection as evidence of procedural trauma. Although this latter approach suggests that at least some of the CSF RBCs are a direct sequela of the LP, it fails to exclude that residual RBCs in the final tube are a result of SAH. Furthermore, intrathecal RBCs introduced by a traumatic tap with inconclusive results can contaminate the pigment analysis on CSF obtained from a repeat LP. Presently, there is no validated standard to confidently determine the etiology of CSF RBCs. However, the presence of erythrophagocytosis in CSF indicates that hemorrhage occurred prior to acquisition.

Tip

The diagnostic dilemmas associated with SAH remain an ongoing debate. CCT is the universal standard as the initial diagnostic test for acute SAH. However, protocol variations exist in the determination of CSF xanthochromia through either visual assessment or spectrophotometry. Despite the lack of consensus, it can be reasonably inferred that properly obtained and interpreted brain imaging followed by LP and CSF analysis when the imaging is non-diagnostic will correctly identify the vast majority of patients with SAH.

With the currently available technology, some general conclusions can be made regarding the work-up of alert patients that present with signs and symptoms suggesting possible SAH:

1. If less than 6 hours from symptom onset and CCT is negative, CSF analysis adds little diagnostic value.

2. If 6–12 hours from symptom onset and CCT is negative, CSF analysis should be performed. However, LP should be delayed 12 hours from symptom onset to allow adequate time for CSF bilirubin formation and xanthochromia detection. An MRI could be performed in the interim and, if an explanatory etiology is identified, LP may not be necessary.

3. If more than 12 hours from symptom onset and CCT is negative, CSF analysis should be performed as soon as possible.

4. MRI may be useful as the initial diagnostic test for patients presenting late.

In the case above, the patient's symptoms are suggestive of SAH but could also be consistent with other etiologies of thunderclap headache. Given her late presentation, the unremarkable CCT does not exclude SAH. CSF analysis is indicated. It would have been reasonable to have performed an MRI with and without gadolinium contrast including GRE and FLAIR sequences and MR angiography (MRA) as the initial imaging modality if rapidly available. This may have identified SAH or an alternate diagnosis and obviated the need for LP.

Pitfalls in the etiologic diagnosis of confirmed SAH

Case 3

A 45-year-old man presented to the ED with a headache. He reported no medical history. Initial evaluation revealed headache and low back pain. During the neurologic examination the patient became comatose and responded only to noxious stimuli with flexor posturing. CCT showed diffuse SAH within the basal cisterns and Sylvian fissures. Obstructive hydrocephalus was present and an external ventricular drainage catheter was placed. A flash of CSF was reported to be "under pressure" upon initial entry into the ventricular system and the patient's responsiveness subsequently improved. He was taken for a repeat CCT after EVD placement and CTA was also performed, which revealed no evidence of intracranial aneurysm. The patient was sent for urgent four-vessel cerebral DSA, which demonstrated a 5 mm left posterior communicating artery aneurysm (Figure 16.8).

Discussion

The prompt and accurate diagnosis of SAH is paramount. However, another critical consideration is the etiology that caused such hemorrhage. The majority of non-traumatic SAH occurs due to ruptured saccular intracranial aneurysms. Using different detection methods, intracranial aneurysms can be found in up to 6% of the general population [7]. Evaluation for intracranial aneurysms can be performed using multiple neurovascular imaging modalities including MRA, CTA, and DSA. Despite improvements in non-invasive techniques, DSA remains the gold standard for diagnosing aneurysms of all sizes. Meta-analyses comparing CTA and MRA to DSA for aneurysms with a diameter greater than 3 mm have been performed. The overall sensitivity and specificity of CTA is reported to be 95% and 96.2%, respectively. Thin slices using 16-detector or greater CT scanners and high flow contrast injections yield the best results. MRA is reported to have a 95% sensitivity and 89% specificity, although it may be lower for ruptured aneurysms when using field strength magnets less than 3 Tesla [33,34]. Moreover, false negatives and false positives have been reported with MRA. These are most commonly seen with aneurysms at the skull base and middle cerebral arteries and may be due to the dynamic nature of flow and local turbulence within the aneurysm, which can adversely affect the signal

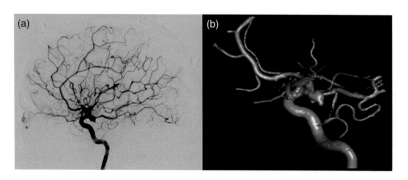

Figure 16.8 (a) DSA showing 5 mm left PCOM aneurysm; (b) DSA reconstruction showing 5 mm left PCOM aneurysm.

required for MRA [33]. Meta-analysis supports 3 mm as a practical cutoff point for aneurysm detection with non-invasive vascular imaging modalities. The sensitivity for aneurysm detection with CTA decreases from 95% to 61% and with MRA from 95% to 38% for aneurysms with diameters less than or equal to 3 mm [35]. It can be generally concluded that at the present time CTA and MRA can be used to detect aneurysms greater than 3 mm, but those smaller in diameter require DSA. This may be more practically applicable to screening for unruptured intracranial aneurysms rather than etiologic assessment of patients with SAH. When small unruptured intracranial aneurysms are identified and followed prospectively, they bleed infrequently. However, many ruptured aneurysms are paradoxically small and may go undetected by non-invasive imaging modalities. DSA offers the added advantages of more detailed assessment of aneurysm geometry and the potential for treatment with endovascular techniques.

Tip

The case illustrates several important diagnostic and management considerations regarding aSAH. First, prompt diagnosis of SAH and immediate management of its acute consequences such as hydrocephalus can be life-saving. Additionally, some ruptured intracranial aneurysms may not be detected by non-invasive neurovascular imaging and DSA is required. Finally, DSA facilitates expeditious endovascular aneurysm obliteration in many cases. Although beyond the scope of this chapter, endovascular aneurysm treatment, when technically feasible, is generally preferred as it has been associated with fewer delayed ischemic neurological deficits due to vasospasm and better functional outcomes compared to craniotomy and microsurgical aneurysm clipping.

Case 4

A 25-year-old woman presented to the ED with a persistent headache and neck pain that began suddenly 24 hours earlier. Her past medical history included migraine and depression. She stated that this headache was nothing like her typical migraines and she was extremely nauseous. Neurologic examination was unremarkable. Prochlorperazine was given on presentation, which provided mild relief of the pain. Given the unique characteristic of the patient's headache, CCT was performed and showed a hyperdense collection surrounding the basis pontis (Figure 16.9). Cerebral DSA was unremarkable.

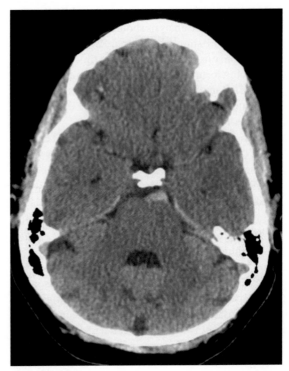

Figure 16.9 CCT showing a hyperdense collection surrounding the basis pontis.

Discussion

Approximately 15% of all patients presenting with SAH have no demonstrable intracranial vascular pathology including aneurysm on DSA. The most common type of angiographically negative SAH is perimesencephalic (pSAH). The typical distribution of pSAH is anterior to the midbrain or pons, with or without extension to the ambient cistern or basal Sylvian fissure. At most, there may be incomplete filling of the anterior interhemispheric fissure and no extension to either lateral Sylvian fissure or intraventricular hemorrhage [36]. Although the imaging pattern of pSAH can suggest aSAH, making this distinction on the basis of CCT findings alone may not be possible. The typical clinical presentation includes thunderclap headache, neck stiffness, and nausea with preservation of consciousness and lack of cranial nerve deficit and sensorimotor signs. Sentinel headache is generally not reported with pSAH. Patients with pSAH are usually classified as Hunt and Hess grades 1 or 2. Vasospasm risk is only 1–5% [37]. The diagnosis is made on the basis of CCT or MRI findings but DSA is indicated to assess for the presence of a posterior circulation aneurysm, which is found in 2–16% of cases [36]. If the initial DSA does not disclose a bleeding source, repeat neurovascular imaging in one week should be considered, as some aneurysms may initially elude detection. Whether or not follow-up imaging should be with DSA or noninvasive neurovascular imaging is debatable and will depend on local technological imaging capabilities and protocols. Assessment for spinal cord vascular malformations (SCVM) should also be considered when the presentation includes neck pain at onset and SAH is present at the level of the foramen magnum. Myelopathic signs and symptoms are not invariably present with SCVM. The etiology of pSAH is unknown but hypothesized to be due to a ruptured ependymal vein. The prognosis is usually favorable even in the presence of delayed cerebral ischemia and good outcomes are reported in 96–100% of cases. Recurrent bleeding is uncommon [36].

Tip

The clinical presentation and imaging findings in the above case are suggestive of pSAH. However, other etiologies must be considered. The presence of neck pain is consistent with pSAH but also raises the possibility of a cervical vertebral arterial dissection extending to the intradural segment where anatomical changes in the structure of vertebral artery wall render it prone to a transmural defect and extravasation of blood. Additionally, the caudal portions of the CCT must be carefully scrutinized for SAH within the cervicomedullary region, raising concern for a spinal vascular malformation. If present, spinal imaging with MRI and DSA in selected cases may be indicated.

Case 5

A 40-year-old healthy man presented to the ED with a 2-day history of severe headache, nausea, and vomiting. He had run a marathon one day prior to symptom onset. In the ED, blood pressure was 100/56 mmHg and pulse 112 beats per minute. Neurologic examination revealed mild lethargy, bilateral papilledema, and diffuse hyperreflexia. Laboratory values were remarkable for an elevated BUN and creatinine. CCT showed a right frontal convexity SAH. Subsequently, MRI and MR venography revealed signal changes consistent with extensive cerebral venous sinus thrombosis (CVST) within the sagittal, transverse, and straight sinuses (Figure 16.10).

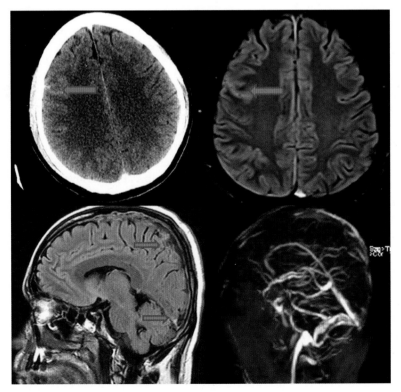

Figure 16.10 Cranial computed tomography (upper left) showing convexity subarachnoid hemorrhage; T2-weighted magnetic resonance imaging (lower left); and magnetic resonance venography (lower right) showing cerebral venous sinus thrombosis.

Discussion

SAH of the convexity (cSAH) is an under-described phenomenon that comprises 5% of all SAH. Etiologies are diverse including trauma, bleeding diathesis due to thrombocytopenia, coagulopathy, or antithrombotic medication, infectious aneurysms, transmural arterial dissection, cerebrovascular malformations, cortical or sinus venous thrombosis, infectious and non-infectious vasculitis, RCVS, cerebral amyloid angiopathy, and posterior reversible encephalopathy syndrome [38]. It is rarely associated with aneurysmal rupture. The characteristic distribution of hemorrhage is within one or more adjacent cortical sulci in the absence of blood at the base of the brain. In a retrospective review of 34 consecutive patients with cSAH, etiology was attributed to RCVS or cerebral amyloid angiopathy in nearly 60% of cases. The latter was more common among those with age greater than 70 years. [39]. The clinical presentation differs from that of aSAH. Only 30% of patients present with thunderclap headache, and only 5% have nuchal rigidity [40]. Seizures (20–58%) and focal neurologic deficits (35–42%) are more commonly reported with cSAH compared to aSAH [40–42]. Neuroimaging evaluation includes both CCT and MRI. CCT is the acute diagnostic imaging modality of choice; however, subacute presentations are common. MRI is recommended if patients present more than 5 days from symptom onset [40]. In addition, MRI can demonstrate many cSAH etiologies. DSA has a limited role but should be considered when MRI is non-diagnostic and there is suspicion for etiologies such as a small vascular malformation, vasculitis, vasculopathy, or infectious aneurysms. CSF analysis should also be considered to support specific diagnoses such as infectious and non-infectious vasculitis. Clinical outcome after cSAH depends on the underlying etiology. Hydrocephalus, cerebral vasospasm, and delayed cerebral ischemia are rare. Overall, outcomes after cSAH are superior to those with aSAH, with 75% of patients returning to their premorbid condition prior to discharge [40].

Tip

The patient in the case above has CVST likely due to dehydration as suggested by his history, exam, and laboratory findings. Given the depressed level of consciousness and signs of elevated ICP, endotracheal intubation should be strongly considered. He should receive hydration with isotonic saline, and hypertonic saline for ICP lowering may be considered depending on his serum sodium level. Until he has been fluid resuscitated, mannitol should be avoided as it may exacerbate his dehydration and thrombosis. Anticoagulation with unfractionated intravenous heparin should be considered as reports suggest that anticoagulation improves outcome even in the presence of hemorrhage although the data is limited. Neither further neurovascular imaging with DSA nor CSF analysis is indicated.

Case 6

A healthy 3-year-old girl with normal development was brought to the hospital after a syncopal episode. The parents reported that the child was standing in the living room when she suddenly screamed in pain while pointing to her back. She abruptly lost consciousness and had urinary incontinence. On arrival at the ED, she was lethargic and hallucinating. She had decreased lower extremity tone and strength, and bilateral Babinski signs were present. CCT showed SAH and blood in the fourth ventricle. Spinal MRI revealed a mass-like structure with multiple flow voids dorsal to the thoracic spinal cord (Figure 16.11). Selective spinal cord angiography demonstrated a left T11 pial arteriovenous fistula. Selective embolization was performed and the child made a full recovery.

Discussion

Non-traumatic spinal subarachnoid hemorrhage (sSAH) is a rare and clinically distinct form of SAH. The most common cause is an SCVM. SCVMs comprise 5–9% of all central nervous system (CNS) malformations and include dural arteriovenous fistula, pial arteriovenous fistula (pAVF), arteriovenous malformation, cavernous malformation, and epidural arteriovenous fistula [43]. Clinical presentations include localized back pain, thunderclap headache, nuchal rigidity, radicular pain, myelopathy, and bowel or bladder dysfunction. In contrast to other spinal cord pathologies that present more indolently, sSAH presents within hours and typically reaches its nadir within a day. SCVMs have a predilection for lower spinal segments. Therefore, most presentations include the lower extremities and spare more rostral function. However, sSAH can extend above the foramen magnum with SAH visible on CCT or brain MRI, making distinction between it and aSAH or other intracranial

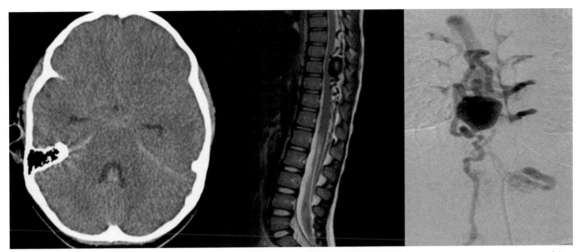

Figure 16.11 Cranial computed tomography (left) showing intraventricular hemorrhage; T2-weighted magnetic resonance imaging of the thoracic spine (center) showing multiple flow voids with varix; and spinal digital subtraction angiography (right) showing pial arteriovenous fistula.

etiologies challenging. SCVMs can also become symptomatic due to ischemia and mass effect. The diagnostic approach includes spinal MRI and MRA and selective DSA of spinal arteries. T2-weighted MRI may display distinct flow voids dorsal or ventral to the spinal cord. A multidisciplinary approach is recommended for diagnosis and treatment, including those with expertise in vascular neurology, neuroradiology, endovascular therapy, microsurgical techniques, and rehabilitation. Prognosis varies and depends on the underlying type of vascular malformation and the surgical technique employed. In general, treatment of the underlying pathology results in a favorable prognosis.

Tip

The case describes a rare occurrence of sSAH from a pAVF. Despite SAH on CCT, the sudden onset of severe back pain with signs of myelopathy predominantly affecting the lower extremities led to rapid spinal imaging with MRI. This revealed the source of bleeding as an SCVM. DSA permitted further characterization of the SCVM as a pAVF and facilitated endovascular treatment. Since arteriovenous fistulae may cause spinal cord edema and signal change on MRI, it is important to distinguish them from inflammatory spinal cord conditions causing transverse myelitis. Corticosteroids are usually given for inflammatory disorders but can exacerbate the neurologic deficits from SCVM.

Pitfalls in the diagnosis of subarachnoid hemorrhage in patients presenting with severe cardiopulmonary dysfunction

Case 7

A 50-year-old man was brought to the ED by paramedics after collapsing at home. His wife stated that he was making noises and shaking uncontrollably at the onset. She reported no significant past medical history, but noted that he had been complaining of a sudden headache 2 weeks earlier. In the ED, he was unresponsive, hypoxemic, and hypotense, requiring endotracheal intubation and resuscitation measures for cardiogenic shock. Chest X-ray showed fulminant pulmonary edema. Diffuse left ventricular hypokinesis with left ventricular ejection fraction of 15% was seen on transthoracic echocardiography. After stabilization with oxygenation and positive end-expiratory pressure with the ventilator, norepinephrine, and milrinone, his neurologic examination revealed GCS of 3 (eye = 1, verbal = 1, motor = 1), anisocoria, and left vitreal hemorrhage. CCT demonstrated diffuse thick subarachnoid blood in the suprasellar cistern, and interhemispheric and Sylvian fissures. Intraventricular clot and obstructive hydrocephalus were also present (Figure 16.12). An EVD was placed and his responsiveness improved.

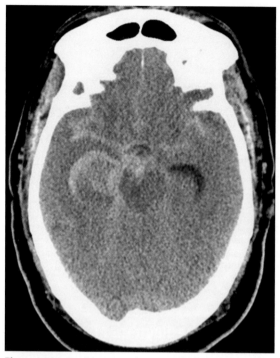

Figure 16.12 Cranial computed tomography showing aneurysmal subarachnoid hemorrhage.

He was able to localize noxious stimulation in all four extremities. A DSA demonstrated a 12 mm posterior communicating artery aneurysm ipsilateral to the larger pupil, which was successfully coiled.

Discussion

Cardiopulmonary abnormalities after aSAH commonly occur and can be life-threatening. ECG changes are most frequently seen. Nearly 67% of patients experience repolarization abnormalities including QT prolongation, T wave inversion, and ST segment changes. Those with ST depression have the poorest outcomes [44]. Serious ventricular and supraventricular arrhythmias can occur. Approximately 10% of patients with aSAH experience acute left ventricular dysfunction, elevated cardiac enzymes, and diffuse T wave abnormalities on ECG [45]. About 3% of patients with SAH will present in cardiac arrest. In contrast to acute myocardial infarction, ventricular wall motion abnormalities after aSAH do not correlate with specific vascular territories. Histologically, there is contraction band necrosis within the distribution of cardiac sympathetic nerve terminals rather than coagulation necrosis typical

of ischemic myocardial infarction. Excessive catecholamine release at these sympathetic terminals is believed to mediate the injury [45]. The left ventricular dysfunction from neurogenic myocardial injury can be severe and is typically out of proportion to the modestly increased cardiac enzymes. The incidence of pulmonary abnormalities varies depending on the definition used. An increased A-a gradient is seen in most patients but frank pulmonary edema occurs in only a minority. Neurogenic pulmonary edema has been proposed; however, distinguishing a neurogenic from a cardiogenic cause is difficult as pulmonary artery catheters are seldom used in the modern era. The precise etiology has little impact on the management. Although hypoxemia and neurogenic myocardial injury are associated with higher grade aSAH and worse outcomes, the ventricular dysfunction usually resolves over several weeks in survivors.

Tip

After successful resuscitation, a thorough neurological history and examination is imperative as neuroimaging is indicated in those with sudden headache, neck stiffness, papilledema, visual disturbances, focal neurologic deficits, or persistently altered sensorium. Up to half of these patients can regain full functional independence with aggressive treatment [46]. In the case described, the patient's presentation could have been attributed to a cardiac arrest from coronary artery disease had close attention not been paid to funduscopy and his neurologic exam findings. These abnormalities prompted CCT and a diagnosis of SAH. Early EVD placement led to rapid improvement in neurologic function. Coil embolization of the aneurysm prevented early mortality from recurrent bleeding. It also facilitates treatment with hypertensive therapy if delayed ischemic deficit from vasospasm subsequently develops.

References

1. Go AS, Mozaffarian D, Roger VL, et al. Heart disease and stroke statistics–2014 update: a report from the American Heart Association. *Circulation* 2014;129:e28.

2. Linn FHH, Rinkel GJ, Algra A, van Gijn J. Incidence of subarachnoid hemorrhage: role of region, year, and rate of computed tomography: a meta-analysis. *Stroke* 1996;27:625–9.

3. Vermeulen, M. Subarachnoid haemorrhage: diagnosis and treatment. *J Neurol* 1996;243:496–501.

4. Vlak MHM, Algra A, Brandenburg R, Rinkel GJ. Prevalence of unruptured intracranial aneurysms, with emphasis on sex, age, comorbidity, country, and time period: a systematic review and meta-analysis. *Lancet Neurol* 2011;10:626–36.

5. Wiebers DO. Unruptured intracranial aneurysms: natural history, clinical outcome, and risks of surgical and endovascular treatment. *Lancet* 2003;362:103–10.

6. Bromberg JE, Rinkel GJ, Algra A, et al. Subarachnoid haemorrhage in first and second degree relatives of patients with subarachnoid haemorrhage. *BMJ* 1995;311:288.

7. Schievink WI. Intracranial aneurysms. *N Engl J Med* 1997;336:28–40.

8. Kowalski RG, Claassen J, Kreiter KT, et al. Initial misdiagnosis and outcome after subarachnoid hemorrhage. *JAMA* 2004;291:866–9.

9. Beck J, Raabe A, Szelenyi A, et al. Sentinel headache and the risk of rebleeding after aneurysmal subarachnoid hemorrhage. *Stroke* 2006;37:2733–7.

10. Edlow JA, Caplan LR. Avoiding pitfalls in the diagnosis of subarachnoid hemorrhage. *N Engl J Med* 2000;342:29–36.

11. Friedman BW, Lipton RB. Headache in the emergency department. *Curr Pain Headache Rep.* 2011;15:302–7.

12. Marks DR, Rapoport AM. Practical evaluation and diagnosis of headache. *Semin Neurol* 1997;17:307–12.

13. Linn FHH, Wijdicks EF, van der Graaf Y, Weerdesteyn-van Vliet FA, Bartelds AI, van Gijn J et al. Prospective study of sentinel headache in aneurysmal subarachnoid haemorrhage. *The Lancet.* 1994;344:590–3.

14. Lipton RB, Bigal ME, Steiner TJ, Silberstein SD, Olesen J. Classification of primary headaches. *Neurology* 2004;63:427–35.

15. Jakobsson K-E, Säveland H, Hillman J, et al. Warning leak and management outcome in aneurysmal subarachnoid hemorrhage. *J Neurosurg* 1996;85:995–9.

16. Brilstra EH, Rinkel GJ, Algra A, van Gijn J. Rebleeding, secondary ischemia, and timing of operation in patients with subarachnoid hemorrhage. *Neurology* 2000;55:1656–60.

17. Linn FHH, Rinkel GJ, Algra A, van Gijn J. Headache characteristics in subarachnoid haemorrhage and benign thunderclap headache. *J Neurol Neurosurg Psychiatry* 1998;65:791–3.

18. McCarron MO, Alberts MJ, and McCarron P. A systematic review of Terson's syndrome: frequency and prognosis after subarachnoid haemorrhage. *J Neurol Neurosurg Psychiatry* 2004;75:491–3.

19. Fahmy JA. Symptoms and signs of intracranial aneurysms with particular reference to retinal haemorrhage. *Acta Ophthalmol* 1972;50:129.

20. Kassell, Neal F, Torner JC, Jane JA, Haley EC Jr., Adams HP et al. The International Cooperative Study on the Timing of Aneurysm Surgery: Part 1: Overall management results. *Journal of Neurosurgery.* 1990;73:18–36.

21. Van der Wee N, Rinkel GJ, Hasan D, van Gijn J. Detection of subarachnoid haemorrhage on early CT: is lumbar puncture still needed after a negative scan?. *J Neurol Neurosurg Psychiatry* 1995;58:357–9.

22. Sames TA, Storrow AB, Finkelstein JA, Magoon MR. Sensitivity of new-generation computed tomography in subarachnoid hemorrhage. *Acad Emerg Med* 1996;3:16–20.

23. Backes D, Rinkel GJ, Kemperman H, Linn FH, Vergouwen MD. Time-dependent test characteristics of head computed tomography in patients suspected of nontraumatic subarachnoid hemorrhage. *Stroke* 2012;43:2115–19.

24. Yuan M-K, Lai PH, Chen JY, et al. Detection of subarachnoid hemorrhage at acute and subacute/chronic stages: comparison of four magnetic resonance imaging pulse sequences and computed tomography. *J Chin Med Assoc* 2005;68:131–7.

25. Roost KT, Pimstone NR, Diamond I, Schmid R. The formation of cerebrospinal fluid xanthochromia after subarachnoid hemorrhage. Enzymatic conversion of hemoglobin to bilirubin by the arachnoids and choroid plexus. *Neurology* 1972;22:973–7.

26. UK National External Quality Assessment Scheme for Immunochemistry Working Group. National guidelines for analysis of cerebrospinal fluid for bilirubin in suspected subarachnoid haemorrhage. *Ann Clin Biochem* 2003;40:481–8.

27. Edlow JA, Bruner KS, Horowitz GL. Xanthochromia: a survey of laboratory methodology and its clinical implications. *Arch Pathol Lab Med* 2002;126:413–15.

28. Petzold A, Keir G, Sharpe LT. Spectrophotometry for xanthochromia. *N Engl J Med* 2004;351:1695–6.

29. Petzold A, Keir G, Sharpe TL. Why human color vision cannot reliably detect cerebrospinal fluid xanthochromia. *Stroke* 2005;36:1295–7.

30. Vermeulen M, Hasan D, Blijenberg BG, Hijdra A, van Gijn J. Xanthochromia after subarachnoid haemorrhage needs no revisitation. *J Neurol Neurosurg Psychiatry* 1989;52:826–8.

31. Perry JJ, Sivilotti ML, Stiell IG, et al. Should spectrophotometry be used to identify xanthochromia in the cerebrospinal fluid of alert patients suspected of having subarachnoid hemorrhage?. *Stroke* 2006;37:2467–72.

32. Shah, Kaushal H, Edlow JA. Distinguishing traumatic lumbar puncture from true subarachnoid hemorrhage. *The Journal of Emergency Medicine*. 2002;23:67–74.

33. Sailer AMH, Wagemans BA, Nelemans PJ, de Graaf R, van Zwam WH. Diagnosing intracranial aneurysms with MR angiography: systematic review and meta-analysis. *Stroke* 2014;45:119–26.

34. Menke J, Larsen J, Kallenberg K. Diagnosing cerebral aneurysms by computed tomographic angiography: meta-analysis. *Ann Neurol* 2011;69:646–54.

35. White PM, Wardlaw JM, Easton V. Can noninvasive imaging accurately depict intracranial aneurysms? A systematic review. *Radiology* 2000;217:361–70.

36. Rinkel GJ, Wijdicks EF, Vermeulen M, et al. Nonaneurysmal perimesencephalic subarachnoid hemorrhage: CT and MR patterns that differ from aneurysmal rupture. *Am J Neuroradiol* 1991;12:829–34.

37. Schwartz TH, Solomon RA. Perimesencephalic nonaneurysmal subarachnoid hemorrhage: review of the literature. *Neurosurgery* 1996;39:433–40.

38. Rinkel GJ, Van Gijn J, Wijdicks EF. Subarachnoid hemorrhage without detectable aneurysm. A review of the causes. *Stroke* 1993;24:1403–9.

39. Bruno VA, Lereis VP, Hawkes M, Ameriso SF. Nontraumatic subarachnoid hemorrhage of the convexity. *Curr Neurol Neurosci Rep* 2013;3:1–3.

40. Refai D, Botros JA, Strom RG, Derdeyn CP, Sharma A, Zipfel GJ. Spontaneous isolated convexity subarachnoid hemorrhage: presentation, radiological findings, differential diagnosis, and clinical course: clinical article. *J Neurosurg* 2008;109:1034–41.

41. Spitzer C, Mull M, Rohde V, Kosinski CM. Non-traumatic cortical subarachnoid haemorrhage: diagnostic work-up and aetiological background. *Neuroradiology* 2005;47:525–31.

42. Kumar S, Goddeau RP Jr., Selim MH, et al. Atraumatic convexal subarachnoid hemorrhage. Clinical presentation, imaging patterns, and etiologies. *Neurology* 2010;74:893–9.

43. Jahan R, Viñuela F. Vascular anatomy, pathophysiology, and classification of vascular malformations of the spinal cord. *Semin Cerebrovasc Dis Stroke* 2002;2:186–200.

44. Sakr YL, Lim N, Amaral AC, et al. Relation of ECG changes to neurological outcome in patients with aneurysmal subarachnoid hemorrhage. *International Journal of Cardiology*. 2004;96:369–73.

45. Banki, Nader M, Kopelnik A, Dae MW, et al. Acute neurocardiogenic injury after subarachnoid hemorrhage. *Circulation*. 2005;112:3314–19.

46. Toussaint LG III, Friedman JA, Wijdicks EF, et al. Survival of cardiac arrest after aneurysmal subarachnoid hemorrhage. *Neurosurgery*. 2005;57:25–31.

Managing hemorrhagic stroke

Katharina Maria Busl

This chapter focuses on the management of hemorrhagic stroke. Eight cases of different types of hemorrhagic stroke are discussed, including hypertensive intracerebral hemorrhage, coagulopathy-related intracerebral hemorrhage, cerebral venous sinus thrombosis, cerebral amyloid angiopathy, arteriovenous malformation, and infectious intracranial hemorrhage. Each case guides the reader through initial presentation and imaging findings as a first step towards diagnosis and treatment. Immediate management considerations are reviewed, differential diagnoses discussed, and treatment options addressed. Depending on the individual case, aspects of disease pathophysiology and background are highlighted. Each case offers potential pitfalls throughout the course, the review and understanding of which will equip the reader with useful tips for their own clinical practice.

Case 1. Hypertensive intracranial hemorrhage

Case description

A 47-year-old man with a 30 pack-year history of smoking was found by his wife on the floor of their living room. He was weak on the left side, and unable to get up without help. Furthermore, his wife noted that his speech was slurred. His blood pressure on arrival at the emergency department was 205/115 mmHg. He was awake, and was attempting to speak; however he was drooling excessively and unintelligible due to pronounced dysarthria. He was found to have a left central facial palsy and left-sided hemiplegia, as well as a mild right-sided paresis. An emergent computed tomography (CT) scan of the brain showed a brainstem hemorrhage (Figure 17.1). On return from the CT

scanner, he had gurgling sounds when breathing. His oxygen saturation level declined to 75% as detected by continuous oxygen level monitoring. Large amounts of saliva and mucus were suctioned out of his mouth, and the degree of his cough reflex was found to be severely reduced. After deep suctioning and supply of oxygen through a high-flow face mask, his oxygen level improved to 92%, but the gurgling respiratory sounds persisted and he remained unable to clear any of his secretions. He was intubated, and mechanical ventilation was initiated. Blood pressure control was initiated by a continuous intravenous infusion of nicardipine with a target goal blood pressure of 160/90 mmHg.

Discussion

Immediate management

This case illustrates several issues that commonly arise in the immediate management of patients with a new neurological deficit consistent with a stroke. Immediate distinction between ischemic and hemorrhagic stroke is of utmost importance as treatment differs substantially. While certain clinical features are more typical for a hemorrhagic stroke – such as headache, nausea, vomiting, abrupt onset of symptoms with maximum of symptoms at onset – these are by no means sensitive and specific enough to establish the etiology. The diagnostic test of choice usually is non-contrasted CT scan of the head: this imaging modality is fast, readily available, and very sensitive in identification of an acute intracranial hemorrhage (ICH). In managing patients with ICH, one immediate goal of treatment should always be kept in mind: minimizing the risk of ongoing or expanding hemorrhage.

The arterial blood pressure is often elevated in patients with ICH, especially in patients who carry a

---

Common Pitfalls in Cerebrovascular Disease: Case-Based Learning, ed. José Biller and José M. Ferro. Published by Cambridge University Press. © Cambridge University Press 2015.

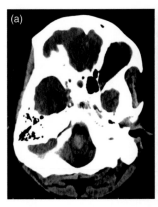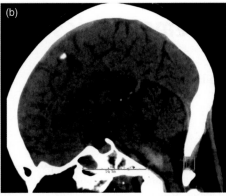

Figure 17.1 CT scan of the head demonstrating an acute intracranial hemorrhage in the medulla (a, axillary image), extending into the lower pons (b, sagittal image). The remainder of the brain parenchyma was normal.

diagnosis of arterial hypertension and in whom the ICH occurred due to hypertension. However, elevated blood pressure is also often noted in patients who are not known to have hypertension and for whom a different etiology of the ICH may be found. Controlling high blood pressure is one of the immediate treatment goals. High blood pressure in ICH has been shown to be linked to hematoma growth, as well as long-term negative impact on outcomes [1]. Therefore, the current guidelines of the American Heart Association (AHA) advise lowering the blood pressure at least to <180 mmHg for systolic blood pressure (SBP) or 130 mmHg for mean arterial pressure (MAP), with consideration of further modest reduction to a MAP of 110 mmHg or a target blood pressure of 160/90 mmHg.

Apart from blood pressure control, it is important to consider other factors that need immediate attention: a bleeding diathesis should always be excluded, and the basic vital functions need to be assessed. In this patient, difficulty with respiration due to bulbar musculature weakness and consequent poor airway protection were exacerbated by lying flat for the neuroimaging test. Potential inability to lie flat should always be considered in patients with neurological deficits involving the lower cranial nerves, especially when obtaining imaging studies that take longer to complete than a simple non-contrasted CT of the head – a magnetic resonance imaging (MRI) of the brain, for example. Some patients may even have to be intubated for the purpose of safely acquiring imaging studies. Early recognition of dysphagia in stroke patients is very important, as it is common and a major risk factor for aspiration pneumonia. Pneumonia contributes substantially to the morbidity amongst stroke patients. In order to guarantee appropriate monitoring of vital

parameters in patients with ICH, the AHA guidelines recommend "initial monitoring and management of ICH patients in an intensive care unit with physician and nursing neuroscience intensive care expertise (Class I; Level of Evidence: B)" [2].

Diagnostic considerations

In a 47-year-old patient with a history of hypertension, the most likely differential diagnosis for an ICH is hypertensive etiology. While the brainstem, mainly the pons, is affected in 5–12% of spontaneous ICH, more common locations for hypertensive ICH are the putamen, the cerebellum, and the thalamus. The reason for these locations is that hypertensive ICHs occur preferentially in the areas of small penetrating arteries that branch off of the major intracranial arteries, often at 90 degree angles. If there is any suspicion that the ICH could be due to a reason other than hypertension – for example due to an unusual shape, location or extent of the ICH, presence of surrounding edema, or an atypical clinical constellation, vascular imaging should be considered. This patient's ICH was located very low in the brainstem, in the medulla, which is not among the most typical locations for a hypertensive hemorrhage. Additionally, he presented at a relatively young age and was not known to carry a history of arterial hypertension. Therefore, a CT angiography of the head and neck vessels was obtained. This revealed dolichoectasia of the vertebrobasilar system, but no vascular malformations. Over the course of his hospitalization, the patient required four oral blood pressure lowering agents in order to reach a well-controlled state of normotension. This is a typical feature of patients presenting with hypertensive ICH. Often, blood pressure controlling medication regimens need to be continually adjusted in the outpatient setting.

Tip

Immediate management of an ICH includes blood pressure control and assessment of respiratory safety, especially if the level of consciousness or the cranial nerves are affected. Difficulty with respiration is often exacerbated during the recumbent position such as for imaging studies, and may not be as overt when positioned with the head of bed elevated at least 30 degrees as is generally recommended for patients at risk of aspiration.

Case 2. Hypertensive intracerebral hemorrhage

Case description

A 39-year-old manager of a grocery store experienced sudden onset of headache while sitting at her desk. Shortly thereafter, her staff noted that she appeared confused and unable to communicate coherently. She was taken to an emergency room, where her blood pressure was found to be 240/160 mmHg. On initial neurological examination, she was awake, appeared alert, but was unable to follow commands due to receptive aphasia. She was attempting to speak, but fluency of language was also disturbed. She had a left gaze preference, but was able to cross midline with her gaze to the right side under visual guidance. She would spontaneously move all extremities, but displayed a mild lag of activation of her right limbs and a drift of her right arm. Her sister, who was her closest relative and listed as emergency contact, reported that she had been diagnosed with arterial hypertension. However, she had not been taking medications in an effort to control her blood pressure by diet and physical exercise. A non-contrasted head CT was performed urgently (Figure 17.2), and showed a large left parietal lobar ICH with diffuse cerebral edema as evidenced by effacement of the cortical sulci, and the finding of pseudo-subarachnoid hemorrhage.

A continuous intravenous infusion of nicardipine was started to lower the blood pressure to an initial goal of SBP of 180 mmHg, as recommended in the AHA guidelines for management of ICH [2]. Coagulation parameters and platelet count were normal. Given the diffuse cerebral edema on head CT, the physician team discussed whether to evacuate the hematoma surgically or whether to first insert an intracranial pressure (ICP) monitor to both assess the intracranial pressure and guide the initial blood pressure management. However, while discussing treatment options with the patient's sister, the patient proceeded to develop a marked right-sided hemiparesis on repeat neurological examination. Her blood pressure was 182/94 mmHg at that time. A CT of the head was repeated, showing the ICH stable in size. On return from the radiology suite, she abruptly deteriorated. She became obtunded, and the right pupil was found markedly dilated at 8 mm and nonreactive to light, as opposed to the left pupil which remained 3 mm in size and reactive to light. She was emergently intubated and taken to the operating room for hematoma evacuation. A postsurgical CT of the head is shown in Figure 17.3.

Discussion

This patient presents in hypertensive crisis with an acute ICH. Immediate management consists of initiating blood pressure control in order to lower the risk of continued hematoma growth as well as the systemic effects of a hypertensive crisis. Prior to aggressively lowering the blood pressure, one must consider whether the ICP might be elevated. If that is the case, blood pressure lowering may lower the cerebral perfusion pressure and therefore be detrimental (by hypoperfusion of brain parenchyma) rather than beneficial. While this patient was awake and alert on initial presentation, her CT scan showed a large (48 mL) parietal hematoma with mass effect as evidenced by effacement of the cerebral sulci. Therefore, a discussion about surgical evacuation and ICP monitoring was initiated. However, deterioration in this patient happened abruptly and rapidly. The features of this deterioration, loss of consciousness and a dilated pupil, indicated an uncal herniation syndrome rather than cerebral hypoperfusion. Emergent hematoma evacuation became necessary.

This patient had a large ICH with profound mass effect, as shown in the upper panel in Figure 17.2. Even in the more caudad parts of the brain, the intracranial pressure was elevated. This is evidenced by the so-called pseudo-subarachnoid hemorrhage shown in Figure 17.2, lower panel. The subarachnoid spaces are narrowed by the elevation in ICP and cerebral edema, resulting in cerebrospinal fluid (CSF) displacement. CSF usually appears hypodense on CT scan, so that with its displacement, a larger proportion of relatively

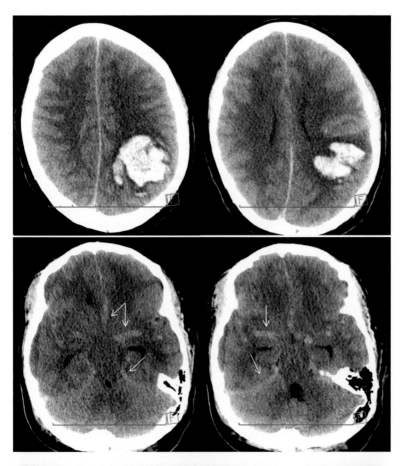

Figure 17.2 Non-contrast CT of the head, axial images. Upper panel: lobulated intraparenchymal hematoma in the left posterior parietal lobe. Diffuse effacement of the cortical sulci. Lower panel: increased attenuation within the basal cisterns and hyperdense appearance of the circle of Willis and the tentorium, consistent with pseudo-subarachnoid hemorrhage.

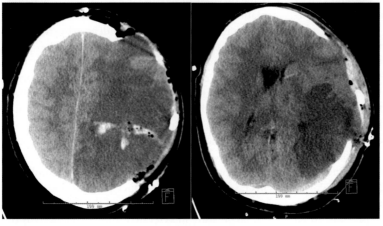

Figure 17.3 Non-contrast CT of the head, axial images, showing postsurgical changes after a left hemicraniectomy with residual left parietal hematoma, and large area of parenchymal hypodensity in the left cerebral hemisphere. There is marked protrusion of brain parenchyma through the skull defect.

hyperdense structures – meninges and blood vessels – become visible, causing the increased attenuation on CT imaging [3]. This may be interpreted as the presence of subarachnoid hemorrhage, while its true meaning is the presence of marked cerebral edema.

One might ask: why was surgical evacuation not performed immediately upon the patient's arrival? On arrival, this patient was awake with a good mental status, and without clinical signs of herniation. Therefore, possible treatment options were evaluated without anticipation of such a rapid deterioration. Based on currently available data, surgical ICH evacuation remains controversial. On the one hand, surgery may limit the mechanical compression of brain; on the other hand, there are surgical risks, especially when the progression of the hemorrhage has not ceased yet. The best-known study evaluating a possible benefit of surgical evacuation, the STICH trial, concluded that for patients with a superficial ICH (extending to 1 cm or closer to the cortical surface) there might be a benefit of surgery within 96 hours. This interpretation is based on a statistical trend towards a better outcome, but did not reach statistical significance (odds ratio 0.69; 95% confidence interval 0.47–1.01) [4]. However, one of the major critiques of that study was that young patients deemed at risk of herniation were likely not enrolled in the study. This pertained to our patient: given the large size of the ICH and the imaging findings indicative of mass effect throughout the brain parenchyma, the risks of increase of ICP and herniation were recognized, and therefore surgical options were discussed, however, not expecting such a drastic deterioration early on. The current AHA guidelines for treatment of ICH suggest considering evacuation by standard craniotomy for patients with lobar ICH >30 mL and within 1 cm of the surface (Class IIb; Level of Evidence: B), but also to have in mind that very early craniotomy may be harmful due to increased risk of recurrent bleeding [2].

The postoperative images (Figure 17.3) of this patient show the left hemisphere largely hypodense, reflecting a combination of cerebral edema and infarcted parenchyma. Furthermore, there is impressive protrusion of the brain parenchyma through the skull defect. Both findings point out under how much pressure the brain parenchyma was prior to the hemicraniectomy. Due to the rigidity of the skull, downward herniation of brain parenchyma is the only way for brain parenchyma to expand, prior to relieving pressure by opening dura and skull.

During her further hospital course, this young woman was diagnosed with renal artery stenosis, which explained her malignant arterial hypertension. She eventually was discharged to a rehabilitation facility, awake, aphasic, and densely hemiplegic on the right side, but able to participate in a rehabilitation program for her left hemispheric stroke syndrome.

Tip

This case highlights one of the most feared complications of ICH: early deterioration. In this situation, the deterioration was immediately life-threatening due to downward herniation, and the only available and life-saving treatment was emergent hemicraniectomy. While data on the benefit of surgical evacuation of ICH are overall still controversial, it should be considered for patients with large ICH who are deemed at risk of herniation.

Case 3. Coagulopathy-related ICH with expansion

Case description

This 51-year-old man developed sudden weakness of his right arm while at home watching TV. He was able to pick up the phone and notify emergency medical services, however with difficulty in speaking. On initial evaluation in the local emergency department, his blood pressure was 164/93 mmHg. He was found to be awake and alert, but had a right-sided facial droop, was severely dysarthric, had a flaccid plegia of his right arm, and a mild paresis of his right leg. His medical history included arterial hypertension, diabetes mellitus, heart failure, atrial fibrillation, and coronary artery disease. Due to his atrial fibrillation, he was anticoagulated with warfarin. Additionally, he had undergone a coronary catheter angiogram 2 months prior for angina pectoris. Coronary atherosclerosis and stenosis was found, and he had had inserted two drug-eluting coronary stents, for which he was now additionally taking aspirin and clopidogrel.

A CT of the brain showed a small hemorrhage in the left basal ganglia (Figure 17.4a). His platelet count was 265 000/μL, and his International Normalized Ratio (INR) was 2.6. He was given 10 mg of vitamin K intravenously, as well as a transfusion of 2 units of fresh frozen plasma (FFP). This reversal therapy was completed 2 hours after his arrival at the emergency room. Repeat testing of the coagulation parameters an hour later showed an INR of 1.8. Two more units of FFP were given, with the follow-up INR reported as 1.4, now 6 hours after initial presentation. However, just upon completion of the transfusions, the patient had a deterioration on his neurological examination. He developed global aphasia and right hemiplegia. A head CT was repeated urgently and showed an expansion of the ICH from 11 to 28 mL (Figure 17.4b).

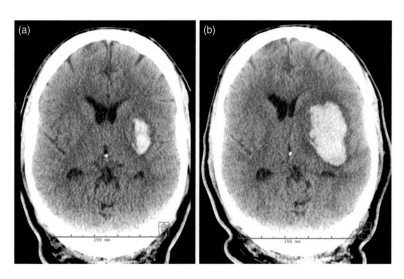

Figure 17.4 Non-contrast CT of the head, axial images. (a) Small hemorrhage in the left basal ganglia. (b) Interval enlargement of the left basal ganglia hemorrhage.

Discussion

In managing patients with ICH, one immediate goal of treatment is to minimize the risk of ongoing or expanding hemorrhage. This patient had a risk factor for hemorrhage expansion that needed immediate attention: his medication-related coagulopathy. While many patients with ICH cannot provide a history due to their neurological deficits, this patient was able to provide a detailed treatment history of his anticoagulant and antiplatelet medications. Even if patients do not or cannot provide a history relevant to risk of hemorrhage or impaired coagulation, the basic laboratory parameters assessing hemostasis (platelet count, prothrombin time (PT), activated partial thromboplastin time (aPTT)) should immediately be checked, as underlying coagulopathy or thrombocytopenia are potentially treatable culprits for expansion of an ICH. Rapid action is the key: rapid reversal of an elevated INR in patients with ICH has been shown to reduce hemorrhage progression and mortality [5]. Normalizing the INR as soon as possible is also a very important determinant for the success of the INR reversal; every 30 minutes of delay in the first dose of FFP in one study was associated with a 20% decreased odds of INR reversal within 24 hours [6]. A target INR of 1.2–1.5 is usually considered adequate reversal [7,8]. If a patient presents with a subtherapeutic INR, it is less clear whether and how much their risk of hemorrhage expansion is increased. The bulk of experience is derived from patients with therapeutic or supratherapeutic INR values. Data regarding the risk of bleeding with subtherapeutic INR are very limited.

Pharmacologic options for INR reversal include the administration of vitamin K, FFP, prothrombin complex concentrates (PCC), and recombinant activated factor VII (rFVIIa). While FFP used to be the standard therapeutic, there are several unfavorable factors that lead to exploration of different reversal strategies: FFP is a blood product with risk of transfusion reactions; the process of obtaining and thawing FFP prior to infusion often results in a longer time to reversal than desired – this was the case for this patient. Even if FFP is ordered immediately, there will be a delay before receiving and administering it. Furthermore, FFP transfusions lead to considerable amounts of volume being given to a patient. For patients with heart failure, this can lead to increased congestion and respiratory problems. PCC have recently been introduced to reversal protocols, and available data so far are favorable. PCC have several advantages: they can be readily administered, are of low fluid volume, and their effect on INR reversal is faster than that of FFP. The most feared side effects of PCC are thromboembolic complications. With all reversal agents, vitamin K should always be given as an additional therapeutic to boost production of coagulation factors. Given its slower time of onset, it is not sufficient to serve as the only therapy. For newer anticoagulants, such as direct thrombin inhibitors (e.g., dabigatran) or direct Xa inhibitors (e.g., rivaroxaban, apixaban, edoxaban), there are no specific reversal agents and experience in patients with ICH taking these medications is limited. There is some evidence that PCCs may have limited effectiveness in reversing the effect of rivaroxaban but not of dabigatran [9]. The use of rFVIIa in ICH patients on dabigatran has shown theoretical potential [10].

For antiplatelet therapy, data vary regarding the impact on hematoma expansion and outcome for patients presenting with ICH. Overall, increased risk of hematoma growth while on these agents is suggested [11]. However, there are no clear data on whether and how to treat patients who are known to take antiplatelet medication, but have a normal platelet count. Practice for utilization of platelet transfusions or other therapeutics varies widely. Possible therapeutics for reversal of antiplatelet therapy include platelet transfusions, desmopressin, and rFVIIa [12]. The current AHA guidelines state that "the usefulness of platelet transfusions in ICH patients with a history of antiplatelet use is unclear and is considered investigational" [2]. A complicating factor may be the risk that is imposed on a patient when an attempt is made to reverse the antiplatelet effect. The patient in our case example had had recent drug-eluting coronary stents placed. Treatment with antiplatelet therapy is usually necessary for several months due to a risk of stent thrombosis. With reversal of anticoagulation and antiplatelet therapy, this possible complication has to be considered, and the patient needs to be monitored appropriately.

Tip

Anticoagulation-induced coagulopathy is a risk factor for hemorrhage expansion in ICH. Rapid reversal is of utmost importance. As a general rule, coagulation parameters and platelet count should be checked immediately for all patients presenting with an ICH.

Case 4. Infective endocarditis

Case description

This 61-year-old man had undergone bioprosthetic aortic valve replacement surgery for heart failure 2 months prior to presentation. He had since then resided at a rehabilitation facility where he continued to make progress with physical therapy; however, he was still too weak to walk without assistance. Other relevant medical problems included arterial hypertension, coronary artery disease, and chronic kidney disease. For the heart disease, he had been maintained on dual antiplatelet therapy with aspirin and clopidogrel. During his stay at the rehabilitation facility, he developed shortness of breath along with fever of 39.5°C and was transferred to a community hospital for evaluation. Findings were consistent with pneumonia, and treatment was initiated with antibiotics. However, his respiratory condition worsened and he became lethargic and confused, eventually requiring intubation and mechanical ventilation. Neurological examination at that time was limited by sedation in the setting of mechanical ventilation, but had revealed a markedly depressed level of alertness and attention, suggestive of delirium, and a mild right hemiparesis. For further evaluation, a CT of the head was performed (Figure 17.5), which showed an acute hematoma in the left precentral gyrus as well as several smaller

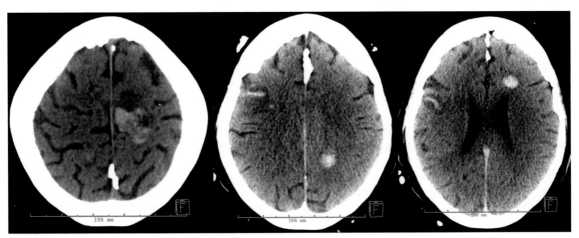

Figure 17.5 CT of the head, non-contrasted. Axial images. Acute hematoma in the left precentral gyrus, several smaller intracranial hemorrhages, and scattered small areas of subarachnoid hemorrhage in both hemispheres.

hemorrhagic foci. The patient's blood pressure and coagulation parameters were within normal limits.

This unexpected imaging result prompted referral and transfer from the community hospital to a tertiary center with a neurological intensive care unit. Physical examination on arrival after transfer showed an ill-appearing, afebrile male who was intubated and obtunded. General physical examination revealed a sternotomy scar that was erythematous and mildly swollen, but without dehiscence or drainage. There was a systolic murmur over the left sternal border. On his right foot, there were raised, erythematous lesions on his second and third toe. On neurological examination, he would open his eyes spontaneously, but would not look at the examiner and had a right gaze preference. He was not able to follow commands. Corneal, oculocephalic, and gag reflexes were intact. He displayed some spontaneous movement of his left arm, but no movements were observed in the other limbs. There was minimal withdrawal of his limbs to external stimulation.

Discussion

This patient appears very ill, and has a markedly abnormal neurological examination. The findings on brain imaging show several small intracranial hematomas. These per se would not be expected to cause such fundamental neurological impairment. In a clinical scenario like this, such global neurologic dysfunction could more likely be caused by a severe medical disease such as sepsis or metabolic derangement, or non-convulsive status epilepticus. In a patient with prior heart surgery, especially valve replacement, and intracranial hemorrhage, a diagnosis of septic bacterial endocarditis needs to be investigated and ruled out. Diagnostic work-up will include an echocardiogram and microbiologic blood culture data. If a transthoracic echocardiogram is not revealing, it should be followed by a transesophageal echocardiogram. In this patient, the transthoracic echocardiogram showed large vegetations on both aortic and mitral valves as well as a new dehiscence of the prosthetic valve. Blood cultures grew methicillin-sensitive *Staphylococcus aureus*. Diagnosis of infective endocarditis is based on the Duke criteria, which define the likelihood of presence of infective endocarditis based on pathologic and major and minor clinical criteria [13]. According to the new modified Duke criteria, our patient displayed two major clinical criteria fulfilling a diagnosis of definite infective

endocarditis: blood cultures were positive for infective endocarditis with a typical microorganism on two separate occasions drawn more than 12 hours apart, and he had a positive echocardiogram. He also fulfilled four of the minor criteria: he had a known predisposing heart condition, a fever with temperature greater than 38°C, and Osler's nodes (tender, erythematous subcutaneous raised lesions that are located on the pulp of the digits of hands or feet, and caused by immune complex depositions), and he was found to have intracranial hemorrhages.

Neurologic complications in patients with infective endocarditis include strokes, intracerebral hemorrhage, brain abscess, meningitis, encephalitis, seizures, and encephalopathy. Their occurrence is common: up to 35% have symptomatic cerebrovascular complications [14], but up to 80% may be found to have cerebrovascular complications on imaging studies. Hemorrhagic strokes can be the consequence of embolic strokes, septic necrotic arteritis, or ruptured mycotic aneurysms. Mycotic aneurysms arise from penetration of septic emboli through the vessel wall which then may rupture and cause ICH or SAH [15]. Identification of neurologic involvement, especially of cerebrovascular disease, often starts with a CT scan of the head, as in our patient. MRI is more sensitive than CT scan, particularly for the detection of small infarcts and microhemorrhages [15]. The appearance of microhemorrhages found in infective endocarditis is different from those in cerebral amyloid angiopathy or hypertensive vasculopathy: Infective endocarditis leads to mostly homogeneous microhemorrhages predominantly located in cortical areas and of small (<5 mm) size. While the mainstay of treatment is systemic antibiosis, urgent cardiac surgery may become necessary if antibiotic therapy fails to stop embolic events, in the setting of heart failure or large abscesses or vegetations. Due to the requirement of cardiopulmonary bypass with heparinization for cardiac surgery, surgery usually has to be postponed for at least a month after occurrence of an ICH. If a patient requires cardiac surgery, screening for microhemorrhages and mycotic aneurysms is usually recommended even in the absence of overt ICH. In a case with presence of ICH, identification of possible mycotic aneurysms is mandatory for treatment planning. Mycotic aneurysms can be detected by both CT angiography and MR angiography (MRA) with high sensitivity (90–95%). While unruptured aneurysms commonly shrink and eventually disappear with antibiotic therapy, ruptured aneurysms require neurosurgical or endovascular treatment in most cases.

Infective endocarditis is a severe illness that often is fatal. The presence of neurologic complications heightens morbidity and mortality in patients with infective endocarditis. This applies especially to staphylococcus endocarditis with neurologic complications, as was the case in our patient, with an estimated mortality of higher than 70%.

Tip

This case example illustrates two important points. First, the brain imaging findings did not explain the severity of the patient's clinical and neurological presentation – a discrepancy that should prompt further work-up. Second, in the differential diagnosis for intracranial hemorrhage, infective endocarditis should always be considered, especially in the presence of fever and predisposing cardiac conditions.

Case 5. Cerebral venous sinus thrombosis

Case description

This 72-year-old man had a long and complicated medical history. Eighteen months prior to the current presentation, he had been diagnosed with colon cancer, and had undergone colon resection with ileostomy placement and chemotherapy. He was believed to be cancer-free after those treatments. During the

hospitalization for treatment of his colon cancer, he had developed a pulmonary embolism, for which anticoagulation with warfarin had been started. Two months prior to the current presentation, he developed difficulty in walking, with unsteady gait, and was reported to experience episodes of confusion and slow speech. He was found to have subacute subdural hematomas, and anticoagulant treatment was placed on hold. One week prior to the current presentation, he underwent surgical evacuation of the subdural hematomas. However, after the surgery, he had several generalized seizures without awakening in between or afterwards. Treatment for status epilepticus was initiated with anticonvulsants and sedative medications, requiring continuation of mechanical ventilation beyond the operative period. Neurological examination was limited by sedation. His gaze was conjugate, pupils were reactive bilaterally, and oculocephalic; cough and gag reflexes were present. Postsurgical imaging was obtained and is shown in Figure 17.6. Apart from the expected findings related to the presence of subdural hematomas and their evacuation, there were small areas of ICH and a hypodense area in different lobar territories.

The combination of hemorrhagic foci and areas of cerebral edema in the setting of new status epilepticus raised the suspicion of cerebral venous sinus thrombosis, and further imaging was obtained. His MRI of the brain with MR venogram is shown in Figure 17.7. The combination of areas of cerebral edema, multiple small hemorrhages, and absent flow in superior sagittal and transverse sinus confirmed the presence of symptomatic cerebral venous sinus thrombosis.

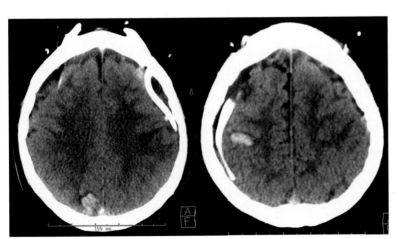

Figure 17.6 Non-contrast CT of the head, axial images. Two small areas of intracranial hemorrhage in right frontal and right occipital lobes. Hypodense area in the left parietal lobe. Expected findings of postsurgical subdural fluid collections, subdural drains and burr holes bilaterally in the skull.

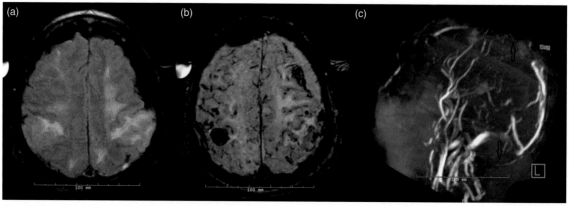

Figure 17.7 MRI of the brain. (a) Axial FLAIR sequence. Cerebral edema in bilateral parietal and occipital lobes. (b) Axial susceptibility weighted sequence. Left frontal and right parietal as well as multiple smaller areas of hemorrhage. (c) Venogram, view from posterior left. Venous sinus thrombosis in superior sagittal sinus and right transverse sinus extending into left transverse sinus (arrows).

Discussion

This is a complicated case, as several disease processes are ongoing at the same time. While seizures can be the presenting symptom of subdural hematomas or occur at any stage of their treatment, new onset status epilepticus after evacuation of a subdural hematoma should prompt repeat imaging. The potential pitfall here is to fail to investigate because of a given possible explanation for seizures. However, while quite possible, new occurrence of seizures or even status epilepticus after uncomplicated evacuation of subdural hematomas is not an expected course. The newly found areas of cerebral edema and hemorrhagic strokes on imaging should raise the suspicion for cerebral venous sinus thrombosis. Both cerebral edema and hemorrhage are the consequence of increased venous pressure: increased venous pressure leads to increased capillary pressure and eventually to a decrease in perfusion with subsequent cytotoxic edema, disturbance of the blood–brain barrier with resulting vasogenic edema, or capillary rupture with hemorrhage. There are many risk factors for the development of cerebral venous sinus thrombosis [16]. This patient carries two of the well-recognized risk factors: malignancy and head injury requiring neurosurgery. At least one risk factor can be identified in more than 85% of adult patients with cerebral venous sinus thrombosis; a prothrombotic state is the most common one [17]. As for clinical presentation of cerebral venous sinus thrombosis, headache often is the first symptom, and may remain the only manifestation, especially in milder cases. In severe cases with widespread thrombosis such

as in our patient, focal symptoms and seizures, as well as disturbance of consciousness are common manifestations. Compared to other stroke subtypes, cerebral venous sinus thrombosis is more likely to present with seizures. Furthermore, the occurrence of status epilepticus in patients with venous sinus thrombosis contributes significantly to early mortality in these patients [18].

For diagnosis, either CT or MR venography can be performed to visualize the thrombosed venous sinus. However, even a plain head CT can offer diagnostic clues. Multifocal hemorrhagic lesions, especially when combined with hypodense lesions that are not located in typical arterial territories, as in this patient, should prompt an investigation for venous sinus thrombosis. The so-called "cord sign," a linear hyperdensity over the cerebral cortex that reflects a thrombosed cortical vein, is another possible finding. In this patient, there was a cord sign; however, this was only recognized in hindsight. On initial review of the axial CT images, this was misinterpreted as acute hemorrhage in the subdural space (Figure 17.8).

Treatment of cerebral venous sinus thrombosis with anticoagulation aims to prevent extension of the thrombosis as well as eventual recanalization of the occluded venous sinuses. If anticoagulation fails, an endovascular approach for either thrombolysis or mechanical clot removal can be considered.

Tip

This case points out the possible pitfall of attributing new findings to pre-existing diseases and

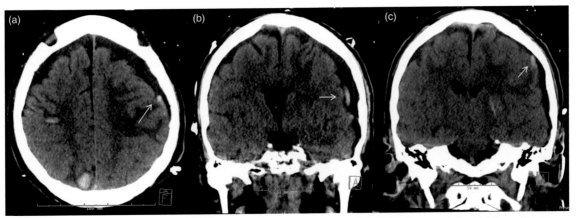

Figure 17.8 Non-contrast CT of the head. (a) Axial image, showing hyperdensity over left frontal cortex (arrow). (b and c) Coronal images, showing cord sign.

conditions. First, attribution of seizure occurrence to present pathology (subdural hematoma); second, misinterpretation of the multifocal cerebral edema and hemorrhagic areas as metastatic disease and omission of vascular imaging; third, misinterpretation of present signs of cerebral vein thrombosis (cord sign in Figure 17.8) in the context of pre-existing brain pathology.

Case 6. Arteriovenous malformation (AVM)

Case description

A 19-year-old healthy young woman developed a sudden headache. There was no preceding trauma or strenuous activity. Following the onset of headache, she rapidly became unresponsive and was found to be apneic on arrival of emergency personnel. Examination on arrival at the emergency room showed an intubated young woman who appeared generally healthy. She was comatose, with anisocoria and an unreactive 7 mm large left pupil. She had no spontaneous movements of her limbs, and only minimal withdrawal of the left limbs to external stimuli. A head CT scan showed a cerebellar ICH (Figure 17.9).

Discussion

Immediate management

This patient presents with a rapidly deteriorating neurological examination and a large cerebellar ICH that compresses the brainstem. She will require

emergent neurosurgical treatment with suboccipital craniotomy (or craniectomy) and hematoma evacuation [2]. It is important to understand that in such a clinical situation, placement of a ventricular drain may not be beneficial – but in fact harmful – due to the risk of upward herniation. Figure 17.10 shows the sagittal view of the patient's ICH. It is apparent that the hemorrhage produces mass effect onto the tentorium (arrow) and the brainstem (arrowhead). If a ventricular drain was placed and the ventricle decompressed, the mass effect onto the brainstem, especially the upper part, could increase. Therefore, drain placement alone, as opposed to surgical hematoma evacuation, is not recommended as treatment [2].

Diagnostic considerations

This is a young and previously healthy woman. The differential etiologies for ICH that pertain to a majority of hemorrhagic strokes in adult or elder patients, namely arterial hypertension, cerebral amyloid angiopathy, hemorrhagic conversion of an ischemic stroke, or hemorrhagic metastasis, are less likely to be found in a young patient. In fact, vascular malformations are the most common underlying etiology in spontaneous childhood ICH [19], while overall, AVMs only constitute 1–2% of all strokes. The typical age of presentation with an AVM lies between the ages of 10 and 40. The gold standard for diagnosis is conventional digital subtraction angiography, as this modality allows for dynamic assessment of flow patterns in addition to delineating the actual malformation. This patient's angiographic image is shown in Figure 17.11.

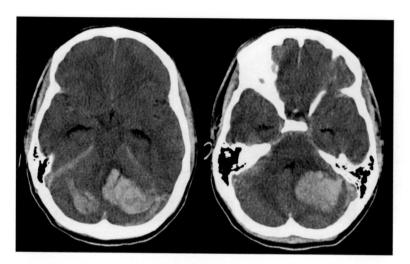

Figure 17.9 Non-contrast CT head, axial images. Large cerebellar ICH, centered in the left hemisphere, extending into the right hemisphere, with mass effect onto the brainstem.

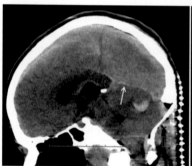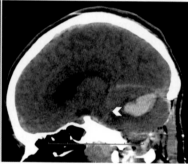

Figure 17.10 Non-contrast CT head, sagittal images. Large cerebellar ICH with mass effect: upward bowing of the tentorium cerebelli (thin arrow), anterior mass effect onto brainstem (thick arrowhead).

This AVM was found to feed from the left posterior inferior cerebellar artery. The hematoma was evacuated and the AVM resected. Due to the rapid initial intervention with suboccipital craniectomy and relief of pressure, the patient recovered well and eventually was transferred to a rehabilitation hospital, awake, conversant, and able to stand up with two-person assistance.

Tip

The most likely diagnosis of a spontaneous ICH in children and adolescents is a vascular malformation. Vascular imaging is a must. If the ICH is located in the posterior fossa, immediate concern is for brainstem compression, and the life-saving measure is a suboccipital craniectomy or craniotomy to relieve pressure. Placement of a ventricular drain should not be the only intervention, as there is a risk of upward herniation and further deterioration.

Case 7. Thrombolysis-related ICH

Case description

A 79-year-old woman was sitting with family around the dinner table when she suddenly became limp, fell over to the right and out of the chair. She was awake and attempting to talk, but could only make grunting sounds. Her family noted her "eyes were rolled back," before she became unconscious. The paramedics emergently intubated her as she was severely dyspneic with poor oxygen saturation. Blood pressure was 190/97 mmHg, and heart rate was 116. Her past medical history was remarkable for heart failure and a myocardial infarction 10 months prior, for which she was taking daily aspirin, and bilateral cataract surgery. On arrival at the emergency room, cardiac rhythm was noted to be atrial fibrillation. Examination in the setting of sedatives given for intubation showed an elderly unresponsive female with a right scalp hematoma. She

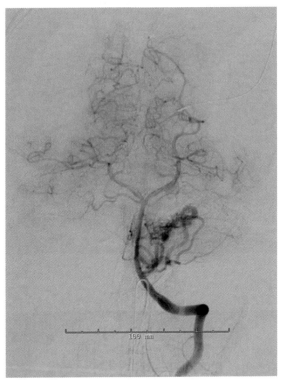

Figure 17.11 Digital subtraction angiography. Coronal view, left vertebral artery injection. Large arteriovenous malformation; feeding artery is left posterior inferior cerebellar artery.

was comatose with no eye opening or command following, and her gaze was noted to be dysconjugate with the right eye pointing outwards and downwards. Her pupils were irregular and small. She had extensor posturing in the arms and triple flexion in the legs. A head CT scan did not reveal intracranial hemorrhage or findings of a large territory acute stroke. Constellation of symptoms was felt to be most consistent with a brainstem stroke, possibly secondary to basilar artery embolus or occlusion, and intravenous thrombolysis with tissue plasminogen activator (tPA) was administered. A contrast-enhanced CT of the head with CT angiography was obtained in order to visualize the posterior circulation. The angiography revealed a thrombus in the right posterior cerebral artery. The contrasted head CT is shown in Figure 17.12. There were multifocal hypodense areas with gyral enhancement.

While intravenous access lines were placed by the intensive care team, the patient's right pupil was noted to dilate and she became bradycardic with a heart rate of 30. A CT of the head was urgently repeated (see

Figure 17.13). Within a short period of time, there had been a drastic change in appearance, with expanding multifocal hemorrhage as well as intraventricular hemorrhage in all ventricles. There was brainstem herniation, which explained the change of examination with pupil dilatation and bradycardia. Due to the grave condition, the patient's family opted for non-escalation of care, and the patient died shortly thereafter.

Discussion

This patient developed symptomatic ICH after intravenous thrombolysis. The first CT scan showing the hemorrhagic areas was a contrasted scan which was obtained for the purpose of vascular imaging just after completion of tPA infusion. In post-contrast studies, it can be very difficult or even impossible to distinguish between contrast extravasation and acute blood. In this case (Figure 17.12), the findings were attributed to contrast enhancement of ischemic infarctions. Progression and new neurological signs prompted further imaging that showed widespread hemorrhage shortly thereafter. A newer imaging modality, dual-energy computed tomography, has become available in advanced radiologic centers. This imaging modality can assist in distinction of hemorrhage and contrast extravasation [20].

The rapid expansion of the hemorrhagic areas in this case underlines the importance of initiation of reversal of coagulopathy in the setting of thrombolysis as quickly as possible when symptomatic hemorrhage has occurred. Baseline laboratory parameters that should be checked immediately include platelet count, prothrombin time, activated partial thromboplastin time, fibrinogen level, and a type and cross test. If the tPA infusion is still in process, it should be stopped immediately. For tPA reversal, guidelines suggest the replacement of clotting factors as well as platelets [21]. Cryoprecipitate is used by many hospital protocols for reversal of intravenous tPA, as it provides the highest content of fibrinogen, and counteracts the fibrinogen depletion that is induced by tPA.

Tip

If symptomatic ICH after thrombolysis is confirmed, tPA should be stopped immediately, if the infusion is still ongoing. If the hemorrhage is detected after the tPA infusion has finished, reversal of tPA includes cryoprecipitate and platelets.

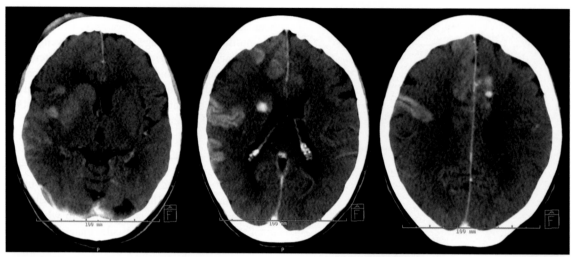

Figure 17.12 CT head with intravenous contrast, axial images. Gyral enhancement of multifocal infarcts as well as a scalp hematoma overlying the right frontal bone.

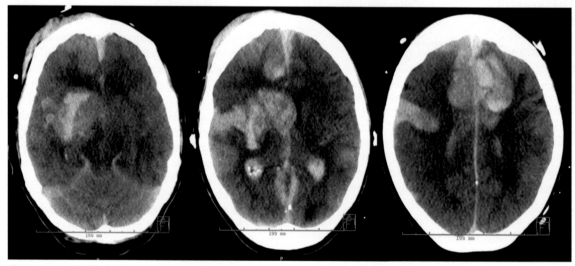

Figure 17.13 CT of the head, non-contrast, axial images. Increased multifocal hyperdensities in both hemispheres, consistent with multifocal ICH, as well as pan-intraventricular hemorrhage, with midline shift and herniation. Increase in size of right frontal scalp hematoma.

Case 8. ICH due to cerebral amyloid angiopathy (CAA)

Case description

A 67-year-old man with no known medical problems presented with difficulty speaking. He felt that he had difficulty finding words and was not able to pronounce them correctly, and drove himself to the emergency room. On presentation to the emergency department, his blood pressure was 202/106 mmHg.

He was in no apparent physical distress, but alert and frustrated due to his inability to communicate. He was alert, but unable to state his age or month. Further language testing showed a mixed aphasia. While he was able to follow simple commands, he was unable to follow three-step commands. He spontaneously produced fluent nonsensical speech. A medication list he provided included aspirin 81 mg daily, but no other blood thinners. A CT scan of the head was performed (Figure 17.14) and showed an ICH in the left opercular area.

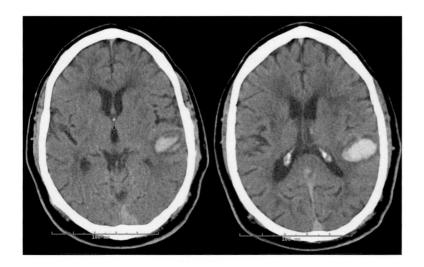

Figure 17.14 Non-contrast CT head, axial images. Intracerebral hematoma centered in the cortex on the left at the junction of the left posterior frontal, temporal, and parietal lobes. There is mild surrounding edema.

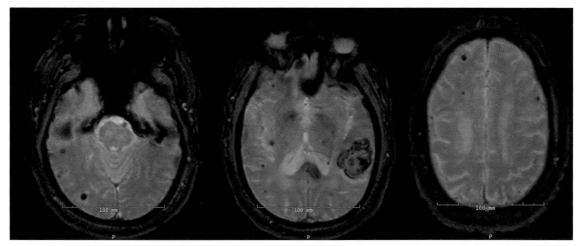

Figure 17.15 MRI brain, axial images, gradient echo sequence. Acute ICH in the left parietal-temporal cortex. Multiple microhemorrhages in both cerebral hemispheres and in the cerebellum.

Discussion

This 67-year-old man presented with a lobar ICH. In patients older than 60 years, the most likely etiology for a spontaneous lobar hemorrhage is cerebral amyloid angiopathy (CAA). In the given clinical scenario with markedly elevated blood pressure, the most likely differential diagnosis to consider is a hypertensive hemorrhage. CAA refers to the deposition of β-amyloid in the media and adventitia of small and mid-sized arteries of the cerebral cortex and the leptomeninges. While hemorrhages due to CAA are not pathophysiologically linked to high blood pressure, many patients have coexisting arterial hypertension or elevated blood pressure on presentation. This patient's blood pressure normalized soon after his arrival at the emergency room, and remained within normal limits throughout his subsequent hospital stay.

Spontaneous lobar ICH is the most common clinical manifestation of CAA. CAA is not associated with systemic amyloidosis. The preponderance of lobar location of amyloid-related hemorrhages is based on the distribution of vascular amyloid deposits in cortical vessels. White matter, deep gray matter, and brainstem are largely spared. Often, the ICH in CAA is located in the posterior lobes. Firm diagnosis of CAA is not easy. A definite diagnosis is only possible by postmortem brain tissue analysis. Therefore, criteria for a probable diagnosis of CAA by imaging or biopsy samples have been established [22]. The imaging modality of choice is a gradient echo or T2-weighted sequence of MR imaging. These sequences detect hemosiderin depositions, breakdown products indicative of prior hemorrhages, as little as 2 mm. In the work-up of this patient's ICH, an MRI was performed, and is shown in Figure 17.15. Besides the acute left opercular ICH, there were multiple cortical microhemorrhages in different vascular territories.

The distribution of these microhemorrhages extended through cortex and grey-white junction, while sparing regions considered "typical" for a hypertensive hemorrhage, such as the basal ganglia, thalamus, and pons. In combination with the clinical setting of a spontaneous hemorrhage at the age of 67 years, in the absence of other explanations, the patient was diagnosed with "probable CAA."

CAA is a disease for which, as of yet, there is no cure. Therefore, the main effort lies in reducing the risk of recurrent hemorrhages. While this patient's blood pressure remained normal after his initial examination, it is important to realize that in the age group after 55 years, arterial hypertension is very prevalent, and may often coexist. Furthermore, blood pressure control has been shown to reduce the risk of a CAA-related hemorrhage by 77% [23]. Another question that often arises in the management of patients with CAA is whether antiplatelet and anticoagulant medications can be resumed – many patients, as with hypertension, are taking one or several of these medications due to coexisting medical conditions that are prevalent in this age group, such as coronary artery disease, or atrial fibrillation. Due to the high recurrence rate of CAA-related hemorrhages, it is generally recommended to avoid anticoagulant and antiplatelet agents once diagnosed with CAA. This may pose a difficult clinical situation, for example if someone with a mechanical heart valve, requiring full anticoagulation, is diagnosed with CAA. Aspirin increases the risk of recurrent hemorrhage less than anticoagulation, but still substantially: in a cohort of patients with primary lobar ICH, aspirin was associated with a near fourfold increased risk of ICH recurrence [24]. Nonetheless, aspirin use can be considered in selected patients with CAA, if they have a strong indication for antiplatelet therapy, such as a coronary stent placement.

Tips

(1) Hypertension is very prevalent in the age group of patients with CAA, and optimal blood pressure control may reduce the risk of CAA-related hemorrhages substantially. (2) Antiplatelet and anticoagulant medications are usually not recommended for patients with CAA. It is important to counsel patients on the potential increased risk of bleeding recurrence when taking over-the-counter nonsteroidal inflammatory drugs as well.

References

1. Willmot M, Leonardi-Bee J, Bath PM. High blood pressure in acute stroke and subsequent outcome: a systematic review. *Hypertension* 2004;43:18–24.

2. Morgenstern LB, Hemphill JC, 3rd, Anderson C, Becker K, Broderick JP, Connolly ES, Jr., Greenberg SM, Huang JN, MacDonald RL, Messe SR, Mitchell PH, Selim M, Tamargo RJ. Guidelines for the management of spontaneous intracerebral hemorrhage: a guideline for healthcare professionals from the American Heart Association/American Stroke Association. *Stroke* 2010;41:2108–29.

3. Given CA, 2nd, Burdette JH, Elster AD, Williams DW, 3rd. Pseudo-subarachnoid hemorrhage: a potential imaging pitfall associated with diffuse cerebral edema. *AJNR Am J Neuroradiol* 2003;24:254–6.

4. Mendelow AD, Gregson BA, Fernandes HM, Murray GD, Teasdale GM, Hope DT, Karimi A, Shaw MD, Barer DH. Early surgery versus initial conservative treatment in patients with spontaneous supratentorial intracerebral haematomas in the international Surgical Trial in Intracerebral Haemorrhage (STICH): a randomised trial. *Lancet* 2005;365:387–97.

5. Ivascu FA, Howells GA, Junn FS, Bair HA, Bendick PJ, Janczyk RJ. Rapid warfarin reversal in anticoagulated patients with traumatic intracranial hemorrhage reduces hemorrhage progression and mortality. *J Trauma* 2005;59:1131–7; discussion 1137–9.

6. Goldstein JN, Thomas SH, Frontiero V, Joseph A, Engel C, Snider R, Smith EE, Greenberg SM, Rosand J. Timing of fresh frozen plasma administration and rapid correction of coagulopathy in warfarin-related intracerebral hemorrhage. *Stroke* 2006;37:151–5.

7. Oyama H, Kito A, Maki H, Hattori K, Noda T, Wada K. Acute subdural hematoma in patients with medication associated with risk of hemorrhage. *Neurol Med Chir (Tokyo)* 2011;51:825–8.

8. Panczykowski DM, Okonkwo DO. Premorbid oral antithrombotic therapy and risk for reaccumulation, reoperation, and mortality in acute subdural hematomas. *J Neurosurg* 2010;114:47–52.

9. Eerenberg ES, Kamphuisen PW, Sijpkens MK, Meijers JC, Buller HR, Levi M. Reversal of rivaroxaban and dabigatran by prothrombin complex concentrate: a randomized, placebo-controlled, crossover study in healthy subjects. *Circulation* 2011;124:1573–9.

10. Oh JJ, Akers WS, Lewis D, Ramaiah C, Flynn JD. Recombinant factor VIIa for refractory bleeding after cardiac surgery secondary to anticoagulation with the direct thrombin inhibitor lepirudin. *Pharmacotherapy* 2006;26:569–77.

11. Thompson BB, Bejot Y, Caso V, Castillo J, Christensen H, Flaherty ML, Foerch C, Ghandehari K, Giroud M, Greenberg SM, Hallevi H, Hemphill JC, 3rd, Heuschmann P, Juvela S, Kimura K, Myint PK, Nagakane Y, Naritomi H, Passero S, Rodriguez-Yanez MR, Roquer J, Rosand J, Rost NS, Saloheimo P, Salomaa V, Sivenius J, Sorimachi T, Togha M, Toyoda K, Turaj W, Vemmos KN, Wolfe CD, Woo D, Smith EE. Prior antiplatelet therapy and outcome following intracerebral hemorrhage: a systematic review. *Neurology* 2010;75:1333–42.

12. Powner DJ, Hartwell EA, Hoots WK. Counteracting the effects of anticoagulants and antiplatelet agents during neurosurgical emergencies. *Neurosurgery* 2005;57:823–31.

13. Li JS, Sexton DJ, Mick N, Nettles R, Fowler VG, Jr., Ryan T, Bashore T, Corey GR. Proposed modifications to the Duke criteria for the diagnosis of infective endocarditis. *Clin Infect Dis* 2000;30:633–8.

14. Roder BL, Wandall DA, Espersen F, Frimodt-Moller N, Skinhoj P, Rosdahl VT. Neurologic manifestations in *Staphylococcus aureus* endocarditis: a review of 260 bacteremic cases in nondrug addicts. *Am J Med* 1997;102:379–86.

15. Ferro JM, Fonseca AC. Infective endocarditis. *Handb Clin Neurol* 2013;119:75–91.

16. Saposnik G, Barinagarrementeria F, Brown RD, Jr., Bushnell CD, Cucchiara B, Cushman M, deVeber G, Ferro JM, Tsai FY. Diagnosis and management of cerebral venous thrombosis: a statement for healthcare professionals from the American Heart Association/ American Stroke Association. *Stroke* 2011;42:1158–92.

17. Ferro JM, Canhao P, Stam J, Bousser MG, Barinagarrementeria F. Prognosis of cerebral vein and dural sinus thrombosis: results of the International Study on Cerebral Vein and Dural Sinus Thrombosis (ISCVT). *Stroke* 2004;35:664–70.

18. Masuhr F, Busch M, Amberger N, Ortwein H, Weih M, Neumann K, Einhaupl K, Mehraein S. Risk and predictors of early epileptic seizures in acute cerebral venous and sinus thrombosis. *Eur J Neurol* 2006;13:852–6.

19. Beslow LA, Licht DJ, Smith SE, Storm PB, Heuer GG, Zimmerman RA, Feiler AM, Kasner SE, Ichord RN, Jordan LC. Predictors of outcome in childhood intracerebral hemorrhage: a prospective consecutive cohort study. *Stroke* 2009;41:313–18.

20. Phan CM, Yoo AJ, Hirsch JA, Nogueira RG, Gupta R. Differentiation of hemorrhage from iodinated contrast in different intracranial compartments using dual-energy head CT. *AJNR Am J Neuroradiol* 2012;33:1088–94.

21. Broderick J, Connolly S, Feldmann E, Hanley D, Kase C, Krieger D, Mayberg M, Morgenstern L, Ogilvy CS, Vespa P, Zuccarello M. Guidelines for the management of spontaneous intracerebral hemorrhage in adults: 2007 update: a guideline from the American Heart Association/American Stroke Association Stroke Council, High Blood Pressure Research Council, and the Quality of Care and Outcomes in Research Interdisciplinary Working Group. *Circulation* 2007;116:e391–413.

22. Greenberg SM. Cerebral amyloid angiopathy: prospects for clinical diagnosis and treatment. *Neurology* 1998;51:690–4.

23. Arima H, Tzourio C, Anderson C, Woodward M, Bousser MG, MacMahon S, Neal B, Chalmers J. Effects of perindopril-based lowering of blood pressure on intracerebral hemorrhage related to amyloid angiopathy: The PROGRESS trial. *Stroke* 2010;41:394–6.

24. Biffi A, Halpin A, Towfighi A, Gilson A, Busl K, Rost N, Smith EE, Greenberg MS, Rosand J, Viswanathan A. Aspirin and recurrent intracerebral hemorrhage in cerebral amyloid angiopathy. *Neurology* 2010;75:693–8.

Chapter 18

Managing patients or managing the results of ancillary tests?

José M. Ferro

Most of neurology practice relies on the interview of the patient and his/her relative or proxy. The interview is complemented by the general physical and neurological examination. While for many patients it is necessary to formulate a detailed diagnosis, for other people seen in outpatient clinics it is only necessary to explain their symptoms and relieve their worries. This simple part of the patient–doctor relationship, consisting of separating the "sick" from the "non-sick" and labeling the different classes of "sick," has become increasingly precise and complex, but also more time consuming and costly, due to the availability of ancillary diagnostic procedures. These diagnostic procedures are in general performed by another doctor, or by a technician, sometimes working in a different institution. Communication between the attending physician and his colleague executing the diagnostic tests is usually limited to referral notes and reports, sometimes to a phone call, rarely to a face-to-face meeting. Diagnostic tools initially consisting of blood tests, electrocardiogram (ECG), and chest X-rays have expanded enormously, and opened a new era in our possibility to diagnose neurologic disorders. Different sectors of hospitals and diagnostic clinics are now dedicated to laboratory tests, including genetics, pathology, neurophysiology, nuclear medicine, neuroradiology, and neuropsychology.

An experienced neurologist has an implicit knowledge of the limitations of interviewing patients. The sequence of the interview is guided not only by the symptoms reported by the patient, but also by the working diagnosis, which the neurologist is formulating as he encounters the patient and starts to ask questions. The doctor may fail to ask some relevant questions. The patient may fail to provide an accurate answer, because he no longer remembers the facts well, or because his own concept of his symptoms may distort the answers.

In other instances, the patient may not be aware of the whole or part of his current medical history because of a consciousness disorder, a memory defect, or a mental trouble. The testimony of a relative, proxy, or witness is valuable, but his report may also be inaccurate or biased. During the interview, as the neurologist interacts with the patient and his proxy, he is mentally reconstructing the succession of events and the details of his patient history and weighting the accuracy of the information he is extracting.

General physical and neurologic examination appears to be more objective. However, comparing the results of neurological examination performed by two different neurologists can provide discrepant results. The interobserver agreement is particularly imperfect for items such as higher nervous functions, eye movements, and sensory examination [1,2]. Diagnostic tools, in particular neuroimaging, have taught us that the diagnostic value, i.e., the accuracy, of important classic neurological signs is limited [3]. This means that in the neurological examination the possibility of false positive and false negative results has to be considered.

Ancillary diagnostic procedures are somehow a "technological application" extending history taking and the classic neurological examination. Despite our contemporary "blind" belief in technology, most of the correct diagnoses are already established before performing ancillary diagnostic tests. Ancillary diagnostic procedures increase or decrease the probability of a working diagnosis formulated while taking the history or performing the physical examination. Unfortunately, today many diagnostic tests are performed simply because they are part of the diagnostic "panel" or are listed in the comprehensive work-up of a clinical condition. Junior doctors in particular rarely

Common Pitfalls in Cerebrovascular Disease: Case-Based Learning, ed. José Biller and José M. Ferro. Published by Cambridge University Press. © Cambridge University Press 2015.

think "Why did I order this test?" and even less "What will I do with the results of this test?"

David Sackett and co-workers [4] thoughtfully listed the eight conditions to value the usefulness of a diagnostic test:

1. Was the new test "blindly" compared with the "gold-standard" diagnostic test?
2. Was the new test evaluated in the whole spectrum of each disease (e.g., severity, sex, age)?
3. Was the evaluation performed in different settings (e.g., primary, ambulatory vs. hospital, inpatient)?
4. Were the precision (reproducibility) and inter- and intraobserver reliability studied?
5. What were the definition and cutoff values for "normal" results?
6. Was the test evaluated as a single test or as part of a cluster or sequence of tests?
7. Were the techniques for carrying out the test described?
8. Was the utility of the test determined?

The guideline development method GRADE [5] states that recommendations regarding diagnostic tests need to provide evidence that performing diagnostic tests modifies patient-relevant outcomes, an area where the evidence is rather limited. Finally, health-care providers and payers will ask for the cost of diagnostic tests and for the added value (cost-effectiveness and cost–utility analysis) [6] of performing a new diagnostic test, before implementing it and/or reimbursing it.

Case 1. Recurrent vertigo or recurrent TIA?

Case description

A 47-year-old masseuse was referred to the neurology outpatient clinic by an ear, nose, and throat (ENT) specialist because her brain magnetic resonance imaging (MRI) showed "multiple strokes" (Figure 18.1). Her current complaints consisted of gait unsteadiness and brief episodes of vertigo related to changes in body/head position for the previous 4 weeks. She described episodes lasting for about 1 minute of a sudden and violent spinning sensation, which more often occurred when she bent to pick up something from the floor or raise her head to reach an object on a top shelf. The same symptoms were also frequent at night, a few moments after she got into bed, when she turned from side to side, and in the morning when she got up. During and shortly after the episode she felt nauseated, cold, and sweaty. She had no other symptoms such as double vision, numbness, limb weakness, dysarthria, hearing loss, tinnitus, or hiccups. The number of daily episodes was variable, but always multiple. Between the episodes she felt unstable, but she denied falls. She was a smoker of a pack of cigarettes a day since her teens. Otherwise she was healthy, apart from asthma, from which she had suffered since childhood and which was well controlled with medical treatment.

On examination pulse was regular. Sitting blood pressure (BP) was 105/70 mmHg, with no orthostatic changes. General physical and neurologic examinations

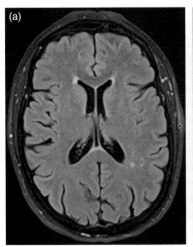 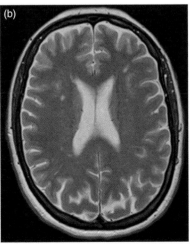

Figure 18.1 Case 1. Brain MRI FLAIR (a) and T2 sequences (b) showing punctate subcortical white matter lesions. None were located on the cerebellum or in the cerebellar or vestibular pathways.

were unremarkable; examination of the V, VII, and VIII cranial nerves was normal and there were no vestibular or cerebellar signs. There was no base widening or side deviations while walking, but the patient was cautious and felt uncomfortable walking with eyes closed. The Dix–Hallpike maneuver with the head rotated to the right side produced intense vertigo, nausea, and sweating, reproducing the symptoms the patient reported during her spells. Vertigo started a few seconds after the patient lay down, lasted for about 20 seconds, and was accompanied by a rotational geotropic nystagmus, as the top pole of the eyes rotated towards the undermost ear. A similar, although less intense, vertigo was noticed when the patient returned to the seating position. Vertigo became less intense and of shorter duration, with repetitive testing.

Canalith repositioning was successfully attempted using the Epley maneuver. The patient was instructed not to sleep completely flat for 2 days, to use dimenhydrinate 50 mg if too nauseated, and to start a home program of vestibular rehabilitation exercises. She was strongly advised to quit smoking.

Discussion

This active healthy woman complained of multiple daily episodes of vertigo and gait unsteadiness for a period of 4 weeks. She was diagnosed as having multiple transient ischemic attacks (TIAs). MRI was ordered and spotty subcortical white matter changes were read as "small strokes." There are several arguments making the diagnosis of TIA implausible in this case: (1) the patient is a young adult and has just one vascular risk factor, she was not diabetic and her blood pressure was normal; (2) the temporal pattern of the episodes does not suggest a vascular cause, as there were multiple daily episodes for a period of 4 weeks. Multiple TIAs can occur, but in general are spaced by days or weeks. A clustered pattern (cluster or crescendo TIA) is also possible in the capsular and pontine warning syndromes [7–9], showing repetitive episodes of hemiplegia, but only for a few days; (3) the spells consisted only of vertigo and the corresponding unsteadiness, plus profuse vegetative symptoms, which point to a peripheral, vestibular origin of the symptoms. Diplopia, numbness, dysphagia, dysarthria, hiccups, or other intra-axial symptoms indicating brainstem ischemia were not reported. Restricted cerebellar infarcts presented isolated vertigo [10], with abnormal vestibular signs on neurological examination. In this case

neurological examination was normal between the episodes. Isolated transient episodes of vertigo should not be considered as due to transient brainstem ischemia, unless accompanied by other brainstem, cerebellar, or occipital symptomatology [11].

Neurologic examination between episodes was normal. However, the Dix–Hallpike maneuver replicated the symptoms experienced by the patient and provided evidence in favor of a peripheral vestibular disorder. In fact, vertigo and nystagmus appeared only when the head was rotated to the right side, there was a latency of seconds before their onset, they faded away spontaneously, and their intensity decreased as the maneuver was repeated, i.e., nystagmus was fatigable. This observation, taken together with the patient's complaints, is sufficient to establish the diagnosis of benign paroxysmal positional vertigo (BPPV) caused by cupololithiasis of the posterior semicircular canal. As its name indicates, BPPV is a benign and frequent condition, which causes recurrent attacks of positional vertigo. A repositioning maneuver is the recommended treatment in the acute phase [12].

MRI showed a few punctate subcortical white matter lesions (WML). Diffusion-weighted imaging (DWI) was negative. WML were interpreted as lacunar infarcts. None were located in the cerebellum or in the vestibular nuclei or pathways. Therefore, WML could not be responsible for the patient's symptomatology. These punctate lesions are smaller than lacunar infarcts and correspond to areas of gliosis. They represent a perivascular reduction in myelin content with atrophy of the neuropil and seem to constitute a negligible extent of tissue damage from low permeability of thickened arteriolar walls [13]. Their frequency increases with age, especially after 60, but they are often detected in MRIs of younger adults, in particular if they have vascular risk factors or migraine. Large cohort studies clearly showed that these punctate lesions (grade 1 in Fazekas' scale) do not increase with time, in contrast to the progression to more extensive lesions seen in early confluent (grade 2) or confluent (grade 3) WML [14,15]. Antiplatelets are not recommended for patients with WML without stroke or TIA. There is no evidence that quitting smoking prevents progression of WML, but quitting smoking definitively reduces the risk of further vascular events including stroke. Any medical encounter is an opportunity to advise smokers to quit their "suicidal" habit.

Tip

Recurrent attacks of intense vertigo with nausea triggered by head or body movement to one side were rather suggestive of BPPV. The characteristic response on the Dix–Hallpike maneuver confirmed the diagnosis.

Pitfall

The ENT specialist failed to perform the appropriate physical examination of a patient with vertigo, which should include the Dix–Hallpike maneuver. Instead he asked for an unnecessary MRI. He misinterpreted benign minor white matter changes as lacunar stroke. He also did not perform a clinical topographical diagnosis, as none of the visible white matter changes were located in a brain area whose damage would produce vertigo.

Case 2. Iatrogenic CT

Case report

A 46-year-old secretary was referred to the neurology outpatient clinic because of "silent strokes." She had no known vascular risk factors, although she did not

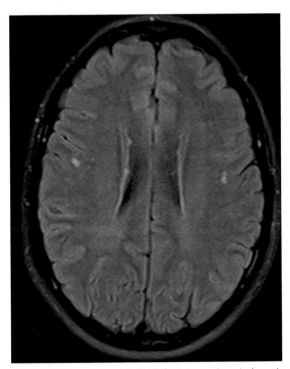

Figure 18.2 Case 2. Brain MRI FLAIR depicting periventricular and punctate subcortical white matter lesions.

check her BP. Her past medical history was unremarkable, except for a long-standing history of tension headache, without analgesic abuse, and recent complaints of job-related anxiety and dry mouth. She had no episodes of sudden focal neurologic deficits, suggesting TIAs or stroke. Brain imaging was performed at another institution. Brain CT raised question of a sphenoid ridge meningioma and therefore an MRI was ordered. MRI ruled out meningioma, but showed linear T2 hyperintense periventricular white matter lesions and a few frontal punctate subcortical white matter lesions (Figure 18.2). DWI was normal. The resident who first examined the patient found no abnormalities on the neurologic examination, but recorded a sitting BP of 130/85 mmHg. He ordered blood tests, including autoimmunity panel and *Borrelia* serology, extra-and intracranial vascular ultrasound, cervical MR, and visual evoked potentials. All these tests gave negative or normal results. An ambulatory 24-hour BP recording was later recorded, which showed that the patient was a non-"dipper." She was started on a beta-blocker.

Discussion

As in the previous case, MRI showed white matter changes, both periventricular and in the deep white matter. Periventricular white matter lesions can be shown in T2 and Fluid Attenuated Inversion Recovery (FLAIR) sequences at the ventral and dorsal limits of the lateral ventricles and have the shape of a cap. They can also appear as a smooth linear halo on the lateral margins of the lateral ventricles. Periventricular caps are characterized pathologically by loosely arranged fine-fiber tracts with low myelin and high extracellular fluid content. Patchy loss of the ependyma with astrocytic gliosis is frequently observed. Smooth periventricular halo has been linked to the disruption of the ependymal lining with subependymal gliosis and subsequent loss of myelin. It has also been found to be related to venous congestion due to noninflammatory periventricular venous collagenosis [13,16,17]. This means that these lesions can hardly be considered of ischemic vascular origin.

MR findings were unrelated to the tension headaches which brought the patient to the consultation. This incidental finding provoked the request of a series of other tests which fortunately were all normal. Otherwise, other or confirmatory tests would be performed, increasing exponentially the risk of new incidental findings. The cost and worries for the patient were not negligible. All tests were ordered to exclude remote possible diagnoses, not taking into consideration the very low pre-test probability of a positive result. As vascular white matter lesions are a manifestation of small vessel disease, ultrasound or angiographic evaluation of the extracranial vessels usually gives normal results or shows minimal stenosis or plaques. The presence and intensity of white matter changes does not have any relationship to the degree of carotid stenosis eventually found in carotid ultrasound [18]. In other words, performing carotid ultrasound in patients with WML has a yield similar to performing it in "normal" individuals. Considering laboratory tests, Lyme disease should not be considered in the differential diagnosis of hyperintense T2 foci in middle-aged and elderly patients, except if clinically suspected [19]. Dry mouth might raise the possibility of Sjögren's syndrome with cerebral involvement, although other features (dry eye, arthralgias) were absent and dry mouth could be interpreted in the context of anxious symptomatology. WML are not more frequent in Sjögren's syndrome than in age-matched controls. Even in Sjögren's syndrome WML are associated with increasing age, diabetes, and hypertension [20]. Several community- and hospital-based studies have established that increasing age, diabetes, and hypertension are the most important risk factors for the appearance of WML. Fasting or casual glycaemia and hemoglobin A_{1c} were performed to detect diabetes. Measurement of blood pressure during outpatient consultation showed borderline values and she would be classified as prehypertensive. Ambulatory 24-hour monitoring of blood pressure revealed that she was a non-dipper, as her BP failed to decrease during sleep. After this result she was started on an antihypertensive, to decrease her risk of vascular events, mainly of stroke. Subcortical white matter lesions are a marker of hypertensive end-organ damage. Its presence has been related to casual or 24-hour BP values, to non-dipper and inverted dipper patterns, to blood pressure surge in the morning, and to blood pressure variability [21].

Tip

Discrete punctate age-related WML do not need extensive ancillary investigation looking for vasculitis and demyelinating disorders. Ambulatory 24-hour BP monitoring is more sensitive than casual office BP measurement to detect hypertension.

Pitfall

WML of vascular origin are associated with small vessel disease. Ultrasound or angiography of the carotids and vertebral arteries, searching for a significantly hemodynamic stenosis, is only recommended when the lesions have a watershed spatial distribution pattern, i.e., when they are located between two cerebral arterial territories.

Case 3. A painful experience

Case report

A 46-year-old nurse, with a previous history of migraines without aura since adolescence and treated hypertension, came to the emergency room (ER) because of aphasia of sudden onset, which had started half an hour before. She suddenly experienced difficulty in recalling the names of common objects and she produced a few made-up words. She was fully aware of the defect and had no trouble understanding language. Examination confirmed anomia in visual confrontation naming with the production of some neologistic paraphasias. No other abnormalities were found. The pulse was regular, sitting BP was 135/80 mmHg and no carotid or cardiac murmurs were heard. While in the ER, she started experiencing a severe throbbing right-sided temporo-orbital headache, with photophobia and sonophobia. She felt nauseated. The headache was similar to her usual migraine. Two hours later the speech defect started to improve, but it was followed by a binocular disturbed vision, which she described as scintillating "white squares." One hour later, all her symptoms had gone. A brain CT did not reveal any early infarct changes or any other lesion except for some diffuse subcortical white matter hypodensities. A brain MRI was then ordered. DWI did not show any area of restricted diffusion. MRI confirmed the presence of scattered T2 and FLAIR hyperintense images in the frontal and subcortical white matter (Figure 18.3). There were no such lesions either on the temporal lobe or on the occipital lobe. The resident on duty admitted the patient for further evaluation, with the possible diagnosis of vasculitis. All ancillary procedures performed were normal, including angio-MR, cervical vascular ultrasound, echocardiography, Holter, blood tests (hematology, biochemistry, syphilis, HIV, hepatitis and *Borrelia* serologies, and prothrombotic and immunological screening panels). Lumbar puncture (LP) revealed a normal cerebrospinal fluid with

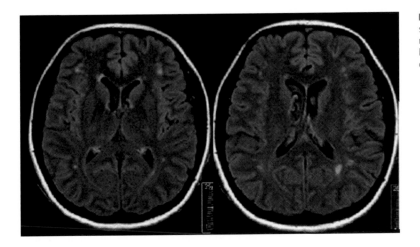

Figure 18.3 Case 3. Brain MRI showing frontal and periventricular and non-confluent subcortical white matter lesions. None of them are located in the occipital lobe.

no increased cell number or oligoclonal bands. Spine MRI and multimodal evoked potential were also normal. The patient was discharged on her previous antihypertensive medication with a diagnosis of migraine with aura.

Discussion

This hypertensive middle-aged nurse had an episode of migraine with aura with some less usual features, which increased the uncertainty about the diagnosis of her current event. Uncertainty leads to a series of unnecessary, costly, and painful experiences including hospital admission and LP. Less common features of the migraine attack included first episode of aura after a long history of migraine without aura, and aura which had an apparently sudden onset and was somewhat prolonged. It is not uncommon that a migraineur who has always had only migraine without aura experiences by his forties–fifties a few or a series of migraine auras, often without headache. These episodes often raise the suspicion of TIA/ischemic stroke. Auras usually have a progressive onset and last a median of half an hour. These are the central values of a biological normal distribution. The extremes of such a distribution are the cases with rapid onset or lasting a few hours. Otherwise this nurse's headache was typical of migraine and was similar in quality and intensity to her previous attacks [22]. The aura, although prolonged, had a typical progression. In fact, as the speech defect cleared, a transient binocular scintillating scotoma appeared.

In 1980, Miller-Fisher presented 120 cases with what he coined late-life migrainous accompaniments

resembling TIAs [23]. In 1986, 85 further cases examined over 5 years were described, supporting the concept advanced previously [24]. In general, the cases had auras with a variable combination of visual disturbances, paresthesias, or speech disturbance. He stressed that "The ages ranged from 40 to 73 years. Headache occurred in association with the episodes in only 40% of cases" and concluded that "The condition can justifiably be regarded as benign. Migrainous accompaniments account for some of the cases of transient ischemia with normal angiograms. Knowledge of the condition helps in the planning of rational management." The current case confirms the accuracy of his detailed observations and judicious remarks.

As MRIs started to be performed in patients with migraine for a variety of reasons (often unnecessary…), it became evident that WMLs were frequent in these patients. A meta-analysis showed that the WML were 3.9 times more frequent in people with migraine [25]. Some studies found an association with duration of migraine history and with the frequency of attacks. Right-to-left shunt does not increase this lesion load. In the ARIC study migraine was associated with white matter hyperintensity (WMH) volume cross-sectionally but not with WMH progression over time [26]. This suggests that the association between migraine and WMH is stable in older age and may be primarily attributable to changes occurring earlier in life. Therefore antiplatelet drugs should not be prescribed to migraineurs because of WMLs mislabeled as "small strokes."

Tip

Subcortical white matter changes are very common in migraineurs. These white matter changes do not represent strokes, vasculitis, or demyelinating disorders and do not warrant any ancillary investigation.

Pitfall

None of the WMLs could explain the symptoms reported by the patient. They were MRI incidental findings.

Case 4. Stroke in an army officer, with multiple causes

Case report

A 45-year-old army officer noticed left-sided hand weakness and blurred vision on his left side on awakening. He was a smoker of 15 cigarettes a day but had no other risk factors. He had been on a military training mission in Angola a month before. He denied head or cervical trauma. When seen at the clinic a month later, neurologic examination showed decreased position sense and tactile hypoesthesia in his right hand with pseudoathetotic posturing of the right fingers. A discharge note from another hospital described a left lower quadrantanopsia, which was no longer detected. A right parietal infarct was apparent on brain CT. CT angiography was also performed and no occlusion or stenosis was identified (Figure 18.4). Additionally, two small internal carotid artery aneurysms, one on each carotid, measuring on the right carotid 2.8 mm and 3.3 mm on the left carotid, were

reported. Blood analysis were normal except for a cholesterol level of 221 mg/dL and positive anticardiolipin IgG (41 GPLU/mL) and antiβ-2 glycoprotein (34 UA/mL). Hepatitis, syphilis, and HIV serologies were negative. Chest X-ray, ECG, and transthoracic and transesophageal echocardiogram were unremarkable. He was discharged on aspirin and atorvastatin. We ordered a brain MRI, which showed two right hemispheric ischemic infarcts with hemorrhagic transformation, a parietal one already visible on CT and a second one located in the parieto-frontal white matter (Figure 18.5). These infarcts were located in the "watershed" areas between the middle cerebral, anterior cerebral, and posterior cerebral artery territories. MR angiography showed decreased diameter and slow flow on the petro-cavernous segment of the right internal carotid and failed to detect the aneurysms, previously shown on CT angiography (Figure 18.6). Repeated testing for antiphospholipid antibodies showed very high titers for lupus anticoagulant, anticardiolipin (104 UGPL/mL), and antiβ-2 glycoprotein (54 UA/mL). Immunological screening for vasculitis and lupus was negative. Because of the twice positive results for antiphospholipid antibodies, the patient was started on warfarin. Considering the probable need for prolonged anticoagulation in a patient harboring two unruptured aneurysms, and the contradictory results of CT and MR angiographies, an intra-arterial angiography was requested. No aneurysms were found but a stenosis of the supraclinoid segment of the right carotid artery was apparent (Figure 18.7). The patient stopped smoking, warfarin was continued, and non-invasive follow-up of the carotid stenosis was planned.

(a)

(b)

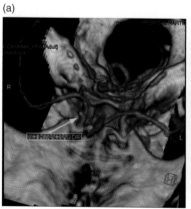
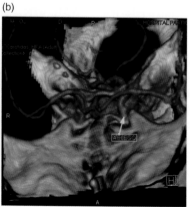

Figure 18.4 Case 4. CT angiography, showing small "aneurysms" in both intracranial carotid arteries.

(a) 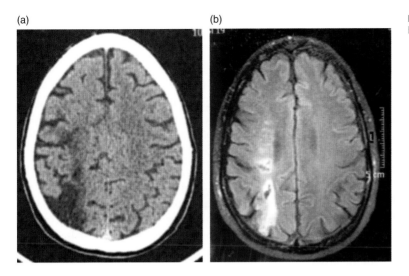 (b)

Figure 18.5 Case 4. Watershed right hemispheric infarcts (CT and MR).

(a) 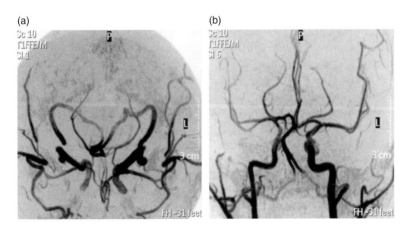 (b)

Figure 18.6 Case 4. MR angiography. No aneurysms. Decreased flow signal on the right intracranial carotid artery.

(a) 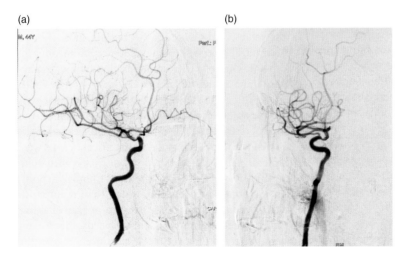 (b)

Figure 18.7 Case 4. Intra-arterial angiography. Right intracranial carotid stenosis with decreased ipsilateral cerebral flow. No aneurysms.

Discussion

This young, physically active smoker suffered a right hemispheric stroke on awakening. The CT and MRI territorial distribution of the infarct was located in the boundaries of the middle cerebral, posterior cerebral, and anterior cerebral artery territories. These "watershed infarcts" have usually a hemodynamic mechanism, due to a severe stenosis or occlusion of a proximal artery, in general the ipsilateral internal carotid. Less often "watershed" infarcts are caused by microembolism. CT angiogram failed to identify any extra or intracranial arterial stenosis or occlusion. Also no cardiac or aortic cause of embolism was detected. Two images, read as small unruptured carotid aneurysms, were incidentally discovered by CT angiography. On the other hand the pursuit of an etiology for the stroke led to the diagnosis of antiphospholipid syndrome, based on high titers of antiphospholipid antibodies on two different measurements. Antiphospholipid syndrome carries a high risk of recurrent thrombotic events and prolonged oral anticoagulation is recommended to decrease such risk. Anticoagulation was started, but further investigation was carried on, exploring the possibility of treatment of the carotid aneurysms, despite their small size, considering the need for prolonged anticoagulation. Neither angio-MR nor intra-arterial angiography confirmed the "aneurysms" seen on CT angiograms, which were probably false images produced by vessel overlap or angulation. On the other hand angio-MR raised the suspicion of a stenosis of the petro-cavernous segment of the internal carotid, which was confirmed by intra-arterial angiography. The nature of the intracranial stenosis cannot be defined beyond doubt. Partially recanalized dissection, congenital stenosis, and intracranial atheroma are etiologic possibilities. The first two entities have a very low risk of progression or embolism. Intracranial carotid stenosis has a high risk of recurrent stroke. Neither warfarin nor endovascular treatment do better than a single antiplatelet regimen to decrease such risk [27]. Warfarin was continued because of the antiphospholipid syndrome [28].

CT and MR angiography have replaced intra-arterial angiography in the evaluation of ischemic stroke, moving it to a second-line diagnostic procedure for doubtful cases or when endovascular or revascularization neurosurgery is planned. However, both CT and MR angiography have a lower precision than intra-arterial angiography [29–31], and can produce either false negative (no intracranial stenosis) or false positive (aneurysms) diagnoses, as this case exemplifies.

Tip

When multiple causes for an ischemic stroke are found, the cause of the current stroke may not be the one with the higher risk of recurrence.

Pitfall

When taking a clinical decision that will affect the patient, it is mandatory to realize the limitations of diagnostic techniques, namely their sensitivity, specificity, and most common false positive and false negative results.

Case 5. Microbleeds and atrial fibrillation

Case report

A 75-year-old retired teacher suffered a transient episode of slurred speech and anomia which lasted for about 5 minutes. He had hypertension and diabetes which were under control with diet and oral medication. General physical examination was unremarkable except for an irregular pulse. On neurologic examination there were no mental status changes and no articulatory or language limitations. No facial asymmetry or hemiparesis could be detected. Gait was somewhat slow and reflexes were brisker in the lower than the upper limbs. Muscular tone was normal and plantar responses flexor. Postural reflexes were preserved. Blood tests were unremarkable with a hematocrit of 42.2%, fasting glycemia 118 mg/dL, normal liver test values, and creatinine 0.8 mg/dL. ECG showed atrial fibrillation with a rate of 80 per minute, but no ischemic changes. Ultrasound examination of extracranial and intracranial vessels was unremarkable. Echocardiogram showed hypertrophy of the left ventricular wall, with good function. Brain MRI showed no areas of restricted diffusion on DWI. On T2 and FLAIR sequences confluent frontal symmetrical WMLs were evident. On T2-weighted gradient-recalled-echo (GRE) MRI sequences of some small rounded hypointense lesions were detected, which were reported as microbleeds (Figure 18.8). Because of fear of intracranial bleeding from the microbleeds the patient was discharged on aspirin 100 mg, once a day. At the

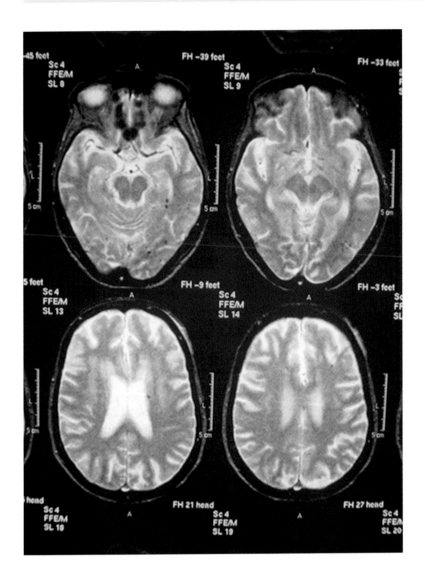

Figure 18.8 Case 5. Multiple small rounded hyperintense lesions (microbleeds) located both in subcortical and cortical regions. Notice also confluent frontal subcortical white matter lesions.

neurological consultation a month later, alternatives relative to antithrombotic treatment (aspirin, warfarin, new oral anticoagulants) were discussed with the patient. Aspirin was stopped and dabigatran 110 mg every 12 h was prescribed.

Discussion

This patient had a TIA without brain infarct associated with atrial fibrillation. Patients with atrial fibrillation who have suffered a TIA or stroke have a high risk of recurrent cerebral embolism. Prolonged oral anticoagulation is the most effective intervention to decrease such risk significantly [32]. When deciding to start anticoagulation, its benefits (prevention of recurrent

vascular events) and risks (serious bleeding, including intracranial ones) need to be balanced. Currently, the CHAD2DS2-VASc and HAS-BLED scores (Table 18.1) are used to quantify such risks [33–35]. Results of CT or MRI, namely microbleeds, are not included in these scores. How do these scores apply to the current patient? The patient has a CHAD2DS2-VASc score of 6 points and a HAS-BLED score of 2 points. Patients with a CHAD2DS2-VASc score ≥2 are high-risk patients for subsequent thromboembolism and must receive prolonged oral anticoagulation [33]. A HAS-BLED score of >3 points indicates a high risk of bleeding, which is fortunately not the case in this patient who had only a score of 2 points. So no doubt this patient should be

Table 18.1 Case 5: CHAD2DS2-VASc and HAS-BLED scores

	Points	Patient
CHAD2DS2-VASc score		
Congestive heart failure/left ventricular dysfunction	1	
Hypertension	1	1
Age ≥75	2	2
Diabetes	1	1
Stroke/TIA/thromboembolism	2	2
Age 65–74	1	
Female	1	
HAS-BLED score		
Hypertension	1	1
Abnormal liver and renal functions tests	1 (each)	
Stroke	1	
Bleeding	1	
Labile INRs	1	
Elderly (age >65)	1	1
Drugs (ASA or NSAID) or alcohol	1 point (each)	

ASA, acetylsalicylic acid. NSAID, nonsteroidal anti-inflammatory drug.

started on oral anticoagulants. Should we consider microbleeds a contraindication for anticoagulation? For future patients, should we advise performing MRI to exclude microbleeds before starting anticoagulation?

Microbleeds are common in elderly patients and frequent in those with cerebrovascular disease. Prevalence data from 5200 subjects and a systematic review of 9073 subjects [36,37] showed the following figures on the prevalence of cerebral microbleeds: elderly without cerebrovascular disease: 5–5.7%; patients with intracerebral hemorrhage: 60–68%; patients with cerebrovascular disease: 34–40%; with lacunes, leukoaraiosis: 57%; with atherothrombotic stroke: 22%; with cardioembolic stroke: 0 –30%. The prevalence of microbleeds is higher (odds ratio 2.7) in anticoagulated patients who have suffered an intracranial bleeding. They are also much more frequent (odds ratio 12.1) in those with recurrent intracranial hemorrhages [38]. However, microbleeds are also more frequent in patients with recurrent ischemic stroke. Microbleeds can be considered markers of small vessel disease when they are located subcortically, and

of amyloid angiopathy if they are located cortically [39]. The association of microbleeds with current or previous antithrombotic therapy was investigated in several studies, producing contradictory results [40]. Trials of warfarin and of new oral anticoagulants excluded patients with history of intracranial bleeding but not those with microbleeds, if they were an incidental finding in brain imaging. Trials also did not exclude patients with neuroimaging results indicating cerebral small vessel disease, such as multiple silent lacunes and confluent white mater lesions. Extensive white matter lesions also increase the risk of intracranial bleeding on anticoagulants [41]. An observational cohort study (CROMIS-2) will investigate the value of MRI markers of small vessel disease, including cerebral microbleeds, in assessing the risk of oral anticoagulation-associated intracerebral hemorrhage [42]. Meanwhile, based on current available evidence, microbleeds should not prevent starting anticoagulation in the current patient. From the public health point of view, performing MRI before starting anticoagulation would have rather negative consequences. Globally, MRI is not readily accessible in the majority of medical centers and GP clinics worldwide. Recommending performing MRI to exclude microbleeds before starting anticoagulation would delay and decrease the proportion of atrial fibrillation patients who are anticoagulated. The net result would be a decrease in the effectiveness of prolonged oral anticoagulation in atrial fibrillation patients.

The main barrier to the prescription of anticoagulants in patients with atrial fibrillation is fear of bleeding. However, physicians' fears of the risk of bleeding are often exaggerated and unfounded [43]. Concerns about the risks of bleeding appear to prevail over stroke prevention. Patients on the contrary are more afraid of stroke than of eventual bleeding [44]. They prefer preventing a stroke, even if it means taking the risk of major bleeding.

Tip

To choose the most appropriate antithrombotic regimen for secondary stroke prevention in an individual patient with atrial fibrillation consider (a) guideline algorithms, (b) the individual thromboembolic risk, and (c) the individual bleeding risk. Use validated scales to grade the thromboembolic and the bleeding risks and to balance benefits and risks of prolonged oral anticoagulation.

Pitfall

Facing a therapeutic dilemma we should consider not only the results of clinical trials but also their inclusion and exclusion criteria. In trials of oral anticoagulants, for the preventions of vascular events in patients with atrial fibrillation, MRI of the brain was not a mandatory baseline examination.

Case 6. Should we treat the angiography?

Case report

A 64-year-old man was referred for a generalized tonic-clonic seizure preceded by white flashes on his left-sided visual field. He had experienced a similar seizure 30 years before which was investigated in another hospital. A "brain lesion" was identified but no surgery was recommended. He suffered from coronary heart disease and had undergone three myocardial revascularization procedures. Neurologic examination was normal with no evidence of visual field defect. A brain CT and an MRI disclosed a calcified right occipital arteriovenous malformation (AVM), with no evidence of recent bleeding (Figure 18.9). CT angiography confirmed a 3 cm occipital AVM without associated aneurysms and no deep venous drainage (Figure 18.10). After discussing the case with a neurosurgeon and explaining the therapeutic alternatives to the patient, a conservative management was decided on, with periodical clinical follow-ups. Valproate, which had been prescribed for the seizure, was continued.

Discussion

Treatments aim at modifying the natural history of diseases for the benefit of the patients. The natural history of AVMs cannot be totally understood because AVMs can only be diagnosed by neuroimaging, surgery, or autopsy. AVMs can be incidental findings or discovered during the investigation of symptoms that may or may not be due to the AVM. The symptoms include headaches, focal deficits, and seizures. The "natural" history will be different in each of these scenarios. Furthermore there are very few well-conducted population-based epidemiological studies investigating the prevalence and outcome of AVMs [45]. The same applies for randomized clinical trials comparing different treatment modalities [46]. Most of the evidence relies on single or multicenter case

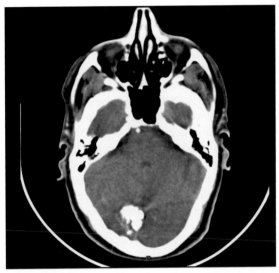

Figure 18.9 Case 6. Calcified occipital arteriovenous malformation.

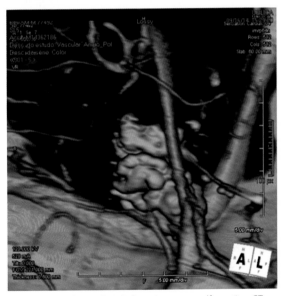

Figure 18.10 Case 6. Occipital arteriovenous malformation: CT angiography, oblique view.

series and nonrandomized comparisons with non-blind evaluation of outcomes from centers specializing in the treatment of AVMs [47]. Because of referral bias, due to the selective referral of more serious and difficult cases, these studies tend to overestimate the risk of rupture and bad outcomes. If the evaluation of the outcome after intervention to "treat" AVMs is performed in a non-blind fashion by the same doctor who performed the treatment, the risk of bias by overestimating the success of the intervention and underestimating minor neurological deficits and functional limitations is obvious. Taking together these sources of bias, most studies produced results which inflate the benefit of treatments. Developed from this type of data, there are scales to calculate the approximate risk of rupture and of the surgery for ruptured and unruptured AVMs. The most commonly used is the Spetzler–Martin AVM grading scale [48]. In the current case the AVM will receive 2 points for size 3–6 cm, 1 point for the eloquence of adjacent brain, and 0 points for the absence of deep venous drainage, making a total of 3 points. On the Spetzler–Ponce classification [49] this AVM will be included in Class B, with preference for multimodality treatment and an 18% (95% confidence interval 15–22) chance, i.e., about 1 in 5, of postoperative deficit. However, the few existing and recent population-based studies showed a much lower risk of bleeding for AVMs that had never ruptured (1–2% per year), than previously described (4%) [50]. A systematic review and meta-analysis of interventions to treat AVMs showed high rates of serious adverse events for all treatment modalities (surgery 29%, embolization 25%, and radiotherapy 13%) [47]. The recently completed ARUBA trial [46] comparing conservative versus any modality treatment (surgery, endovascular occlusion, radiosurgery alone or in any combination) of unruptured AVM showed a clear disadvantage (threefold) of treating unruptured AVM, regardless of the modality and type of AVM. This difference was mainly due to the initial risk of neurological deficit related to the treatment. The follow-up in the ARUBA trial was relatively short and a longer follow-up is necessary to verify if this disadvantage is sustained or decreases over time, as the non-treated group eventually experiences more intracerebral bleedings. At present there is no evidence to support treatment by surgery, endovascular occlusion, or radiosurgery of unruptured AVM, unless the patient explicitly wants the AVM to be treated, because his quality of life is negatively influenced by knowing that he lives with what has been popularized as a "mine" or a "bomb" in the brain [50].

Tip

The risk of intracerebral bleeding associated with a non-ruptured AVM is low. All treatment modalities have a non-negligible risk of producing disabling neurological defects in an intact independent patient.

Pitfall

Treatment of this AVM based only on its image, without considering the age of the patient, presenting symptoms, the AVM's natural history, and the scarce evidence from clinical trials, would be an irresponsible decision, most probably causing a permanent visual field defect in this patient.

Conclusions

The six cases described in this chapter exemplify how the results of ancillary tests such as neuroimaging can be misleading. We should master the limitations of diagnostic procedures, namely their sensitivity and specificity and the most common causes and features of false positive and false negative results. Also, highly sensitive diagnostic technologies produce numerous "incidental" findings, which are often unrelated to the patient's complaints and diagnosis. These findings may lead to further unnecessary investigations and expose patients to the risks of needless treatments and erroneous statements about their health problems and outcomes.

References

1. Hand PJ, Haisma JA, Kwan J, et al. Interobserver agreement for the bedside clinical assessment of suspected stroke. *Stroke* 2006;37(3):776–80.

2. Shinar D, Gross CR, Mohr JP, et al. Interobserver variability in the assessment of neurologic history and examination in the Stroke Data Bank. *Arch Neurol* 1985;42(6):557–65.

3. Manschot S, van Passel L, Buskens E, Algra A, van Gijn J. Mayo and NINDS scales for assessment of tendon reflexes: between observer agreement and implications for communication. *J Neurol Neurosurg Psychiatry* 1998;64(2):253–5.

4. Sackett DL, Haynes RB, Tugwell P (eds.). *Clinical Epidemiology. A Basic Science for Clinical Medicine.* Boston/Toronto: Little Brown and Company; 1985.

5. Brozek JL, Akl EA, Jaeschke R, et al. GRADE Working Group, Grading quality of evidence and strength of recommendations in clinical practice guidelines: Part 2 of 3. The GRADE approach to grading quality of evidence about diagnostic tests and strategies. *Allergy* 2009;64(8):1109–16.

6. Post PN, Kievit J, van Baalen JM, van den Hout WB, van Bockel J. Routine duplex surveillance does not improve the outcome after carotid endarterectomy: a decision and cost utility analysis. *Stroke* 2002;33(3):749–55.

7. Donnan GA, O'Malley HM, Quang L, Hurley S, Bladin PF. The capsular warning syndrome: pathogenesis and clinical features. *Neurology* 1993;43(5):957–62.

8. Saposnik G. Noel de Tilly L, Caplan LR. Pontine warning syndrome. *Arch Neurol* 2008;65(10):1375–7.

9. Paul NL, Simoni M, Chandratheva A, Rothwell PM. Population-based study of capsular warning syndrome and prognosis after early recurrent TIA. *Neurology* 2012;79(13):1356–62.

10. Lee H, Cho YW. A case of isolated nodulus infarction presenting as a vestibular neuritis. *J Neurol Sci* 2004;221(1–2):117–19.

11. Fonseca AC, Canhão P. Diagnostic difficulties in the classification of transient neurological attacks. *Eur J Neurol* 2011;18(4):644–8.

12. Shenoy AM. Guidelines in practice: therapies for benign paroxysmal positional vertigo. *Continuum (Minneap Minn)* 2012;18(5 Neuro-otology):1172–6.

13. Fazekas F, Schmidt R, Kleinert R, Kapeller P, Roob G, Flooh E. The spectrum of age-associated brain abnormalities: their measurement and histopathological correlates. *J Neural Transm Suppl* 1998;53:31–9.

14. Schmidt R, Enzinger C, Ropele S, Schmidt H, Fazekas F; Austrian Stroke Prevention Study. Progression of cerebral white matter lesions: 6-year results of the Austrian Stroke Prevention Study. *Lancet* 2003;361(9374):2046–8.

15. Gouw AA, van der Flier WM, Fazekas F, et al. LADIS Study Group. Progression of white matter hyperintensities and incidence of new lacunes over a 3-year period: the Leukoaraiosis and Disability study. *Stroke* 2008;39(5):1414–20.

16. Fazekas F, Schmidt R, Scheltens P. Pathophysiologic mechanisms in the development of age-related white matter changes of the brain. *Dement Geriatr Cogn Disord* 1998;9(suppl 1):2–5.

17. Gouw AA, Seewann A, van der Flier WM, et al. Heterogeneity of small vessel disease: a systematic review of MRI and histopathology correlations. *J Neurol Neurosurg Psychiatry* 2011;82(2):126–35.

18. Potter GM, Doubal FN, Jackson CA, Sudlow CL, Dennis MS, Wardlaw JM. Lack of association of white matter lesions with ipsilateral carotid artery stenosis. *Cerebrovasc Dis* 2012;33 (4):378–84.

19. Agarwal R, Sze G. Neuro-Lyme disease: MR imaging findings. *Radiology* 2009;253(1):167–73.

20. Harboe E, Beyer MK, Greve OJ, et al. Cerebral white matter hyperintensities are not increased in patients with primary Sjögren's syndrome. *Eur J Neurol* 2009;16(5):576–81.

21. Sierra C. Associations between ambulatory blood pressure parameters and cerebral white matter lesions. *Int J Hypertens* 2011;**2011**:478710.

22. Headache Classification Committee of the International Headache Society (IHS). The International Classification of Headache Disorders, 3rd edition (beta version). *Cephalalgia* 2013;33(9):629–808.

23. Fisher CM. Late-life migraine accompaniments as a cause of unexplained transient ischemic attacks. *Can J Neurol Sci* 1980;7(1):9–17.

24. Fisher CM. Late-life migraine accompaniments – further experience. *Stroke* 1986;17(5):1033–42.

25. Swartz RH, Kern RZ. Migraine is associated with magnetic resonance imaging white matter abnormalities: a meta-analysis. *Arch Neurol* 2004;61(9):1366–8.

26. Hamedani AG, Rose KM, Peterlin BL, et al. Migraine and white matter hyperintensities: the ARIC MRI study. *Neurology* 2013;81(15):1308–13.

27. Kernan WN, et al. on behalf of the American Heart Association Stroke Council, Council on Cardiovascular and Stroke Nursing, Council on Clinical Cardiology, and Council on Peripheral Vascular Disease. Guidelines for the prevention of stroke in patients with stroke and transient ischemic attack. A guideline for Healthcare professionals from the American Heart Association/American Stroke Association. *Stroke* 2014.;45(7):2160–236.

28. Arachchillage DR, Machin SJ, Cohen H. Antithrombotic treatment for stroke associated with antiphospholipid antibodies. *Expert Rev Hematol* 2014;7(2):169–72.

29. European Stroke Organisation (ESO) Executive Committee; ESO Writing Committee. Guidelines for management of ischaemic stroke and transient ischaemic attack 2008. *Cerebrovasc Dis* 2008;25(5):457–507.

30. Kokkinis C, Vlychou M, Zavras GM, Hadjigeorgiou GM, Papadimitriou A, Fezoulidis IV. The role of 3D-computed tomography angiography (3D-CTA) in investigation of spontaneous subarachnoid haemorrhage: comparison with digital subtraction angiography (DSA) and surgical findings. *Br J Neurosurg* 2008;22(1):71–8.

31. Lu L, Zhang LJ, Poon CS, et al. Digital subtraction CT angiography for detection of intracranial aneurysms: comparison with three-dimensional digital subtraction angiography. *Radiology* 2012;262(2):605–12.

32. Hart RG, Pearce LA, Aguilar MI. Meta-analysis: antithrombotic therapy to prevent stroke in patients who have nonvalvular atrial fibrillation. *Ann Intern Med* 2007;146(12):857–67.

33. Camm AJ, et al. ESC Committee for Practice Guidelines-CPG; Document Reviewers. 2012 focused update of the ESC Guidelines for the management of atrial fibrillation: an update of the 2010 ESC Guidelines for the management of atrial fibrillation – developed with the special contribution of the European Heart Rhythm Association. *Europace* 2012;14(10):1385–413.

34. Lip GY. Recommendations for thromboprophylaxis in the 2012 focused update of the ESC guidelines on atrial fibrillation: a commentary. *J Thromb Haemost* 2013;11(4):615–26.

35. Pisters R, Lane DA, Nieuwlaat R, de Vos CB, Crijns HJ, Lip GY. A novel user-friendly score (HAS-BLED) to assess 1-year risk of major bleeding in patients with atrial fibrillation: the Euro Heart Survey. *Chest* 2010;138(5):1093–100.

36. Koennecke HC. Cerebral microbleeds on MRI: prevalence, associations, and potential clinical implications. *Neurology* 2006;66(2):165–71.

37. Cordonnier C, Al-Shahi Salman R, Wardlaw J. Spontaneous brain microbleeds: systematic review, subgroup analyses and standards for study design and reporting. *Brain* 2007;130(Pt 8):1988–2003.

38. Lovelock CE, Cordonnier C, Naka H, et al. Antithrombotic drug use, cerebral microbleeds, and intracerebral hemorrhage: a systematic review of published and unpublished studies. *Stroke* 2010;41(6):1222–8.

39. Cordonnier C. Brain microbleeds: more evidence, but still a clinical dilemma. *Curr Opin Neurol* 2011;24(1):69–74.

40. Romero JR, Preis SR, Beiser A, et al. Risk factors, stroke prevention treatments, and prevalence of cerebral microbleeds in the Framingham Heart Study. *Stroke* 2014;45(5):1492–4.

41. Gorter JW. Major bleeding during anticoagulation after cerebral ischemia: patterns and risk factors. Stroke Prevention In Reversible Ischemia Trial (SPIRIT). European Atrial Fibrillation Trial (EAFT) study groups. *Neurology* 1999;53(6):1319–27.

42. Charidimou A, Shakeshaft C, Werring DJ. Cerebral microbleeds on magnetic resonance imaging and anticoagulant-associated intracerebral hemorrhage risk. *Front Neurol* 2012;3:133. eCollection 2012.

43. Man-Son-Hing M, Laupacis A. Anticoagulant-related bleeding in older persons with atrial fibrillation: physicians' fears often unfounded. *Arch Intern Med* 2003;163(13):1580–6.

44. Devereaux PJ, Anderson DR, Gardner MJ, et al. Differences between perspectives of physicians and patients on anticoagulation in patients with atrial fibrillation: observational study. *BMJ* 2001;323(7323):1218–22.

45. van Beijnum J, Lovelock CE, Cordonnier C, et al. SIVMS Steering Committee and the Oxford Vascular Study. Outcome after spontaneous and arteriovenous malformation-related intracerebral haemorrhage: population-based studies. *Brain* 2009;132(Pt 2):537–43.

46. Mohr JP, Parides MK, Stapf C, et al. International ARUBA investigators. Medical management with or without interventional therapy for unruptured brain arteriovenous malformations (ARUBA): a multicentre, non-blinded, randomised trial. *Lancet* 2014;383(9917):614–21.

47. van Beijnum J, van der Worp HB, Buis DR, et al. Treatment of brain arteriovenous malformations: a systematic review and meta-analysis. *JAMA* 2011;306(18):2011–19.

48. Spetzler RF, Martin NA. A proposed grading system for arteriovenous malformations. *J Neurosurg* 1986;65(4):476–83.

49. Spetzler RF, Ponce FA. A 3-tier classification of cerebral arteriovenous malformations. Clinical article. *J Neurosurg* 2011;114(3):842–9.

50. Molina CA, Selim MH. Unruptured brain arteriovenous malformations. Keep calm or dance in a minefield. *Stroke* 2014;45(5):1543–4.

Index

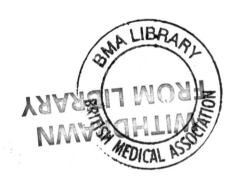